Gesundheit und Gesellschaft

Series Editors
Ullrich Bauer, Fakultät für Erziehungswissenschaft, Universität Bielefeld,
Bielefeld, Germany
Matthias Richter, Institut für Medizinische Soziologie, Martin-Luther-Universität
Halle-Wittenberg, Halle (Saale), Germany
Uwe H. Bittlingmayer, Institut für Soziologie, Pädagogische Hochschule
Freiburg, Freiburg, Germany

D0840063

Der Forschungsgegenstand Gesundheit ist trotz reichhaltiger Anknüpfungspunkte zu einer Vielzahl sozialwissenschaftlicher Forschungsfelder – z. B. Sozialstrukturanalyse, Lebensverlaufsforschung, Alterssoziologie, Sozialisationsforschung, politische Soziologie, Kindheits- und Jugendforschung – in den Referenzprofessionen bisher kaum präsent. Komplementär dazu schöpfen die Gesundheitswissenschaften und Public Health, die eher anwendungsbezogen arbeiten, die verfügbare sozialwissenschaftliche Expertise kaum ernsthaft ab. Die Reihe „Gesundheit und Gesellschaft" setzt an diesem Vermittlungsdefizit an und systematisiert eine sozialwissenschaftliche Perspektive auf Gesundheit. Die Beiträge der Buchreihe umfassen theoretische und empirische Zugänge, die sich in der Schnittmenge sozial- und gesundheitswissenschaftlicher Forschung befinden. Inhaltliche Schwerpunkte sind die detaillierte Analyse u. a. von Gesundheitskonzepten, gesundheitlicher Ungleichheit und Gesundheitspolitik.

More information about this series at http://www.springer.com/series/12229

Luis A. Saboga-Nunes ·
Uwe H. Bittlingmayer ·
Orkan Okan · Diana Sahrai
Editors

New Approaches to Health Literacy

Linking Different Perspectives

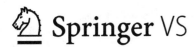 Springer VS

Editors
Luis A. Saboga-Nunes
Institut für Soziologie
Pädagogische Hochschule Freiburg
Freiburg im Breisgau, Germany

Uwe H. Bittlingmayer
Institut für Soziologie I
Pädagogische Hochschule
Freiburg im Breisgau, Germany

Orkan Okan
Fakultat für Erziehungswissenschaft
Universitat Bielefeld
Bielefeld, Germany

Diana Sahrai
Institut für Spezielle Pädagogik und
Psychologie, Pädagogische Hochschule
Fachhochschule Nordwestschweiz
Basel, Switzerland

ISSN 2626-6172 ISSN 2626-6180 (electronic)
Gesundheit und Gesellschaft
ISBN 978-3-658-30908-4 ISBN 978-3-658-30909-1 (eBook)
https://doi.org/10.1007/978-3-658-30909-1

Responsible Editor: Katrin Emmerich
This Springer VS imprint is published by the registered company Springer Fachmedien Wiesbaden GmbH part of Springer Nature.
The registered company address is: Abraham-Lincoln-Str. 46, 65189 Wiesbaden, Germany

Foreword

Over the last twenty years, scientific publications on health literacy have increased exponentially, also including books. The legitimate question arises: Is there a need for another book on health literacy? Even if it were to face the dangers of being lost in a market that has recently been flooded with books dedicated to this topic, the present publication will place itself in a niche that has not been inhabited before. Two arguments underpin this relevance and they will persuade the reader that this book is worth to be taken into consideration:

First, it is essential to raise awareness of the fact that health literacy is far from being the theoretically convincing and empirical, robust concept of public health science referred to in so many publications. Therefore, this book raises questions that are otherwise hard to find within the contemporary mainstream discourse relating to health literacy. Germany has evolved into what seems to be a natural epicenter for further investigating and exploring the debates surrounding the theoretical assumptions and developments regarding health literacy, not only because there is a remarkable growth of attention for the topic in German speaking countries, but there are still very few contributions in English available from within these countries, creating a gap which demands closing. While health literacy is definitely a topic that appeals as a *zeitgeist* topic, this particular discussion aims at stimulating a *brightgeist* discussion related to health literacy.

Second, the explorations of health literacy within this book embrace cultural aspects critical to the concept, which seem peripheral but are in fact most important as they address questions pertaining to health literacy and multiculturalism, inclusion and diversity. In this sense we shift away from the sole focus on the health- and Western-centered discussion to grasp topics and cultures that are not part of the dominant Anglo-Saxon rainbow where health literacy was born and which determines most of the mainstream discourse surrounding health literacy.

In order to do so and widen both the concept and its discussion, both the author and the reader need to have an open mindset towards such thinking, which in particular is what this book wants to facilitate, acknowledge and contribute to. To achieve this, the reader will be provided with unique perspectives on health literacy from Afghanistan and Columbia. The book also contains discussions on the relationship between health literacy and multimodal adapted communication, which is especially important in rapidly changing societies and digitization of health and information. Some contributions to this book set out to challenge the mainstream theoretical model of health literacy, which inherently suggests that being health literate all by itself contributes to informed rational health behaviour, better health decisions and positive health outcomes. Other contributions challenge the measurement and operationalization procedures by which health literacy levels are being assessed, and some contributions endeavor to link the health literacy concept directly to health policy issues.

In short, this book shows the wide range and great diversity of current health literacy research, critically engages with intriguing thinking and emphasizes much needed further debates in the field. The contributions explore the fruitfulness of the health literacy concept as well as its limitations and raises open questions. In this sense, we hope that this book will stimulate further discussion on the topic, contribute to a reflection on the concept of health literacy and facilitate new theoretical developments.

This book is closely linked to the international research network "Health Literacy of Childhood and Adolescence" lead by Ullrich Bauer, Paulo Pinheiro and Orkan Okan from Bielefeld University (www.hlca-consortium.de/en). We are very grateful for their support. Furthermore, we want to thank all the authors for their trust that this endeavor would one day be published successfully. Additionally, we want to thank Katrin Emmerich from Springer VS for her support. Last but not least we want to thank Alla Dinges from University of Education Freiburg for her extraordinary support during the stressful procedure of formatting the contributions under time pressure and Dr. Konrad Jocksch for his reliable and valuable help in proofreading and language editing this book, as publishing in English is still a huge challenge to non-native speakers.

Lisbon, Freiburg, Bielefeld and Muttenz (near Basel) Luis A. Saboga-Nunes
May 2020   Uwe H. Bittlingmayer
                      Orkan Okan
                      Diana Sahrai

Contents

Health Literacy in the Education Setting

Some Cultural Dimensions of Health Literacy

Contributors

Ullrich Bauer Faculty of Educational Sciences, Bielefeld University, Bielefeld, Germany

Isabella C. Bertschi Department of Psychology, University of Zurich, Zurich, Switzerland

Uwe H. Bittlingmayer Institute of Sociology, University of Education Freiburg (Germany), Freiburg, Germany

Eva Maria Bitzer Departement of Public Health and Health Education, University of Education Freiburg (Germany), Freiburg, Germany

Anja Blechschmidt Pädagogische Hochschule FHNW (ISP), Muttenz, Switzerland

Paula Bleckmann Institute of School Pedagogy and Teacher Education, Alanus University of Applied Science, Alfter, Germany

Torsten M. Bollweg Faculty of Educational Sciences, Bielefeld University, Bielefeld, Germany

Dirk Bruland Institute for educational and health-care research in the health sector (InBVG), FH Bielefeld University of Applied Sciences, Bielefeld, Germany

Janine Bröder Deutsche Gesellschaft für Ernährung e. V., Bonn, Germany

M. Ebrahim Jawid Director Shuda Hospital, Shuhada Organization, Ghazny, Afghanistan

Simone Flaig Department of Public Health and Health Education, University of Education Freiburg (Germany), Freiburg, Germany

Shanti George Independent Researcher and Learning for Well-Being Foundation (the Netherlands), The Hague, The Netherlands

Jürgen Gerdes Institute of Sociology, University of Education Freiburg (Germany), Freiburg, Germany

Patricia Graf Faculty of Educational Sciences, Bielefeld University, Freiburg, Germany

Stefanie Harsch Institute of Sociology, University of Education Freiburg (Germany), Freiburg, Germany

Zeynep Islertas Institute of Sociology, University of Education Freiburg (Germany), Freiburg, Germany

Asadullah Jawid Institute of Mathematics and Statistics, American University of Afghanistan, Kabul, Afghanistan

Didier Jourdain UNESCO Chair Global Health & Education—WHO Collaborating Centre for Research in Education & Health, Université Clermont Auvergne, Clermont-Ferrand, France

Rahel Kahlert Ludwig Boltzmann Institute, Health Promotion Research Vienna, Vienna, Austria

Lea Kuntz Department of Public Health and Health Education, University of Education Freiburg (Germany), Freiburg, Germany

Almas Merchant Ludwig Boltzmann Institute, Health Promotion Research Vienna, Vienna, Austria

Thomas Mößle Vice Director of the Criminological Research Institute of Lower Saxony, Hannover, Germany

Orkan Okan Faculty of Educational Sciences, Bielefeld University, Bielefeld, Germany

Gözde Okcu Institute of Sociology, University of Education Freiburg (Germany), Freiburg, Germany

Igor Osipov Institute of Educational Research, Wuppertal University, Wuppertal, Germany

Paulo Pinheiro Faculty of Educational Sciences, Bielefeld University, Bielefeld, Germany

Luis A. Saboga-Nunes Institute of Sociology, Public Health Research Centre, University of Education Freiburg (Germany), Freiburg, Germany

Diana Sahrai School of Education, University of Applied Sciences and Arts Northern Switzerland, Institute of Special Education and Psychology, Muttenz, Switzerland

Agnes Santha Faculty of Technical and Human Sciences, Sapientia Hungarian University of Transylvania, Tirgu Mures, Romania

Hanna E. Schwendemann Departement of Public Health and Health Education, University of Education Freiburg (Germany), Freiburg, Germany

Elise Sijthoff Founder ChildPress.Org, Publishing House Fysio Educatief Amsterdam, Amsterdam, The Netherlands

Anja Stiller Department of Public Health and Health Education, University of Education Freiburg (Germany), Freiburg, Germany

Kristine Sørensen Director of the Global Health Literacy Academy, Risskov, Denmark

Lilliana Villa-Vélez National Faculty of Public Health, University of Antioquia, Medellín, Colombia

Linking Different Perspectives: Some Introductory Remarks

Luis A. Saboga-Nunes

We live in a world that needs a thorough shake-up if we are going to aim at its sustainability. Recent positions of world leaders like the U.N. Secretary-General Antonio Guterres (see Time, 24.06.2019) are just the expression of millions of voices that echoed around the globe calling for the necessary changes to be made. Beneath the surface of the issues addressed, there are profound causes that have common grounds in literacy levels.

Literacy has been recognized as an issue that necessitates a global agenda. For 50 years, UNESCO`s mission (among others) has been to enhance literacy levels of individuals and within entire countries across the world.

Nevertheless, very soon after the acknowledgment that literacy concerns vast domains of human life, the need to explore specific niches arose, where research or best practices implementation could thrive in the context of such complexity.

This is how during the last 20 years a body of knowledge was established around the topic of health literacy. Introducing the broader perspective of literacy into the health domain became a priority for world organizations, such as the WHO. The 9th global conference on health promotion organized by WHO in Shanghai in 2016 is one of many expressions how determined WHO is to push forward the promotion of health literacy. The Shanghai Declaration that evolved from this conference defined health literacy as one of three core pillars in order to accomplish the Agenda for Sustainable Development by 2030.

L. A. Saboga-Nunes (✉)
University of Education Freiburg, Institute of Sociology, Public Health Research Centre, Freiburg, Germany
e-mail: luis.saboga-nunes@ph-freiburg.de

Nevertheless, the problem is that, ultimately, we know very little about health literacy, how it is constructed, how individuals and social contexts shape its contents and how health literacy is actually incorporated into everyday life. In order to accomplish needful changes, this portion of the spectrum of human existence needs to be understood so that it may influence other components of life in a positive way. The constant endeavor to comprehend these issues is what made health literacy a focus of interdisciplinary research.

With particular concern to interdisciplinarity, the Health Literacy in Childhood and Adolescence-Consortium (HLCA) consortium[1] was established, initiated by Ullrich Bauer and Paulo Pinheiro. Considered to be a key component of the life cycle, investigating health literacy for this target age, was considered a relevant strategy to manage what is also considered the complexity of health literacy in all of the human experience.

The HLCA consortium initiated a track of exploration that led to various novel outputs in relation to health literacy. Some of them survived the tunneling process of journal publication, losing in that procedure many of the details or relevant insights. Not surfacing in the dissemination process, many good ideas stayed in the shelves or minds of HLCA members, in the interesting exchanges over coffee and around dinner tables, in corners, during walks in gardens, in undergrounds or airport queues. Impromptu conversations and structured knowledge translations outputs, all expressing how creative the human mind can be, lived shoulder to shoulder with a set of materials that constitute the rich literature in the HLCA consortium!

This book is a contribution to this effort. It is a rescuing mission to save parts of this production from lying hidden from the public that is interested in the topic of health literacy.

The idea for this book was born during the first summer school organized by HLCA in Freiburg, Germany as early as 2016. The richness of exchanges, the spontaneity of many ideas led the organizers to propose to those attending, that some of these thoughts be captured in writing, as they constitute links of a chain of developments in health literacy. The authors are researchers from HLCA or invited guest, participants and speakers of the Freiburg summer school. They came from Germany, Afghanistan, Israel, Colombia or Portugal (just to name some of the many countries that were present at the Summer School).

---

[1]For further details please access www.hlca-consortium.de/en.

Although all participants of the summer school were invited to join the publication and some responded positively, for various reasons not every submission was included in this project.

Chapter 2 of this anthology discusses the state of the art in health literacy research. This Chapter by Uwe H. Bittlingmayer, Stefanie Harsch and Zeynep Islertas puts health literacy in the context of health inequality. As the field evolves so fast, the argument for this state of the art on health literacy from the perspective of health inequality, lays a solid foundation for the purpose of this book, since it calls for a more systematic treatment of the connection between general health disparities on the one hand, and the role of health literacy on the other.

Chapter 3 by Orkan Okan, Torsten M. Bollweg and Janine Bröder reviews research on health literacy in children and adolescents. The authors identify the year 2006 as a starting point from which research increased and evolved rapidly within the past few years. Some of the core topics they deal with are health literacy concepts and definitions, measurement tools and evidence.

Anja Blechschmidt introduces, in the fourth chapter, an interesting perspective on communication and health literacy, arguing that health literacy concerns every member of society, even people with severe disabilities. Therefore, health literacy has a relevant role to play in social inclusion. Called Multimodal Adapted Communication' (MAC), this perspective is reputed to improve health literacy in children. To tackle health literacy communication in all of its forms is fundamental. Consequently, there is a need to consider how adaptation of language can meet the task. Speech therapy and the setting of special education are the background of the discussion of MAC in a multidisciplinary approach. Here it is argued that health-related phenomena are as conceptually accessible by everyone as language is – a fundamental mode of conveying information (e.g. related to health) – understandable to everyone.

There is a tendency to consider health literacy from the individualistic perspective – a tendency that has negative consequences. Therefore, in the fifth chapter, Eva-Maria Bitzer argues that in order to achieve public health goals we must go beyond individual health literacy. This chapter first looks at current definitions, strategies and actions of public health. Since health literacy is a public health goal, three perspectives are used: infectious diseases, population-based cancer screenings and chronic diseases management. In this chapter the discussion of the concept of health literacy responsiveness is introduced and the argumentation is built upon the idea that increasing systems' health literacy responsiveness may be equally or even more important than attempts to increase individual health literacy.

Renewing the Conceptual Framework for Health Literacy: the Contribution of Salutogenesis to Tapered the Health Gap, is the chapter six, introduced by Luis Saboga-Nunes, Didier Jourdain and Uwe H. Bittlingmayer to discuss the inclusion of health literacy (HL) in the development of a comprehensive paradigm that focusses on the origins of health. Health and HL have been mostly discussed from the bio-medical pathogenic perspective. This has had as a consequence serious hindrances to sustainability which is a critical component to human well-being. Breaking apart from traditional bio-medical approaches to health, the salutogenic approach was introduced by Aaron Antonovsky. The novelty of this perspective is that it considers health to be a part of a disease-ease continuum and to be a supply that is dependent on other resources. HL is as one of these other resources that has drawn attention, being today considered a valuable standing reserve to humanity. From the stand point of the Sense of Coherence theory, health literacy is regarded as a Macro Social General Resistance Resource.

The second part of this book addresses health literacy in the educational setting and how this setting can contribute to promote health literacy.

With the seventh chapter Hanna E. Schwendemann, Anja Stiller, Paula Bleckmann, Thomas Mößle and Eva-Maria Bitzer take us on a journey of complex intervention/implementation in the kindergarten setting. The point of departure is screen media usage, generally considered a major public health issue. Research reports an increase in the amount of time children spend with screen media, with negative effects on their physical, emotional and cognitive development. This establishes the need for primary prevention of developmental problems. From this, an intervention to support screen media-sensitive environments in the home and the child care setting was implemented. Considering children's problematic or addictive use of screen media in a multi-setting approach through the targeting of parents, children and teachers in a longitudinal cluster-controlled trial among kindergartens is the ambitious research project, the results of which the team shared with us. They examined practical experiences, looked at the children's bedroom screen media equipment and screen time, and addressed parental perceived need of media education support in the target group and its dependence on actual screen media use and equipment in the family.

A challenging eigth chapter is introduced by a team of authors led by Paulo Pinheiro and Shanti George and co-authored by Orkan Okan, Elise Sijthoff, Uwe H. Bittlingmayer, Rahel Kahlert, Almas Merchant, Dirk Bruland, Janine Bröder and Ullrich Bauer. Here the goal is to de-construct health literacy meanings by giving a voice to children in their meaning making process. This chapter is like looking through a window into a gathering of people discussing at the table: we get the glimpse of insights that were generated in the course of wider exchange with researchers within the network Working together Internationally on Social development and health in Every School and family (WISHES). This chapter depicts what is not often captured on paper, the vibrant exchanges (usually verbal) between researchers working in allied areas, notably at gatherings more open and fluid than those which assemble members of a single entity. In this particular case, WISHES and HCLA were invited to co-host a pre-conference on 'Recognizing Children and Young People as Active Citizens within health literacy: Theory and practice across Europe', at the Third European Health Literacy Conference held in Brussels in November 2015. During this pre-conference, and through the different presentations that were given (largely by the co-authors of this chapter), the researchers concerned, and many other participants felt and expressed the need for new perspectives within research and debate on children's health literacy. This need is here addressed as a result of a debate from a 'liquid network' to recognize young citizens' capacities for meaning-making.

One of the specific targets of the HLCA consortium was mental health literacy. In chapter nine, Dirk Bruland and Patricia Graf explain why we need a different mental health literacy concept. Starting from Anthony Jorm's concept of mental health literacy, common strategies to "assess" mental health literacy are presented and discussed. The concept itself is critically reflected in this chapter and its usefulness is regarded from different perspectives

To finalize this second part of the book, chapter ten by Agnes Santha, Uwe H. Bittlingmayer, Torsten M. Bollweg, Igor Osipov, Jürgen Gerdes, Orkan Okan, Gözde Okcu and Diana Sahrai links directly two almost completely separated discourses and concepts: Health Literacy and Life Skills. This chapter analyses the relationship of the two broad concepts on an empirical basis. The analysis brings to the fore immense differences between German federal states. Assessing this regional difference is the key finding of this study. The analysis underlines the role of family affluence and gender, widely recognized as impacting health literacy, whereas school-related agents such as school type and performance also prove relevant.

The third part of the book, "Some cultural dimensions of health literacy", looks at what propels health literacy internationally today. It opens with the eleventh chapter where Zeynep Islertas invites us to consider the importance of New Media and ehealth-information in the everyday life of female adolescents with Turkish migration backgrounds in Germany. This perspective looks at a „vulnerable group" of migrants, described to have worse health status than the indigenous population. According to recent studies, digital media and especially apps represent a way to encourage adolescents to deal with health-related issues. Study results describing the use of applications by adolescents with a Turkish migration background are hard to find and therefore represent a research desideratum. In order to contribute to closing this gap, this qualitative-ethnographic study assessed the relevance of New Media in the everyday life of female adolescents with a Turkish migration background as well as the relevance of New Media in the health information search of the target group. It is stated that electronic health information processed in a technically and substantively low-threshold manner can be an opportunity to reach female adolescents with a Turkish migration background and furthermore to counteract health inequalities in the Federal Republic of Germany.

Asadullah Jawid, Uwe H. Bittlingmayer, Stefanie Harsch, M. Ebrahim Jawid, Luis Saboga-Nunes, Kristine Sørensen and Diana Sahrai help us travel to the Afghan context in order to grasp health literacy among male Afghans in a quantitative and explorative study. This chapter twelve deals with the fact that health literacy, a popular concept widely discussed in 'Western' countries is little known in low- and middle-income countries or even in conflict and crisis affected states. Nevertheless, this will not decrease the interest of exploring health literacy in these parts of the world, since it is believed that increasing health literacy might directly improve the overall health status of the Afghan population. This is one of the priorities in countries such as Afghanistan. This article aims to contribute to research by exploring health literacy in Afghanistan and the application of the health literacy concept to this country.

Reflections on health literacy in the European and Colombian context, this is the main topic of chapter thirteen that helps us consider the topic of health literacy outside of the western borders also. Isabella Bertschi and Lilliana Villa-Vélez take us to South America. The purpose of this chapter is to present reflections on the concept of health literacy and how it is reflected in public policies in Europe and Colombia. There is an ongoing debate regarding the concept of health literacy and its relation to health education and health promotion that has not yet led to consensus regarding its conceptualization and the use of terminology. In the European Union we witnessed an effort to develop public policies with a focus on health literacy that was channeled by the European Commission (in countries like Scotland, Wales, Austria and Switzerland also NGOs such as NALA and WHO, the various patient organizations and associated bodies of the EU). Colombia, on the other hand, has several policies that very generally mention health education without explications on how it should be developed. It is important to articulate the theory and practice of health literacy and health education. In order to do so, there is a need to look into several issues such as strengthening the training of health professionals in education, improving educational methodology in health education, better aligning the education that is suggested and the one that is practiced, taking into account the particularities of the contexts in which health literacy is sought to improve and reflecting what health and what education aims to promote. Finally, neither health literacy nor health education can be implemented uncritically in any given context without considering the local demands, expectations and developments. This chapter helps to frame the ongoing debate that should continue in order to develop public policies that contribute to healthier and more equitable societies.

"Health literacy in Afghanistan – astonishing insights that provoke a reconsideration of the common concept and measures of health literacy" is the foreteenth chapter of this book presented by Asadullah Jawid, Stefanie Harsch and M. Ebrahim Jawid. Asadullah Jawid and Ebrahim Jawid came from Afghanistan to participate in the summer school and considerably enriched the discussion with their standpoints. Going back home, Asadullah and Ebrahim Jawid went on a mission, not only collecting data but exploring the meaning of health literacy deep inside this country. The study is based on general health data, two main policy programs, and the expertise of practitioners. After describing the relevant data and findings on health literacy, these are compared with the findings by the European Health Literacy Survey (HLS on the same Items).

The final part of this book comprises two chapters that focus on health literacy in the context of policy implications.

The first one, chapter fifteen, by Kristine Sørensen looks at health literacy champions and their leadership. Recognizing the important role of health literacy champions for re-designing and re-orienting health systems towards people-centredness as the World Health Organization pledged to do, this chapter aims to explore how health literacy champions are characterized and nurtured as change-agents for the development of health literate organizations, settings and societies.

The second chapter of this final part, chapter sixteen, closes this book with the explorations by Paulo Pinheiro and Ullrich Bauer from the perspective of the healthy life, using health literacy as a key concept. These authors argue that the recent proliferation of health literacy research has revealed that there is no universal concept but rather a coexistence of different concepts that are linked to different terminologies and conceptual backgrounds. The constituent dimensions of health literacy, therefore, remain disputed, and ways to make them visible through empirical observation vary widely. Subjecting the skill-based view of health literacy to a critical analysis raises some crucial concerns such as a disregard of the social practice, a neglect of social determinants, or a subordination of personal determinants other than skills, such as values, dispositions or beliefs. Within the health literacy discourse, a critical reflection on such concerns has been sparse. Therefore, this paper suggests that important conceptual and methodological issues remain to be addressed and discussed.

With "Linking different perspectives" we hope that the reader will get immersed in the multiple corners of the fabric to which piece by piece new threads and strands are added in the creation of health literacy knowledge. Hopefully by un-revealing some of the in-depth literature of the HLCA consortium, we have recovered some gems that will proliferate, giving rise to new opportunities for enhancing well-being and quality of life as well as to new discussions focusing on the topic of health literacy.

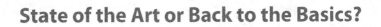

State of the Art or Back to the Basics?

Health Literacy in the Context of Health Inequality – A Framing and a Research Overview

Uwe H. Bittlingmayer, Stefanie Harsch and Zeynep Islertas

1   Introduction

In this chapter we provide a general overview of the current state of health literacy research. Here we have chosen to proceed more selectively and at the same time more broadly than is now usual in the systematic literature reviews based on the PRISMA standard that are customary in specialist journals. One reason is that the field of knowledge in health literacy is presented much more comprehensively than in a methodologically meaningful approach to meta-analysis, which generally involves a compilation of the effectiveness of specific active

In discussions about health literacy – or more generally – about the opportunities of health promotion strategies I hear far too rarely and far too little about the fact that in almost all European countries poverty and social inequality are increasing faster or more strongly than can be compensated for by the best health promotion policy and the best primary prevention. [...] This consistently violates the most important requirements for health literacy and even if we can't change that we have to say it. (Rosenbrock 2015 p. 1)

U. H. Bittlingmayer (✉) · S. Harsch · Z. Islertas
University of Education Freiburg (Germany), Institute of Sociology, Freiburg, Germany
e-mail: uwe.bittlingmayer@ph-freiburg.de

S. Harsch
e-mail: stefanie.harsch@ph-freiburg.de

Z. Islertas
e-mail: zeynep.islertas@ph-freiburg.de

© The Editor(s) (if applicable) and The Author(s), under exclusive license to
Springer Fachmedien Wiesbaden GmbH, part of Springer Nature 2021
L. A. Saboga-Nunes et al. (eds.), *New Approaches to Health Literacy*,
Gesundheit und Gesellschaft, https://doi.org/10.1007/978-3-658-30909-1_2

components or interventions. Rather, for our purposes, we require a more systematic treatment of the connection between general health disparities on the one hand, and the role of health literacy on the other. With this in mind, the framing in this state of research is broader. A selective approach to the literature is still necessary, simply because we can neither reflect the entire international, empirical state of knowledge here – for that would also involve a more detailed discussion of current results of health literacy studies, for example, from Taiwan, Mongolia, Brazil, Australia or Nigeria – nor can we pursue the health literacy concepts in all small-scale differentiations, such as food literacy or diabetes literacy, or discuss all the available measuring tools. In this respect, this chapter does not aim to present a comprehensive research overview on the topic of health literacy, but, more modestly, to formulate a research overview of the state of health literacy research as we see it.

2   Discourse on Health Disparities

In the last ten to fifteen years, a retrospective discourse on health disparities began in the German-speaking countries, which has been established for at least a decade longer in the Anglo-American regions (cf. a.o. Black and Whitehead 1992; Blaxter 1983; Wilkinson 1996; Wilkinson and Marmot 2003). Socio-epidemiological pioneers such as Andreas Mielck (2000, 2005) Helmert (2003; Helmert and Schorb 2006) or Elkeles and Mielck (1997) have gradually contributed to the realisation in Germany, Austria and Switzerland that scandalous health disparities exist in these very wealthy countries with regard to the dependence of (multi-)morbidity and mortality on socio-demographic criteria and in the context of disparities in care (cf. e.g. Bauer et al. 2008; Jungbauer-Gans and Kriwy 2004; Lampert 2016; Richter and Hurrelmann 2006a; Simon 2016; Slotala 2011; Tiesmeyer et al. 2008). Although the findings are not entirely clear, it can be assumed that health disparities have remained stable at least over the last fifteen years. The difference in life expectancy – the strongest indicator for disparities between the poor and affluent populations – was just under nine years for men according to data from the German Socio-Economic Panel (SOEP) from 2001 to 2004 (Lauterbach et al. 2006). Lampert et al. (2007) arrive at a result of 10.8 years in an evaluation of SOEP data for the years 1995 to 2005, and in a more recent study by the WZB [Berlin Social Science Center], the difference in life expectancy between poor and affluent men is also just under 11 years (Habich 2013). The majority of studies, such as those by Kroll (2010) or Rathmann (2015), assume a limited increase in health disparities; however, these link health disparities more strongly with welfare state research in international comparison. Furthermore, Habich's study states a difference in life expectancy of eight years for women, which would be a reduction of almost one year compared to Lauterbach's study, which indicates 8.9 years. The state of research in the German-speaking regions on the dynamics of health disparities must therefore be described as unclear and inconsistent; however, it was already clear in 2006 that there was consensus on the fact that there are massive health disparities in Germany, Austria and Switzerland (Richter and Hurrelmann 2006b), and this is no longer seriously disputed. Thomas Lampert (2016, p. 131), one of the leading experts in health disparity research at the Robert Koch Institute, sums up the developmental dynamics as follows: "The available results, which were obtained primarily on the basis of the health surveys by the Robert Koch Institute and the SOEP, suggest that the observed health disparities have proved to be extremely stable over time and in some cases have even increased."

Since the existence of health disparities is no longer repudiated, increased efforts are now being made to determine the explanatory and development factors. The following list is not intended to suggest completeness, but to outline the large number of differing methods and approaches: In recent years, numerous and varied explanatory approaches have been developed that can be associated with health disparities. On the one hand, general models were constructed with the aim of initiating a complex (multivariate) statistical study (Mielck 2000, 2005; WHO and Europe 2008; cf. also Wilkinson and Marmot 2003) [cf. Fig. 1].

In addition, studies were carried out to analyse the role of individual factors, such as the individual or aggregate social capital (Hartung 2014; Kawachi et al. 1997; Siegrist et al. 2006), the influence of regional differences (by examining socio-demographic features) (Bittlingmayer et al. 2009; Hoffmann et al. 2014; Sundmacher 2016), general inequalities of income (Wilkinson 2005; Wilkinson and Pickett 2010)[1] or the link between general social and health disparities (Hradil 2006; Kroll 2010; Vester 2009). A major part of the studies attempted to determine the precise extent of health disparities, above all by focusing on specific target groups, such as the poor population (congruent with unemployed persons and recipients of *Hartz IV* [German social welfare], groups of ethnic minorities or people with a migrant background or experience of having to flee their homeland (Razum 2006; RKI 2008; Sahrai 2009), women (Babitsch 2009;

---

[1]Cf. also Pickett and Wilkinson (2015), who go as far as to say that disparity of income has a real causal effect on a variety of unequal health outcomes.

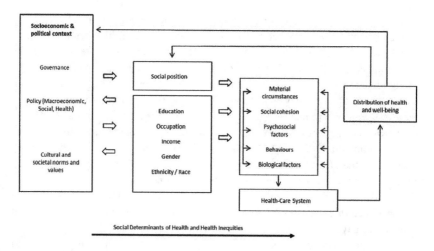

Fig. 1 Conceptual framework of the WHO Commission Social Determinants of Health based on Solar and Irwin 2007 and the WHO Final Report 2008; quoted after Lampert 2016: 130

Babitsch et al. 2017; Kolip 2000; Kuhlmann and Kolip 2008; Sperlich 2009) or children and young people (Rathmann 2015; Richter 2005).

In the context of questions on the connection between social determinants, health literacy and health disparities, research work ultimately plays an important role in attempting to empirically determine the factors that influence a person's individual behaviour towards overarching social structures (cf. Sperlich 2016 and Bittlingmayer 2016) regarding the conceptual level). In the socio-science approach to health disparity research (in contrast to socio-psychological), it is considered in the first instance as undisputed that the structural constraints exert more influence on health disparity than individual health-related behaviour. Giesecke and Müters (2009) show in a secondary analysis of SOEP data that two thirds of the explanation of subjective health status can be attributed to structural aspects and only one third to aspects of individual behaviour.

Nevertheless, from the perspective assumed here of an *analysis of social practices*, distinguishing between social structures and individual behaviour that interact inseparably in the everyday practices of real subjects, can only be a matter of *analytical differentiation*. This becomes clear in the debate about so-called 'healthy lifestyles', which are propagated as a guarantee for maximizing the years of a healthy life. In a study dealing with health disparities, Cockerham et al.

(2006) demonstrate on the basis of Russian data that social class circumstances, age, gender, milieu and living conditions have the capacity to determine health-related individual behaviour in one direction or the other: "The analysis shows that variables in each of the categories were associated with particular health life-style practices and self-rated health" (Cockerham et al. 2006, p. 195).

Such analyses also exist for Germany: "The present empirical analysis of the relationship between class affiliation and three important aspects of individual health behaviour (smoking, obesity, sporting activities) emphatically confirm that socio-structural conditions (material/financial situation, educational resources and occupational position) continue to influence individual health behaviour in Germany". (Helmert and Schorb 2006, p. 137). Individual health-promoting decisions which are made in the living environments of social protagonists and, all in all, constitute a health-promoting lifestyle, are neither the product of a conscious decision, nor can individual actions simply be extracted from social structures. Rather, individual actions – and this also applies to a range of skills – are incontrovertibly permeated by socio-structural framings and combinations of circumstances (Nideröst 2007; Sperlich and Mielck 2003; Vester 2009), as well as by status and power structures in society (Brunnett 2009; Foucault 1983; Kühn 1993).

Even if the significance of disparity structures in society as a whole, for individual health in general and for health disparity circumstances in particular, can hardly be doubted, a stronger trend towards behavioural approaches in dealing with such disparities has been observed in recent years. This trend towards health behaviour is fuelled by role models presented by the mass media, such as the 'autonomous subject as a self-carer for his health' (Schmidt 2017, p. 158). This is because the avoidance of behaviour that is detrimental to health seems to be an attractive and feasible health policy strategy to at least counter rising costs in the health sector or the increase in rates of obesity (even in childhood and adolescence) and to be regarded as successful in the context of smoking rates, which have been declining for years. It is this standpoint of reconstruction and argumentation that lends the health literacy discourse and approach its particular relevance. For, on the one hand, this approach provides – as will become apparent – a fully illustrative and explanatory perspective at the interface between structure and individual behaviour, especially for adolescents (Paakkari et al. 2019), and on the other hand, it particularly suits the current neoliberal health policy, which relies primarily on changing behaviour (cross-disziplinary: Lessenich 2013; Schmidt 2017; Schmidt and Kolip 2007; Simon 2011), because structural disparities can be transformed into deficits in individual competencies (Bittlingmayer and Sahrai 2019). Furthermore, health literacy is also associated with lowering costs in the entire health care sector: "Overall, the long-held promise of health literacy is that improved health literacy will produce improvements in health status – ideally at lower costs" (Pleasant et al. 2018).

At all events, there is wide consensus in current public health research and practice that health literacy is a promising approach that can identify disparities in care provision, prevention or health promotion, which are causes of inequity in a different way than in the socio-epidemiological presentation of significant correlations pointing to social disparity, and also that health literacy is closely associated with the topic of health disparity (Mantwill 2015; Paasche-Orlow and Wolf 2010). Furthermore, the concept increasingly serves as a promising starting point for prevention and health promotion. The National Action Plan Health Literacy in Germany was presented recently in Berlin, which along with the proximity of the health literacy concept to health policy, also highlights the importance of prevention and health promotion (Schaeffer et al. 2019). Furthermore, the Interdisciplinary Centre for Health Literacy Research at the University of Bielefeld was opened in 2019. As a result of the proven link between health literacy and various negative health outcomes, such as lower self-assessment of health, more frequent use of health services and difficulties in interacting with health professionals, a health policy based on population-wide health literacy empowerment is expected to contribute significantly to health equality. Accordingly, the WHO Shanghai Declaration was formulated in 2016 as a call to all relevant players to improve health literacy (see Box 1).

Box 1: WHO Shanghai Declaration (Excerpt)

Health Literacy Empowers and Drives Equity
Health literacy empowers individual citizens and enables their engagement in collective health promotion action. A high health literacy of decision-makers and investors supports their commitment to health impact, co-benefits and effective action on the determinants of health. Health literacy is founded on inclusive and equitable access to quality education and life-long learning. It must be an integral part of the skills and competencies developed over a lifetime, first and foremost through the school curriculum.
We commit to

- recognize health literacy as a critical determinant of health and invest in its development;
- develop, implement and monitor intersectoral national and local strategies for strengthening health literacy in all populations and in all educational settings;

- increase citizens' control of their own health and its determinants, through harnessing the potential of digital technology;

Ensure that consumer environments support healthy choices through pricing policies, transparent information and clear labelling.

4 Definitory Approaches to Health Literacy

In spite of this broad consensus on the importance of health literacy, there is by no means any agreement in sight when it comes to a precise definition of health literacy; on the contrary, the debate on the correct definition of health literacy is described as contested terrain (Mackert et al. 2015; Pleasant et al. 2018; Pleasant and McKinney 2011). And in spite of the greatly increasing research interest in health literacy, there is much uncertainty about the dimensions it contains. There is so far no generally accepted definition of health literacy; on the contrary, there are various approaches to describing the concept (Abel 2008; Berkman et al. 2010; Coulter and Ellins 2007; Frisch et al. 2012; Kickbusch 2009; Wills 2009). Mancuso (2009, p. 88) already stated ten years ago, "The concept of health literacy is not entirely straightforward and the term is defined broadly and in a variety of ways in the literature". Current contributions to health literacy research also lean in the same direction. For instance, in the words of one of the most renowned researchers, Diane Levin-Zamir, health literacy research is still a 'work in progress' and remains a dynamic construct (Levin-Zamir, Leung, Dodson, and Rowlands 2017, p. 133); to date, no gold standard has been established with regard to methodically inquiring about and measuring health literacy (Nguyen et al. 2017, p. 190). At present there are more than 150 different measurement methods for health literacy (Okan et al. 2017; an overview of existing health literacy tools can be found at http://healthliteracy.bu.edu/). In view of the large number of health literacy operationalisations, we wish to associate the following presentation with only a curtailed claim: to trace, in more detail, important developments in the definitory approach to the term health literacy.

An early definition from the important journal *Das Gesundheitswesen* describes health literacy as "the degree to which individuals have the capacity to obtain, process, and understand basic health information and services needed to make appropriate health decisions" (Parker et al. 2003, p. 147). Health literacy is thus seen as a set of individual skills regarding the recognition of medical vocabulary, the comprehension of written text and numeracy skills which allow a person to acquire and use new information from the field of health. This definition has been problematised many times because it conceives health literacy more or less exclusively as a construct at the individual level (Berkman et al. 2010). This runs the risk of contextualising low levels of health literacy as a deficit on the part of the patients, thus attaching the responsibility for corrective action in the case of poor health literacy exclusively on to the person (Bernhardt et al. 2005; Freedman et al. 2009).

The Shanghai Declaration attempts to counteract this problem, for example, by having the health literacy of professionals described as an independent health system dimension (see Box 1 above; cf. for health literacy perspectives not referring to individuals, etc.) (Bruland et al. 2017; Dodson et al. 2015).

A modified version of the definition of Parker and colleagues was proposed by Nancy Berkman's team from the Agency for Health Care Research and Quality: Health literacy is, according to them, "[t]he degree to which individuals can obtain, process, understand, and communicate about health-related information needed to make informed health decisions" (Berkman et al. 2010, p. 16). Oral communication is explicitly emphasized here as an essential feature of health literacy. The reformulation of "have the capacity to" to "can" is intended to counter the criticism described above of understanding health literacy exclusively as an individual construct. The focus should be placed on knowhow which people can acquire instead of speaking of a more or less primordial skill in the sense of cognitive abilities. This was meant to lead to a more dynamic understanding of health literacy. Similar approaches, such as that of David Baker (2006), understand health literacy as a variable construct depending on the current medical problem, the healthcare professional(s), and the health system. In this concept, health literacy refers only to a specific treatment situation and may be expressed differently in the same person under different conditions. An analogous formulation emphasizes the potential for variability by defining health literacy as "the wide range of skills and competencies that people *develop* to seek out, comprehend, evaluate and use health information and concepts to make informed choices, reduce health risks and increase quality of life" (Zarcadoolas et al. 2005 196 f.). What is important about this approach is the relationship between health literacy and the dimension of quality of life. Through this dimension, health literacy is moved out of the care-related setting and connected, at least loosely, with motives of everyday lifestyle. However, the inclusion of a person's living environment in aspects of health literacy is already laid out at an earlier stage but is then closely linked to individual educational skills and performance in written language.

The widely-discussed proposal by Nutbeam (2000) for defining health literacy, which we already presented briefly in the introduction, conceives of health literacy as a hierarchical construct and distinguishes three levels: (1) *functional/*

basal health literacy as in having sufficient reading and writing skills to function in everyday situations, (2) *interactive/communicative health literacy,* meaning a combination of competence in reading and writing and social skills, enabling people to obtain information from a variety of communication channels, and (3) *critical health literacy,* meaning: sophisticated cognitive and social skills that enable a critical analysis of health information and thus increased control over one's own life. Creating a clear-cut hierarchy of these three levels enables both a quantitative and a qualitative acquisition of health literacy. Furthermore this concept underlines the possibility of increasing skills in the field of health literacy and the associated gain in autonomy (Nutbeam 2009; Tones 2002).

The close connection between educational skills and health literacy is, on the face of it, extremely plausible because, for example, a large number of empirical studies describe a high correlation between formal education and health literacy in very different countries. A representative study conducted in Japan in 2006, for example, found that people with a lower level of formal education more often have limited communicative and critical health skills in the sense of Nutbeam (Furuya et al. 2013). A recent representative study in Switzerland showed that people with less formal education have a lower average level of health literacy (Schweizerische Akademie der Medizinischen Wissenschaften 2015). Lastly, the Robert Koch Institute also presented a representative study in 2013, which established that within the group of people with less formal education, the percentage of people with inadequate health skills was almost twice as high as in the group of people with high formal educational status (Jordan and Hoebel 2015). However, the close interconnection of health literacy and formal education set out in Nutbeam's model is less self-evident than it seems at first glance (see Bittling-mayer and Sahrai 2019 for details). To use a somewhat polemical example: it is not absolutely essential for a person who does not have higher education and consumes tobacco on a daily basis to first take school-leaving examinations in order to decide to stop smoking (cf. the contributions of Harsch et al. in this volume).

A definition which associates health literacy with skills for promoting and maintaining health without reference to formal educational qualifications has been put forward by the World Health Organization (WHO): "Health literacy represents the cognitive and social skills which determine the motivation and ability of individuals to gain access to, understand and use information in ways which promote and maintain good health" (WHO 2009, p. 10). This is the only definition that takes up the aspect of being motivated to maintain one's health. However, the formulation that health literacy is a prerequisite for the motivation for promoting and maintaining personal health is clumsy and evidentially untrue (Powell et al. 2007).

The largest recent research project in the field of health literacy was the *European Health Literacy Survey (HLS-EU)*, in which research teams from eight European countries participated (Pelikan et al. 2012). Based on a systematic review of definitions and concepts in the field of health literacy, the HLS-EU Consortium defines health literacy very comprehensively as:

"people's knowledge, motivation and competences to access, understand, appraise, and apply health information in order to make judgments and take decisions in everyday life concerning healthcare, disease prevention and health promotion to maintain or improve quality of life during the life course" (Sørensen et al. 2012, p. 3).

This conceptual model establishes a link between health literacy and a person's state of health or quality of life. It also links health literacy to health care in terms of institutions, to disease prevention and to health promotion. It conceives of health literacy as a multi-layered concept that goes far beyond the mere comprehension of medical vocabulary (HLS-EU Consortium 2012; Sørensen et al. 2012; Sørensen and Brand 2014). A similar definition comes from Switzerland:

"Health literacy is the ability to apply knowledge about the maintaining and regaining of physical, mental and social well-being to personal and collective decisions and behaviour in such a way that they have a positive effect on one's own health and the health of others as well as on living and environmental conditions." (Netzwerk Bildung + Gesundheit 2015)

As can be seen from these two comprehensive formulations, efforts are being made to combine the various definitions and to propose the most uniform solution possible (Sørensen et al. 2012). Whether this is feasible at all, however, is viewed with scepticism, as the research context and the goal of knowledge in the various fields of application of health literacy are scarcely comparable (Abel 2008; Berkman et al. 2010; Chinn 2011).

If health literacy, as in the variant of the European Health Literacy Survey, is *freed from the care-related strait jacket* and a definition is chosen which, in addition to informed action in care-related settings, *seeks to cover the areas of prevention and health promotion*, then *the necessary practical reference to the living environment will be linked to the health literacy concept, which moves the concept closer to an everyday sociology of health behaviour.* However, this conceptual proximity between everyday behavioural skills, subjective relevance settings and lifestyle practices and an expanded health literacy definition that is not restricted to the provision of care is not reflected – as will become clear below – in the attempts to operationalise health competence.

5   Measurement or Recording of Health Literacy

Since no uniform definition of the term health literacy exists so far, there are also very different approaches to measuring the construct (Abel 2008; Canadian Council on Learning 2007; Mackert et al. 2015; Pleasant et al. 2018).

Initially, literacy, and thus, indirectly, health literacy, was seen as a direct product of school education, which is why the number of years of education was chosen as the indicator (Berkman et al. 2010). However, since it soon became apparent that reading and writing skills correlate only partially with the duration of education, schooling was rejected as a direct indicator of literacy. For a long period, a strong focus on reading and writing as well as basal numerical skills characterized efforts to measure health literacy (Kutner et al. 2007)[2]. Following several American literacy studies and the International Adult Literacy Survey (IALS) from 1994–1998 (Kirsch 2001), items for measuring health literacy were systematically collected and classified for the first time. The result was the Health Activities Literacy Scale (HALS) (Rudd, Kirsch, and Yamamoto 2004). Due to its length, however, HALS was not suitable for studies in a clinical medical context, which is why shorter tests were developed in this area for recording the comprehension of written texts (Berkman et al. 2004). The first test was the Rapid Estimate of Adult Literacy in Medicine (REALM) (Davis et al. 1993; Murphy et al. 1993). It contains 66 words from the field of medicine, which the person being tested must read aloud. The evaluation is based on the number of correctly read words and gives an assessment of reading skills according to levels of education. A version was also developed for young people, the REALM-Teen (Davis et al. 2006). The second tool, which is mainly used in clinical settings, is the Test of Functional Health Literacy in Adults (TOFHLA) (R. M. Parker et al. 1995). It contains three text passages with 50 reading comprehension tasks and 17 numerical skill items. There is also a short version, the S-TOFHLA (Baker et al. 1999), which contains only two passages of text and four items of arithmetic. Both versions of TOFHLA define the results using three levels of health literacy: inadequate, marginal and adequate. The reading comprehension tasks were validated for use with adolescents (Chisolm and Buchanan 2007). The Brief Health Literacy Screen (BHLS) (Chew et al. 2004; Wallston et al. 2014), which

---

[2]It should be mentioned only in passing that the approach of Social Literacy or New Literacy Studies (cf. Street 1984, 2003), which adopts a different view of literacy skills than is usual in the now predominant PISA tradition of competence, has found virtually no entry into existing health literacy research.

contains only three items, and the Newest Vital Sign (NVS) (Weiss et al. 2005) with six questions, are also very short. Both these tests are intended for use as screening instruments in medical settings and, in line with Nutbeam (2009), measure "health-related literacy in clinical settings" (p. 304), which raises doubt about their application in contexts other than medical settings.

The measurement methods presented here clearly show that they all measure skills that are defined in a very limited framework, which does not do justice to today's wide theoretical understanding of health literacy (Levin-Zamir et al. 2017; Pleasant and McKinney 2011). Furthermore, the vast majority of them focus on measuring functional health literacy (for a critical view see, for example, Sørensen et al. 2012). In its efforts to record health literacy as a multi-layered concept, the HLS-EU Consortium (2012) developed the European Health Literacy Study Questionnaire (HLS-EU-Q). It contains 47 questions that record the subjectively perceived difficulty of performing certain health-related tasks. Four levels of health literacy are defined on a scale of 0 to 50 points: inadequate, problematic, sufficient and excellent, with the two lower levels referred to jointly as 'limited health literacy'. An important difference with regard to the other measurement tools presented is the concept of a self-assessment questionnaire. The measurement is therefore subjective when compared to the objective assessments achieved by functional health literacy tests (Sørensen et al. 2012). Here, too, a short version was developed, which was meant to reflect the three dimensions of health literacy using 16 items (HLS-EU 16), but which can no longer differentiate the three factors by factor analysis.

All the tools presented so far measure health literacy quantitatively and have been developed mostly in a clinical medical setting. The aim of the measurements is to obtain an estimate of the existing skills of the person being examined, usually patients, within the shortest possible time. This runs counter to the efforts to adequately reflect the complexity of the concept of health literacy within the measuring tools (Jordan et al. 2010). What is lacking so far are measurement methods that take account of the development of health literacy definitions towards a more strongly socio-scientific perspective.

In reference to this, Mancuso (2009, p. 87) rightly points out:

"Many constraints exist to the assessment of health literacy. (…) Health literacy includes more than word recognition, reading comprehension, and numeracy. The existing measures and screenings do not fully grasp the concept of health literacy in terms of language, context, culture, communication, or technology. Thus, we do not yet possess a measure that takes into account the full set of skills and knowledge associated with health literacy".

This statement makes several criticisms of the tools used so far to measure health literacy:

- Many of today's concepts of health literacy, and thus also the measuring tools based on them, have an individualistic and cognitivist bias. They focus (too) strongly on literacy skills and notions of health behaviour as rational and calculated decision-making (Bittlingmayer and Sahrai 2019; McCormack et al. 2010; Pleasant et al. 2018; Sahrai et al. 2018; van der Vaart et al. 2011).
- The existing instruments are not sufficiently culture-sensitive. This point must also be considered in translations (Levin-Zamir et al. 2017; cf. Nguyen et al. 2017).
- The context of a health-relevant action is not given sufficient attention. As already mentioned several times, most instruments refer explicitly to clinical medical settings (Nguyen et al. 2015).
- The different technologies that could be used to support health communication are not employed. The current test procedures are largely limited to paper-and-pencil questionnaires, although digital media in particular are considered to have great potential in the area of health literacy (Mancuso 2009; Pleasant et al. 2018).
- The communicative context, in which (the application of) health literacy is generally embedded, is given too little consideration. Whether a patient with little knowledge of the national language will actually ask critical questions about his treatment plan during the two-minute visit by the consultant physician will be primarily determined by the social situation – the power asymmetry between doctor and patient, and, for example, the trust in a person with more knowledge in the health-related field will have a significant influence on the behaviour of the patient.
- Due to the history of their origins as screening instruments for inadequate health literacy, the existing measuring tools are deficit-oriented. The primary goal is the identification of a lack of skills (Nguyen et al. 2015; Pleasant et al. 2018). A resource-oriented perspective aimed at making existing health-relevant skills visible and usable has so far been neglected (Bittlingmayer and Sahrai 2019).

What the more complex definitions of health literacy presented here, which are currently at the forefront the of academic discourse (Bröder et al. 2016; Nutbeam 2009; Sørensen et al. 2012), have in common is that they have removed the concept of health literacy from the care-specific context and placed it conceptually in the vicinity of everyday actions and living environments. This has resulted in a methodological shift outside the clinical setting, and from the direct measurement of written language skills to the indirect measurement of self-assessed health literacy.

6   Link Between Health Literacy and Health Outcomes

As already explained in detail, the definition and, to a lesser extent, the recording of health literacy has undergone some significant changes in recent years. This places certain limits on the significance of studies which establish links between the shaping of health literacy and the state of health. It is difficult to arrive at reliable comparable statements on the basis of the different definitions from which they are derived (Mackert et al. 2015). Nevertheless, the available studies provide valuable information on how a possible link between social inequalities and health disparities could be established. The findings presented below underline the importance attributed to health literacy in the context of health disparities, self-responsibility and health-related prevention.

Improving health literacy is seen as an important political and social objective because numerous studies have shown a link between poor health literacy and poorer health outcomes (DeWalt et al. 2004; Statistics Canada and OECD 2005). A review that considered studies from 1980 to 2003 demonstrated that patients with poor health literacy had on average a 1.5 to 3 times greater chance as patients with at least sufficient health literacy of showing a certain negative outcome (DeWalt et al. 2004). Poor health literacy is thus associated with a poorer state of health, the greater use of health services and higher health costs (Canadian Council on Learning 2007; Kindig, Panzer, Nielsen-Bohlman, Committee on Health Literacy, and Board on Neuroscience and Behavioral Health, Institute of Medicine 2004; Statistics Canada and OECD 2005; Weiss 2005). According to the results of the Adult Literacy and Life Skills Survey (ALLS), there are, among other things, connections between poor skills in the field of health literacy and low life satisfaction or health limitations in everyday and social activities. Further studies show that poor health literacy is consistently associated with a higher prevalence of chronic illnesses and poorer skills in coping with these (DeWalt et al. 2004; Rothman et al. 2009; Sarkar et al. 2006; Williams et al. 1998; Zarcadoolas et al. 2009). Other correlations exist between poor health literacy and more frequent hospitalization (Baker et al. 2002; Baker et al. 1998; Cimasi et al. 2013; Fleisher et al. 2014; Schillinger et al. 2002), repeated and major use of emergency services (Griffey et al. 2014; Mancuso and Rincon 2006), less participation in preventative measures (Bennett et al. 2009; Cho et al. 2008), a poorer understanding of package inserts for medication and general health information (Wolf et al. 2007) and poorer adherence to medication taken by the patients themselves (Lin et al. 2014; Rothman et al. 2009; Weiss 1999; Zhang et al. 2014). In Germany at least, older people generally have a lower standard of health literacy (Berens et al. 2016). There is also a negative correlation between health literacy and mortality among older people (Baker et al. 2007; Baker et al. 2008; Bostock and Steptoe 2012; Sudore et al. 2006), as well as in patients receiving outpatient treatment for cardiac insufficiency (McNaughton et al. 2015; Peterson et al. 2011). In an Australian cohort study, poor health literacy was associated with high blood pressure, smoking, diabetes and lack of exercise as well as depression (Appleton et al. 2013). Poor health literacy is not only associated with factors of diminished physical health but can also be linked to poorer mental health (Lee et al. 2010). Among the negative psychological correlates of poor health literacy are diminished psychological well-being (Tokuda et al. 2009 cf. also the contribution of Bruland and Graf in this volume), low self-efficacy (Como 2014; Osborn et al. 2010; Sarkar et al. 2006), a lower perceived quality of life (Mancuso and Rincon 2006; Song et al. 2012) and an increase in depressive symptoms.

Poor health literacy is expressed in difficulties with completing forms in medical contexts, in complying with medication prescription, and especially in physician-patient interaction (Schillinger 2004; Seurer and Vogt 2013) or, for example, failure to ask questions (Katz et al. 2007). A further complicating factor is that it has been shown that people with poor health literacy feel shame for their low skills in this area (Chew et al. 2004; Mancuso 2009). This can lead to attempts to hide difficulties with reading or vocabulary (Parikh 1996). Other studies have also shown that people with poor health literacy are less likely to ask clarifying questions due to embarrassment or even fear, which can hinder the accurate diagnosis of individual health problems (Vernon et al. 2007). In order to ensure access to health care and more equal opportunities in this context, a sensitive recording of health literacy is therefore crucial. Since the importance of health literacy for a range of health outcomes has become apparent, the following section shows more precisely how health literacy is distributed among the population.

7   Distribution of Health Literacy Among the Population

Despite different paradigms in measurement and theoretical conceptualization, poor health literacy is by no means a marginal phenomenon. According to several studies, there is a significant proportion of people with poor health literacy even in high-income countries. For example, the Institute of Medicine came to the conclusion in its somewhat over-optimistically titled report *Health Literacy: A Prescription to End Confusion* that more than 90 million adults in the US do not have the necessary skills to effectively navigate the American healthcare system (Kindig et al. 2004). In common with the Adult Literacy and Life Skills Survey (ALLS), it was found that in many high-income countries less than half of the population reaches adequate health literacy levels (Australian Bureau of Statistics 2008; Rudd 2007). Current figures on the prevalence of poor or sufficient health literacy in Europe can be found in the European Health Literacy Survey (HLS-EU), which was conducted between 2010 and 2012 (cf. Fig. 2).

Throughout all eight participating countries and regions, almost half of the population has limited health literacy. The highest rate of limited health literacy is found in Spain with 58.3 %, the lowest in the Netherlands with 28.7 % (HLS-EU Consortium 2012). The results for Germany show that 54.9 % of the population have limited health skills Schaeffer et al. 2017.

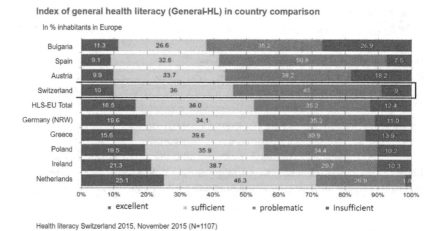

Fig. 2 Index of Health Literacy in Europe (gfs.bern 2016, p. 3)

A study is available for Switzerland, according to which the German-speaking population of Switzerland has a very high level of health literacy: 93.6 % of the persons tested have an appropriate level of health literacy. The differences to the other two other major linguistic regions are striking: in French-speaking Switzerland the proportion of people with adequate health literacy is 83.2 %, in Italian-speaking Switzerland 66.7 %. Health literacy was measured here with the S-TOHFLA, which is why only functional health literacy in the narrower sense can be depicted (Connor et al. 2013). In addition, there is a study that uses the HLS-EU-47 tool and provides comparative figures for Switzerland, showing that Switzerland is in the midfield of European countries (see Fig. 2).

Another large-scale representative survey for Germany provides similarly alarming findings. In this study, which was conducted by Doris Schaeffer and Klaus Hurrelmann, less than half of the population of Germany was shown to have sufficient health literacy, while the other half has limited health literacy (see Table 2). Health literacy was measured here with the self-assessment method using the HLS-EU 47 tool. The results are significantly worse than those of the European survey, in which, however, Germany was represented only by participants from North Rhine-Westphalia.

Source: (Berens et al. 2016, p. 4)

Having been able to illustrate the problems involved in measuring health literacy lacks with standardised tools, we will now investigate more precisely the possible social determinants of poor health literacy and their general association with social and health disparities.

8   Social Determinants of Health Literacy

All the studies cited consistently show links between health literacy and various socio-demographic variables. This inevitably raises questions about social and health disparities in the health system (see in particular Shanghai Declaration 2016; NHS Scotland 2014; Schaeffer et al. 2019). It seems that the lower their level of education, the poorer a person's health literacy will be. In Canada, for example, the ALLS showed a positive correlation between educational levels and health literacy scores (Canadian Council on Learning 2007). This correlation was confirmed in the HLS-EU and, in addition, a lower standard of health literacy was observed in association with membership in a lower social class and lower income levels (Gibney et al. 2020; HLS-EU Consortium 2012).

Health literacy declines with age (Australian Bureau of Statistics 2008; Berens et al. 2016; Rudd 2007; Statistics Canada and OECD 2005). Age even amplifies the differences based on the level of education (Canadian Council on Learning 2007). Children and adolescents are hardly ever examined in a study on health literacy; a fact that has already been criticized many times (DeWalt and Hink 2009; Manganello 2008; Wolf et al. 2009; Yin et al. 2009; Yin et al. 2007). The few studies are usually limited to unrepresentative samples. According to their results, between one tenth and one third of young people have limited to inadequate health literacy. Trout et al. (2014) tested adolescents from an American home for children and young people and concluded that nearly one-third (31 %) had difficulty understanding basic patient information due to their limited health literacy. A study of HIV-infected adolescents from the USA found 20 % with limited health literacy (Navarra et al. 2014). A sample of adolescents in Taiwan showed a significantly lower percentage (9.7 %) with poor health literacy. At the same time, this study confirmed the socio-demographic risk factors for poor health literacy: If adolescents were from ethnic minority families, had a low income or if their parents had not had tertiary education, low levels of health literacy in the children were significantly more frequent (Chang 2011).

A direct connection between ethnicity and the level of health literacy can also be statistically proven by many studies. Ethnic minority groups are disproportionately affected by poor health literacy in the USA (Kutner et al. 2006; Nguyen et al. 2015; Vernon et al. 2007). People with a migrant backgrounds tend to have poorer health literacy readings than those without a migrant background (Abrams et al. 2009; Mensing 2012), although the correlation is not clearly verifiable in all studies (HLS-EU Consortium 2012). In cases when a relationship between migrant status and health literacy can be established, migrants with a mother tongue other than the national language are particularly affected. This circumstance can be explained at least partly by the focus of the measurement tools on written comprehension that are offered in the official language of the country (Australian Bureau of Statistics 2008). Within the migrant population in Switzerland, persons from Kosovo, persons with a low level of education, men and older persons tend to have less knowledge about the symptoms that require a visit to the doctor (Ackermann et al. 2014). In Germany, a representative survey to determine the health literacy level of the adult population did not specifically identify people with a migration background or migrant history (Jordan and Hoebel 2015).

An overview of the findings on health literacy, migration and cultural differences contained many indications that a migrant background is associated with lower compliance, worse outcomes for chronic diseases and less frequent participation in preventative measures such as breast cancer screening. Poor health literacy is cited as an explanation in most studies. This is explained, among other things, by very different ideas and practices regarding health in the countries of origin and by language barriers (Shaw et al. 2008). A new study from the USA has shown that women from low-income minority groups with poor literacy and numeracy skills report major difficulties with contraception. As a result, this population has a high rate of unwanted pregnancies (Yee and Simon 2014). In Switzerland, increases in abortion rates among migrant women have been documented several times (Merten and Gari 2013). Among other things, a survey of well-qualified migrant women mainly from the Latin American cultural sphere, who, however, did not have official documents, showed that 40 % of respondents had experienced at least one unwanted pregnancy and almost half of these had had an abortion (Sebo et al. 2011). In a Swedish study, the health literacy of refugees and their health status were recorded. It was found that a high proportion of refugees have little to inadequate health literacy (Wångdahl et al. 2015, 2018). A systematic review of the literature revealed a correlation between the migration status and the omission of various health protection measures such as vaccinations and preventative medical screening. The main factor cited as an explanation for this is poor health literacy (Kowalski et al. 2014). In contrast to previous correlations, a study from Canada shows that there is a negative correlation between the health literacy level and the health status reported by immigrants themselves. The authors consequently assume that improving the health literacy of migrants could achieve two goals: improving health and improving the knowledge of the local language (Omariba and Ng 2011).

Many of the findings we have presented support the hypothesis that a migrant background can be regarded as a risk factor for lower skills in the area of health literacy. According to Ingleby et al. (2012), however, this view does not go far enough. They advocate the active participation of the migrant population in their integration into Western health systems. The values and thought patterns of those affected must consistently be taken into account in the development and expansion of health care, curation, rehabilitation, prevention and health promotion, rather than pushing migrants into mere assimilation into existing structures by means of programmes aimed at specific target groups. Zou and Parry (2012) or Mergenthal (2014) present similar arguments: it is not enough to state that migrants are difficult to reach for health promotion due to poor health skills and cultural, linguistic and socio-economic barriers. These factors must be consciously born in mind when planning health strategies and programmes. In Switzerland, efforts are being made in this direction within the framework of the National Programme on Migration and Health. Among other things, the Swiss Federal Office of Public Health published a manual on *Migration-Oriented Prevention and Health Promotion* in cooperation with Health Promotion Switzerland.

Overall, studies on the health and health literacy of migrants should conduct balanced surveys and systematically research the, at times, contradictory findings. There is much ambivalence between findings that underline the 'healthy migrant effect' and those that identify migration as a health risk factor, although it is still not fully understood to what extent these different results are also due to statistical artefacts (Makarova et al. 2013; Razum and Rohrmann 2002). It should again be pointed out that the migrant population is by no means a homogeneous group. As has already been noted, there are large health and socio-demographic differences between migrants from different backgrounds. Important factors that influence the link between migration and health include the reasons for migration, the personal experience of the migration process, the legal and social situation in the host country, educational success and specific ethnicity (e.g. as a suppressed minority of a national majority (Kurds, Alevis, Hazara, etc.) (Schenk 2007).

In this contribution, we first tried to appropriately determine the definitional difficulties concerning health literacy and reported measurement problems, some of which were considerable. Subsequently, we presented the importance of health literacy for a number of health outcomes as well as outlined the significant dimensions of limited health literacy. Finally, we identified a number of social determinants that have a significant influence on individual health literacy – always to be understood as literacy tests or self-reports.

References

Abel, T. (2008). Measuring health literacy: Moving towards a health - promotion perspective. *International Journal of Public Health, 53*(4), 169–170. https://doi.org/10.1007/s00038-008-0242-9.

Abrams, M. A., Klass, P., & Dreyer, B. P. (2009). Health literacy and children: Introduction. *Pediatrics, 124*(Suppl 3), 262–264. https://doi.org/10.1542/peds.2009-1162A.

Ackermann Rau, S., Sakarya, S., & Abel, T. (2014). When to see a doctor for common health problems: Distribution patterns of functional health literacy across migrant populations in Switzerland. *International Journal of Public Health, 59*(6), 967–974. https://doi.org/10.1007/s00038-014-0583-5.

Appleton, S., Biermann, S., Hamilton-Bruce, M. A., Piantadosi, C., Tucker, G., Koblar, S. A., et al. (2013). Health literacy (HL) mediates the relationship of socioeconomic status (SES) and stroke in a population sample. *International Journal of Stroke, 8*, 43.

Australian Bureau of Statistics. (2008). *Health Literacy*. Canberra: Australia.

Babitsch, B. (2009). Die Kategorie Geschlecht: Theoretische und empirische Implikationen für den Zusammenhang zwischen sozialer Ungleichheit und Gesundheit. In K. Hurrelmann & M. Richter (Eds.), *Gesundheitliche Ungleichheit: Grundlagen, Probleme, Perspektiven* (2nd Edn., pp. 283–299). Wiesbaden: VS Verlag für Sozialwissenschaften / GWV Fachverlage GmbH Wiesbaden. https://doi.org/10.1007/978-3-531-91643-9_16.

Babitsch, B., Götz, N.-A., & Zeitler, J. (2017). Gender und Gesundheit. In M. Jungbauer-Gans & P. Kriwy (Eds.), *Handbuch Gesundheitssoziologie* (19. Vol., pp. 1–19). Wiesbaden: Springer. https://doi.org/10.1007/978-3-658-06477-8_11-1.

Baker, D. W., Parker, R. M., Williams, M. V., & Clark, W. S. (1998). Health literacy and the risk of hospital admission. *Journal of General Internal Medicine, 13*(12), 791–798. https://doi.org/10.1046/j.1525-1497.1998.00242.x.

Baker, D. W. (2006). The meaning and the measure of health literacy. *Journal of General Internal Medicine, 21*(8), 878–883. https://doi.org/10.1111/j.1525-1497.2006.00540.x.

Baker, D. W., Gazmararian, J. A., Williams, M. V., Scott, T., Parker, R. M., Green, D., et al. (2002). Functional health literacy and the risk of hospital admission among Medicare managed care enrollees. *American Journal of Public Health, 92*(8), 1278–1283. https://doi.org/10.2105/AJPH.92.8.1278.

Baker, D. W., Williams, M. V., Parker, R. M., Gazmararian, J. A., & Nurss, J. (1999). Development of a brief test to measure functional health literacy. *Patient Education and Counseling, 38*(1), 33–42. https://doi.org/10.1016/S0738-3991(98)00116-5.

Baker, D. W., Wolf, M. S., Feinglass, J., & Thompson, J. A. (2008). Health literacy, cognitive abilities, and mortality among elderly persons. *Journal of General Internal Medicine, 23*(6), 723–726. https://doi.org/10.1007/s11606-008-0566-4.

Baker, D. W., Wolf, M. S., Feinglass, J., Thompson, J. A., Gazmararian, J. A., & Huang, J. (2007). Health literacy and mortality among elderly persons. *Archives of Internal Medicine, 167,* 1503–1509. https://doi.org/10.1001/archinte.167.14.1503.

Bauer, U., Bittlingmayer, U. H., & Richter, M. (Eds.) (2008). *Gesundheit und Gesellschaft. Health Inequalities: Determinanten und Mechanismen gesundheitlicher Ungleichheit* (1. Aufl.). Wiesbaden: VS Verlag für Sozialwissenschaften. Retrieved from http://www.socialnet.de/rezensionen/isbn.php?isbn=978-3-531-15612-5.

Bennett, I. M., Chen, J., Soroui, J. S., & White, S. (2009). The contribution of health literacy to disparities in self-rated health status and preventive health behaviors in older adults. *Annals of Family Medicine, 7*(3), 204–211. https://doi.org/10.1370/afm.940.

Berens, E.-M., Vogt, D., Messer, M., Hurrelmann, K., & Schaeffer, D. (2016). Health Literacy among different age groups in Germany: results of a cross-sexctional survey. *BMC Public Health, 16,* 1151. https://doi.org/10.1186/s12889-016-3810-6.

Berkman, N. D., DeWalt, D. A., Pignone, M. P., Sheridan, S. L., Lohr, K. N., Lux, L., & Bonito, A. J. et al. (2004). *Literacy and Health Outcomes: Evidence Report/Technology Assessment*, No. 87. AHRQ Publication. (04-E007-2).

Berkman, N. D., Davis, T. C., & McCormack, L. (2010). Health literacy: What is it? *Journal of Health Communication, 15*(Suppl 2), 9–19. https://doi.org/10.1080/10810730.20 10.499985.

Bernhardt, J. M., Brownfield, E. D., & Parker, R. M. (2005). Understanding health literacy. In J. G. Schwartzberg, J. VanGeest, & C. C. Wang (Eds.), *Understanding Health Literacy: Implications for Medicine and Public Health*. American Medical Association.

Bittlingmayer, U. H. (2016). Strukturorientierte Perspektiven auf Gesundheit und Krankheit. In M. Richter and K. Hurrelmann (Eds.), *Lehrbuch. Soziologie von Gesundheit und Krankheit* (1st Edn., pp. 23–40). Wiesbaden: Springer. https://doi.org/10.1007/978-3-658-11010-9_2.

Bittlingmayer, U. H., Bauer, U., Richter, M., & Sahrai, D. (2009). Die Überund Unterschätzung von Raum in Public Health. *Deutsche Zeitschrift Für Kommunalwissenschaft, 48*(2), 21–34.

Bittlingmayer, U. H., & Sahrai, D. (2019). Health literacy for all? Inclusion as a serious challenge for health: The case of disablity. In O. Okan, U. Bauer, D. Levin-Zamir, P. Pinheiro, & K. Sørensen (Eds.), *International Handbook of Health Literacy: Research, practice and policy across the lifespan* (pp. 689–703). Bristol: Policy Press.

Black, D., & Whitehead, M. (1992). *Inequalities in health: The Black report [and] The health divide* (Reprinted). *Penguin books*. London: Penguin Books.

Blaxter, M. (1983). Peter Townsend and Nick Davidson, Inequalities in Health: the Black Report, Penguin, London, 1982. 240 pp. £2.50. *Journal of Social Policy, 12*(2), 284–285. https://doi.org/10.1017/S0047279400012812.

Bostock, S., & Steptoe, A. (2012). Association between low functional health literacy and mortality in older adults: Longitudinal cohort study. *BMJ (Clinical Research Ed.), 344*, e1602. https://doi.org/10.1136/bmj.e1602.

Bröder, J., Okan, O., Schlupp, S., Bauer, U., & Pinheiro, P. (2016). Figuring out the meaning of health literacy during childhood and adolescence. *European Journal of Public Health, 26*. https://doi.org/10.1093/eurpub/ckw165.067.

Bruland, D., Kornblum, K., Harsch, S., Bröder, J., Okan, O., & Bauer, U. (2017). Schüler mit einem psychisch erkrankten Elternteil und die Mental Health Literacy von Lehrkräften [Students Having Parents with Mental Health Issues and Teachers' Mental Health Literacy]. *Praxis der Kinderpsychologie und Kinderpsychiatrie, 66*(10), 774–790. https://doi.org/10.13109/prkk.2017.66.10.774.

Brunnett, R. (2009). *Die Hegemonie symbolischer Gesundheit: Eine Studie zum Mehrwert von Gesundheit im Postfordismus. Sozialtheorie.* s.l.: Transcript. Retrieved from http://www.content-select.com/index.php?id=bib_viewandean=9783839412770 .

Canadian Council on Learning (2007). *Health Literacy in Canada: Initial Results from the International Adult Literacy and Skills Survey 2007.* Ottawa.

Chang, L.-C. (2011). Health literacy, self-reported status and health promoting behaviours for adolescents in Taiwan. *Journal of Clinical Nursing, 20*(1–2), 190–196. https://doi.org/10.1111/j.1365-2702.2009.03181.x.

Chew, L. D., Bradley, K. A., & Boyko, E. J. (2004). Brief questions to identify patients with inadequate health literacy. *Family Medicine, 36*, 588–594.

Chinn, D. (2011). Critical health literacy: A review and critical analysis. *Social Science and Medicine, 73*, 60–67. https://doi.org/10.1016/j.socscimed.2011.04.004.

Chisolm, D. J., & Buchanan, L. (2007). Measuring adolescent functional health literacy: A pilot validation of the Test of Functional Health Literacy in Adults. *The Journal of Adolescent Health: Official Publication of the Society for Adolescent Medicine, 41*(3), 312–314. https://doi.org/10.1016/j.jadohealth.2007.04.015.

Cho, Y. I., Lee, S.-Y. D., Arozullah, A. M., & Crittenden, K. S. (2008). Effects of health literacy on health status and health service utilization amongst the elderly. *Social Science and Medicine, 66*(8), 1809–1816. https://doi.org/10.1016/j.socscimed.2008.01.003.

Cimasi, R. J., Sharamitaro, A. P., & Seiler, R. L. (2013). The association between health literacy and preventable hospitalizations in Missouri: Implications in an era of reform. *Journal of Health Care Finance, 40*(2), 1–16.

Cockerham, W. C., Hinote, B. P., & Abbott, P. (2006). A Sociological Model of Health Lifestyles. In C. Wendt & C. Wolf (Eds.), *Kölner Zeitschrift für Soziologie und Sozialpsychologie Sonderhefte* (Vol. 46, pp. 177–197)., *Soziologie der Gesundheit: Kölner Zeitschrift für Soziologie und Sozialpsychologie* Wiesbaden: VS Verlag für Sozialwissenschaaften.

Como, J. M. (2014). Health literacy and self-efficacy: Impact on medication adherence and health outcomes in urban cardiology practices. *Dissertation Abstracts International Section B: The Sciences and Engineering, 74*, 11-B (E).

Coulter, A., & Ellins, J. (2007). Effectiveness of strategies for informing, educating, and involving patients. *British Medical Journal, 335,* 24–27. https://doi.org/10.1136/bmj.39246.581169.80.

Davis, T. C., Long, S. W., Jackson, R. H., Mayeux, E. J., George, R. B., Murphy, P. W., et al. (1993). Rapid estimate of adult literacy in medicine: A shortened screening instrument. *Family Medicine, 25*(6), 391–395.

Davis, T. C., Wolf, M. S., Arnold, C. L., Byrd, R. S., Long, S. W., Springer, T., Bocchini, J. A. et al. (2006). Development and validation of the Rapid Estimate of Adolescent Literacy in Medicine (REALM-Teen): A tool to screen adolescents for below-grade reading in health care settings. *Pediatrics, 118*(6), e1707–e1714. https://doi.org/10.1542/peds.2006-1139.

DeWalt, D. A., Berkman, N. D., Sheridan, S., Lohr, K. N., & Pignone, M. P. (2004). Literacy and health outcomes: A systematic review of the literature. *Journal of General Internal Medicine, 19*(12), 1228–1239. https://doi.org/10.1111/j.1525-1497.2004.40153.x.

DeWalt, D. A., & Hink, A. (2009). Health literacy and child health outcomes: A systematic review of the literature. *Pediatrics, 124* (Suppl 3), pp. 265–S274. https://doi.org/10.1542/peds.2009-1162B.

Dodson, S., Good, S., & Osborne, R. H. (2015). Optimizing Health Literacy: Improving health and reducing health inequities. Retrieved from http://apps.searo.who.int/PDS_DOCS/B5147.pdf.

Elkeles, T., & Mielck, A. (1997). Entwicklung eines Modells zur Erklärung gesundheitlicher Ungleichheit. *Das Gesundheitswesen, 59*(3), 137–143.

Fleisher, J. E., Minger, J., Fitts, W., & Dahodwala, N. (2014). Low health literacy: An under-recognized obstacle in Parkinson's disease. *Movement Disorders: Official Journal of the Movement Disorder Society, 29,* 158–159.

Foucault, M. (1983). *Der Wille zum Wissen: Sexualität und Wahrheit, Band 1* (14., durchges., korrig. Aufl.). *Suhrkamp-Taschenbuch Wissenschaft: Vol. 716.* Frankfurt a.M.: Suhrkamp.

Freedman, D. A., Bess, K. D., Tucker, H. A., Boyd, D. L., Tuchman, A. M., & Wallston, K. A. (2009). Public health literacy defined. *American Journal of Preventive Medicine, 36*(5), 446–451. https://doi.org/10.1016/j.amepre.2009.02.001.

Frisch, A.-L., Camerini, L., Diviani, N., & Schulz, P. J. (2012). Defining and measuring health literacy: How can we profit from other literacy domains? *Health Promotion International, 27*(1), 117–126. https://doi.org/10.1093/heapro/dar043.

Furuya, Y., Kondo, N., Yamagata, Z., & Hashimoto, H. (2013). Health literacy, socioeconomic status and self-rated health in Japan. *Health Promotion International, 30*(3), 505–513. https://doi.org/10.1093/heapro/dat071.

Gazmararian, J. A., & Parker, R. M. (2005). Overview of health literacy in health care. In J. G. Schwartzberg, J. VanGeest, & C. C. Wang (Eds.), *Understanding Health Literacy: Implications for Medicine and Public Health*. American Medical Association.

gfs.bern (2016). Bevölkerungsbefragung "Erhebung Gesundheitskompetenz 2015". Retrieved from: https://blog.careum.ch/wp-content/files/152131_GesKomp_SB_def.pdf.

Gibney, S., Bruton, L., Ryan, C., Doyle, G., & Rowlands, G. (2020). Increasing Health Literacy May Reduce HealthInequalities: Evidence from a National Population Survey in Ireland. *International journal of environmental research and public health 17*(16). https://doi.org/10.3390/ijerph17165891.

Giesecke, J., & Müters, S. (2009). Strukturelle und verhaltensbezogene Faktoren gesundheitlicher Ungleichheit: Methodische Überlegungen zur Ermittlung der Erklärungsanteile. In K. Hurrelmann & M. Richter (Eds.), *Gesundheitliche Ungleichheit: Grundlagen, Probleme, Perspektiven* (2. Edn., pp. 353–366). Wiesbaden: VS Verlag für Sozialwissenschaften/GWV Fachverlage GmbH Wiesbaden. https://doi.org/10.1007/978-3-531-91643-9_20.

Griffey, R. T., Kennedy, S. K., McGownan, L., Goodman, M., & Kaphings, K. A. (2014). Is low health literacy associated with increased emergency department utilization and recidivism? *Academic Emergency Medicine, 21*(10), 1109–1115.

Habich, R. (2013). *Pressekonferenz „Datenreport 2013" am 26. November in Berlin. Statement von Dr. Roland Habich (WZB)*. Retrieved from http://www.wzb.eu/sites/default/files/u6/datenreport_statement_habich.pdf.

Hartung, S. (2014). *Sozialkapital und gesundheitliche Ungleichheit*. Wiesbaden: Springer Fachmedien Wiesbaden. https://doi.org/10.1007/978-3-658-04870-9.

Helmert, U. (2003). *Soziale Ungleichheit und Krankheitsrisiken*. Augsburg: Maro.

Helmert, U., & Schorb, F. (2006). Die Bedeutung verhaltensbezogener Faktoren im Kontext der sozialen Ungleichheit von Gesundheit. In M. Richter & K. Hurrelmann (Eds.), *Gesundheitliche Ungleichheit: Grundlagen, Probleme, Perpektiven* (pp. 125–139). Wiesbaden: Springer.

HLS-EU Consortium (2012). *Comparative report of health literacy in eight EU member states*. Online publication: http://www.health-literacy.eu.

Hoffmann, R., Borsboom, G., Saez, M., Mari Dell'Olmo, M., Burström, B., Corman, D., Borrell, C. et al. (2014). Social differences in avoidable mortality between small areas of 15 European cities: An ecological study. *International Journal of Health Geographics, 13*, 8. https://doi.org/10.1186/1476-072X-13-8.

Hradil, S. (2006). Was prägt das Krankheitsrisiko: Schicht, Lage, Lebensstil? In M. Richter & K. Hurrelmann (Eds.), *Gesundheitliche Ungleichheit: Grundlagen, Probleme, Perpektiven* (pp. 33–52). Wiesbaden: VS Verlag für Sozialwissenschaften.

Ingleby, D., Krasnik, A., Lorant, V., & Razum, O. (Eds.). (2012). *Health inequalities and risk factors among migrants and ethnic minorities*. Antwerp: Garant Publishers.

Jordan, J. E., Buchbinder, R., & Osborne, R. H. (2010). Conceptualising health literacy from the patient perspective. *Patient Education and Counseling, 79*(1), 36–42. https://doi.org/10.1016/j.pec.2009.10.001.

Jordan, S., & Hoebel, J. (2015). Gesundheitskompetenz von Erwachsenen in Deutschland : Ergebnisse der Studie "Gesundheit in Deutschland aktuell" (GEDA) [Health literacy of adults in Germany: Findings from the German Health Update (GEDA) study]. *Bundesgesundheitsblatt, Gesundheitsforschung, Gesundheitsschutz, 58*(9), 942–950. https://doi.org/10.1007/s00103-015-2200-z.

Jungbauer-Gans, M., & Kriwy, P. (Eds.). (2004). *Soziale Benachteiligung und Gesundheit bei Kindern und Jugendlichen*. Wiesbaden: VS Verlag für Sozialwissenschaften.

Katz, M. G., Jacobson, T. A., Veledar, E., & Kripalani, S. (2007). Patient literacy and question-asking behavior during the medical encounter: A mixed-methods analysis. *Journal of General Internal Medicine, 22*(6), 782–786. https://doi.org/10.1007/s11606-007-0184-6.

Kawachi, I., Kennedy, B. P., Lochner, K., & Prothrow-Stith, D. (1997). Social Capital, Income Inequality and Mortality. *American Journal of Public Health, 87*(9), 1491–1498.

Kickbusch, I. (2009). Health literacy: Engaging in a political debate. *International Journal of Public Health, 54*(3), 131–132. https://doi.org/10.1007/s00038-009-7073-1.

Kindig, D. A., Panzer, A. M., & Nielsen-Bohlman, L., Committee on Health Literacy, and Board on Neuroscience and Behavioral Health, Institute of Medicine (2004). *Health Literacy: A Prescription to End Confusion*. Washington (DC).

Kirsch, I. (2001). The International Adult Literacy Survey (IALS): Understanding What Was Measured. https://www.ets.org/Media/Research/pdf/RR-01-25-Kirsch.pdf.

Kolip, P. (Ed.). (2000). *Weiblichkeit ist keine Krankheit: Die Medikalisierung körperlicher Umbruchphasen im Leben von Frauen*. Weinheim, München: Juventa.

Kowalski, C., Loss, J., Kölsch, F., & Janssen, C. (2014). Utilization of Prevention Services by Gender, Age, Socioeconomic Status, and Migration Status in Germany: An Overview and a Systematic Review. In C. Janssen, E. Swart, & T. von Lengerke (Eds.), *Health Care Utilization in Germany* (Vol. 74, pp. 293–320). New York: Springer New York. https://doi.org/10.1007/978-1-4614-9191-0_16.

Kroll, L. E. (2010). *Sozialer Wandel, soziale Ungleichheit und Gesundheit: Die Entwicklung sozialer und gesundheitlicher Ungleichheiten in Deutschland zwischen 1984 und 2006*. Wiesbaden: VS Verlag für Sozialwissenschaften.

Kühn, H. (1993). *Healthismus. Eine Analyse der Präventionspolitik und Gesundheitsförderung in den U.S.A.* Berlin: Edition Sigma.

Kuhlmann, E. & Kolip, P. (2008). Die "gemachten" Unterschiede - Geschlecht als Dimension gesundheitlicher Ungleichheit. In U. Bauer, U. H. Bittlingmayer, & M. Richter (Eds.), *Gesundheit und Gesellschaft. Health Inequalities: Determinanten und Mechanismen gesundheitlicher Ungleichheit* (1st Edn., pp. 191–219). Wiesbaden: VS Verlag für Sozialwissenschaften.

Kutner, M., Greenberg, E., Jin, Y., Boyle, B., Hsu, Y., & Eric Dunleavy (2007). *Literacy in everyday life: Results from the 2003 National Assessment of Adult Literacy*. Washington (DC).

Kutner, M., Greenberg, E., Jin, Y., Paulsen, C., & U. S. Department of Education (2006). *The health literacy of America's adults: Results from the 2003 National Assessment of Adult Literacy, NCES 2006–483*.

Lampert, T. (2016). Soziale Ungleichheit und Gesundheit. In M. Richter & K. Hurrelmann (Eds.), *Lehrbuch. Soziologie von Gesundheit und Krankheit* (1st ed., pp. 121–138). Wiesbaden: Springer VS.

Lampert, T., Saß, A.-C., Häfelinger, M., & Ziese, T. (2007). *Armut, soziale Ungleichheit und Gesundheit: Expertise des Robert Koch-Instituts zum 2. Armuts- und Reichtumsbericht der Bundesregierung* (Geänd. Nachdr.). *Beiträge zur Gesundheitsberichterstattung des Bundes*. Berlin: Robert Koch-Inst.

Lauterbach, K., Lüngen, M., Stollenwerk, B., Gerber, A., & Klever-Deichert, G. (2006). *Zum Zusammenhang zwischen Einkommen und Lebenserwartung: Forschungsberichte des Instituts für Gesundheitsökonomie und klinische Epidemiologie der Universität zu Köln* (Studien zu Gesundheit, Medizin und Gesellschaft No. 01/2006). Köln. Retrieved from http://gesundheitsoekonomie.uk-koeln.de/forschung/schriftenreihesgmg/2006-01_einkommen_und_rentenbezugsdauer.pdf.

Lee, S.-Y. D., Tsai, T.-I., Tsai, Y.-W., & Kuo, K. N. (2010). Health literacy, health status, and healthcare utilization of Taiwanese adults: Results from a national survey. *BMC Public Health, 10*, 614. https://doi.org/10.1186/1471-2458-10-614.

Lessenich, S. (2013). *Die Neuerfindung des Sozialen: Der Sozialstaat im flexiblen Kapitalismus* (3rd Edn.). Bielefeld: Transcript.

Levin-Zamir, D., Leung, A. Y. M., Dodson, S., & Rowlands, G. (2017). Health literacy in selected populations: Individuals, families, and communities from the international and cultural perspective. *Information Services and Use, 37*(2), 131–151. https://doi.org/10.3233/ISU-170834.

Lin, H., Sawyer, P., Allman, R. P., Kennedy, R. E., & Williams, C. P. (2014). he association between health literacy and medication selfmanagement in community-dwelling older adults. *Journal of the American Geriatrics Society, 62,* 271.

Mackert, M., Champlin, S., Su, Z., & Guadagno, M. (2015). The Many Health Literacies: Advancing Research or Fragmentation? *Health Communication, 30*(12), 1161–1165. https://doi.org/10.1080/10410236.2015.1037422.

Makarova, N., Reiss, K., Zeeb, H., Razum, O., & Spallek, J. (2013). Verbesserte Möglichkeiten zur Identifikation von Menschen mitMigrationshintergrund für die Mortalitätsforschung am Beispiel Bremens. *Gesundheitswesen (Bundesverband der Ärzte des Offentlichen Gesundheitsdienstes(Germany)) 75*(6), 360–365. https://doi.org/10.1055/s-0032-1321767.

Mancuso, C. A., & Rincon, M. (2006). Impact of health literacy on longitudinal asthma outcomes. *Journal of General Internal Medicine, 21*(8), 813–817. https://doi.org/10.1111/j.1525-1497.2006.00528.x.

Mancuso, J. M. (2009). Assessment and measurement of health literacy: An integrative review of the literature. *Nursing and Health Sciences, 11*(1), 77–89. https://doi.org/10.1111/j.1442-2018.2008.00408.x.

Manganello, J. A. (2008). Health literacy and adolescents: A framework and agenda for future research. *Health Education Research, 23*(5), 840–847. https://doi.org/10.1093/her/cym069.

Mantwill, S. (2015). *Linking health literacy and health disparities: Conceptual implications and empirical results.* Lugano: Università della Svizzera italiana.

McCormack, L., Bann, C., Squiers, L., Berkman, N. D., Squire, C., Schillinger, D., et al. (2010). Measuring health literacy: A pilot study of a new skills-based instrument. *Journal of Health Communication, 15*(Suppl 2), 51–71. https://doi.org/10.1080/10810730.2010.499987.

McNaughton, C. D., Kripalani, S., Cawthon, C., & Roumie, C. L. (2014). The association between health literacy and 90-day re-hospitalization or death: A cohort study of patients hospitalized for heart failure. *Circulation: Cardiovascular Quality and Outcomes, 7.*

McNaughton, C. D., Cawthon, C., Kripalani, S., Liu, D., Storrow, A. B., Roumie, C. L. (2015). Health literacy and mortality: a cohort study of patients hospitalized for acute heart failure. *Journal of the American Heart Association 4*(5). https://doi.org/10.1161/JAHA.115.001799.

Mergenthal, K. (2014). Migrantinnen empowern! *Prävention Und Gesundheitsförderung, 9*(1), 52–59. https://doi.org/10.1007/s11553-013-0415-0.

Merten, S., & Gari, S. (2013). *Die reproduktive Gesundheit der Migrationsbevölkerung in der Schweiz und anderen ausgewählten Aufnahmeländern.* Basel: Swiss Tropical and Public Health Institute.

Mielck, A. (2000). *Soziale Ungleichheit und Gesundheit: Empirische Ergebnisse, Erklärungsansätze, Interventionsmöglichkeiten.* Bern: Huber.

Mielck, A. (2005). *Soziale Ungleichheit und Gesundheit: Eine Einführung in die aktuelle Diskussion.* Bern: Huber.

Murphy, P. W., Davis, T. C., Long, S. W., Jackson, R. H., & Decker, B. C. (1993). Rapid Estimate of Adult Literacy in Medicine (REALM): A quick reading test for patients. *Journal of Reading, 37*(2), 124–130. https://doi.org/10.2307/40033408.

Navarra, A.-M., Neu, N., Toussi, S., Nelson, J., & Larson, E. L. (2014). Health literacy and adherence to antiretroviral therapy among HIV-infected youth. *The Journal of the Association of Nurses in AIDS Care : JANAC, 25*(3), 203–213. https://doi.org/10.1016/j.jana.2012.11.003.

Netzwerk Bildung + Gesundheit Schweiz (2015). Gesundheitskompetenz – compétence en matière de santé.

Nguyen, T. H., Paasche-Orlow, M. K., & McCormack, L. A. (2017). The state of the science of health literacy measurement. *Information Services and Use, 37*(2), 189–203. https://doi.org/10.3233/ISU-170827.

Nguyen, T. H., Park, H., Han, H.-R., Chan, K. S., Paasche-Orlow, M. K., Haun, J., & Kim, M. T. (2015). State of the science of health literacy measures: Validity implications for minority populations. *Patient Education and Counseling.* Advance online publication. https://doi.org/10.1016/j.pec.2015.07.013.

Nideröst, S. (2007). *Männer, Körper und Gesundheit: Somatische Kultur und soziale Milieus bei Männern.* Bern: Huber.

Nutbeam, D. (2000). Health literacy as a public health goal: a challenge for contemporary health education and communication strategies into the 21st century. *Health Promotion International, 15*(3), 259–267. https://doi.org/10.1093/heapro/15.3.259.

Nutbeam, D. (2009). Defining and measuring health literacy: what can we learn from literacy studies? *International Journal of Public Health, 54,* 303–305.

Okan, O., Bollweg, T. M., Bröder, J., Pinheiro, P., & Bauer, U. (2017). Qualitative methods in health literacy research in young children. *The European Journal of Public Health, 27*(suppl_3). https://doi.org/10.1093/eurpub/ckx187.139.

Omariba, D. W. R. & Ng, E. (2011). Immigration, generation and self-rated health in Canada: on the role of health literacy. *Canadian Journal of Public Health = Revue Canadienne De Sante Publique, 102*(4), 281–285.

Osborn, C. Y., Cavanaugh, K., Wallston, K. A., & Rothman, R. L. (2010). Self-efficacy links health literacy and numeracy to glycemic control. *Journal of Health Communication, 15*(Suppl 2), 146–158. https://doi.org/10.1080/10810730.2010.499980.

Paakkari, L. T., Torppa, M. P., Paakkari, O.-P., Välimaa, R. S., Ojala, K. S.A., & Tynjälä, J. A. (2019). Does health literacy explain the link between structural stratifiers and edoles-cent health? *European Journal of Public Health*, 1–6. https://doi.org/10.1093/eurpub/ckz011.

Paasche-Orlow, M. K., & Wolf, M. S. (2010). Promoting health literacy research to reduce health disparities. *Journal of Health Communication, 15*(Suppl 2), 34–41. https://doi.org/10.1080/10810730.2010.499994.

Parikh, N. S., Parker, R. M., Nurss, J. R., Baker, D. W., & Williams, M. V. (1996). Shame and health literacy: the unspoken connection. *Patient Education and Counseling, 27*(1), 33–39. https://doi.org/10.1016/0738-3991(95)00787-3.

Parker, R. M., Ratzan, S. C., & Lurie, N. (2003). Health Literacy: A Policy Challenge For Advancing High-Quality Health Care. *Health Affairs, 22*(4), 147–153. https://doi.org/10.1377/hlthaff.22.4.147.

Parker, R. M., Baker, D. W., Williams, M. V., & Nurss, J. R. (1995). The test of func-tional health literacy in adults. *Journal of General Internal Medicine, 10*(10), 537–541. https://doi.org/10.1007/BF02640361.

Pelikan, J. M., Röthlin, F., & Ganahl, K. (2012). Die Gesundheitskopmetenz der öster-richischen Bevölkerung nach Bundesländern und im internationalen Vergleich. Retrieved from http://old.fgoe.org/projektfoerderung/gefoerderte-projekte/FgoeProject_1412/90528.pdf.

Peterson, P. N., Shetterly, S. M., Clarke, C. L., Bekelman, D. B., Chan, P. S., Allen, L. A., et al. (2011). Health literacy and outcomes among patients with heart failure. *JAMA, 305*, 1665–1701.

Pickett, K. E., & Wilkinson, R. G. (2015). Income inequality and health: A causal review. *Social Science and Medicine, 1982*(128), 316–326. https://doi.org/10.1016/j.socscimed.2014.12.031.

Pleasant, A., Maish, C., O'Leary, C., & Carmona, R. H. (2018). *A theory-based self-report measure of health literacy: The Calgary Charter of Health Liter-acy Scale*. Methodological Innovations: Advance online publication. https://doi.org/10.1177/2059799118814394.

Pleasant, A., & McKinney, J. (2011). Coming to consensus on health literacy measurement: An online discussion and consensus-gauging process. *Nursing Outlook, 59*(2), 95–106. e1. https://doi.org/10.1016/j.outlook.2010.12.006.

Powell, C. K., Hill, E. G., & Clancy, D. E. (2007). The relationship between health literacy and diabetes knowledge and readiness to take health actions. *The Diabetes Educator, 33*(1), 144–151. https://doi.org/10.1177/0145721706297452.

Rathmann, K. (2015). *Bildungssystem, Wohlfahrtsstaat und gesundheitliche Ungleichheit: Ein internationaler Vergleich für das Jugendalter*. Wiesbaden: Springer.

Razum, O. (2006). Migration, Mortalität und der Healthy-migrant-Effekt. In M. Richter & K. Hurrelmann (Eds.), *Gesundheitliche Ungleichheit: Grundlagen, Probleme, Perpek-tiven* (pp. 255–270). Wiesbaden: VS Verlag für Sozialwissenschaften.

Razum, O., & Rohrmann, S. (2002). Der Healthy-migrant-Effekt: Bedeutung von Auswahl-prozessen bei der Migration und Late-entry-Bias. *Das Gesundheitswesen, 64*, 82–88.

Richter, M. (2005). *Gesundheit und Gesundheitsverhalten im Jugendalter: Der Einfluss sozialer Ungleichheit*. Wiesbaden: VS Verlag für Sozialwissenschaften.

Richter, M., & Hurrelmann, K. (Eds.). (2006a). *Gesundheitliche Ungleichheit: Grundlagen, Probleme, Perpektiven*. Wiesbaden: VS Verlag für Sozialwissenschaften.

Richter, M., & Hurrelmann, K. (2006b). Gesundheitliche Ungleichheit: Ausgangsfragen und Herausforderungen. In M. Richter & K. Hurrelmann (Eds.), *Gesundheitliche Ungleichheit: Grundlagen, Probleme, Perpektiven* (pp. 11–31). Wiesbaden: VS Verlag für Sozialwissenschaften.

RKI (2008). Migration und Gesundheit. Retrieved from https://www.rki.de/DE/Content/ Gesundheitsmonitoring/Gesundheitsberichterstattung/GBEDownloadsT/migration. pdf?__blob=publicationFile.

Rosenbrock, R. (2015, October). *Stellungnahme in der Podiumsdiskussion: Gesundheitspolitik für gesunde Wahrmöglichkeiten - Partnerschaften für die Gesundheitsbildung*, European Health Forum Gastein.

Rothman, R. L., Yin, H. S., Mulvaney, S., Co, J. P. T., Homer, C., & Lannon, C. (2009). Health literacy and quality: Focus on chronic illness care and patient safety. *Pediatrics, 124*(Suppl 3), S315–S326. https://doi.org/10.1542/peds.2009-1163H.

Rudd, R. (2007). Health literacy skills of US adults. *American Journal of Health Behavior, 31*, S8–S18.

Rudd, R., Kirsch, I. S., & Yamamoto, K. (2004). *Literacy and Health in America: Policy Information Report*. Princeton, NJ.

Sahrai, D. (2009). Healthy Migrants oder besondere Risikogruppe? *Zur Schwierigkeit des Verhältnisses von Ethnizität, Migration, Sozialstruktur und Gesundheit Jahrbuch Für Kritische Medizin Und Gesundheitswissenschaften, 45*, 70–94.

Sahrai, D., Bertschi, I., & Bittlingmayer, U. H. (2018). Differenz und Anerkennung in der Migration. Eine ethnografische Studie zu gesundheitsbezogenen Alltagspraktiken lateinamerikanischer Familien. *Schweizerische Zeitschrift Für Heilpädagogik, 24*, 32–39.

Sarkar, U., Fisher, L., & Schillinger, D. (2006). Is self-efficacy associated with diabetes self-management across race/ethnicity and health literacy? *Diabetes Care, 29*(4), 823–829.

Schaeffer, D., Berens, E-M., & Vogt, D. (2017). Health Literacy in the German Population: Results of a Representative Survey. *Deutsches Ärzteblatt International 114*(4), 53–60. https://doi.org/10.3238/arztebl.2017.0053.

Schaeffer, D., Hurrelmann, K., Bauer, O., Kolpatzik, K., Gille, S., & Vogt, D. (2019). Der Nationale AktionsplanGesundheitskompetenz – Notwendigkeit, Ziel und Inhalt. *Gesundheitswesen 81*(06), 465–470. https://doi.org/10.1055/a-0667-9414.

Schenk, L. (2007). Migration und Gesundheit-Entwicklung eines Erklärungs- und Analysemodells für epidemiologische Studien [Migration and health–developing an explanatory and analytical model for epidemiological studies]. *International journal of public health, 52*(2), 87–96. https://doi.org/10.1007/s00038-007-6002-4.

Schillinger, D., Bindman, A., Wang, F., Stewart, A., & Piette, J. et al. (2004). Functional health literacy and the quality of physician–patient communication among diabetes patients. *Patient Education and Counseling, 52*(3), 315–323.

Schillinger, D., Grumbach, K., Piette, J., Wang, F., Osmond, D., Daher, C., Bindman, A. et al. (2002). Association of health literacy with diabetes outcomes. *JAMA: The Journal of the American Medical Association, 288*(4), 475–482.

Schmidt, B. (2017). *Exklusive Gesundheit: Gesundheit als Instrument zur Sicherstellung sozialer Ordnung.* Wiesbaden: Springer.

Schmidt, B., & Kolip, P. (Eds.). (2007). *Gesundheitsförderung im aktivierenden Sozialstaat: Präventionskonzepte zwischen Public Health, Eigenverantwortung und Sozialer Arbeit.* Weinheim: Juventa.

Schweizerische Akademie der Medizinischen Wissenschaften (2015). Gesundheitskompetenz in der Schweiz – Stand und Perspektiven. *Swiss Academics Report, 10*(4).

Sebo, P., Jackson, Y., Haller, D. M., Gaspoz, J.-M., & Wolff, H. (2011). Sexual and reproductive health behaviors of undocumented migrants in Geneva: A cross sectional study. *Journal of Immigrant and Minority Health, 13*(3), 510–517. https://doi.org/10.1007/s10903-010-9367-z.

Seurer, A. C., & Vogt, H. B. (2013). Low health literacy: a barrier to effective patient care. *South Dakota Medicine, 66*(2), 51–53.

Shaw, S. J., Huebner, C., Armin, J., Orzech, K., & Vivian, J. (2008). The role of culture in health literacy and chronic disease screening and management. *Journal of Immigrant and Minority Health, 11*, 460–467.

Siegrist, J., Dragano, N., & dem Knesebeck, O. (2006). Soziales Kapital, soziale Ungleichheit und Gesundheit. In M. Richter & K. Hurrelmann (Eds.), *Gesundheitliche Ungleichheit: Grundlagen, Probleme, Perpektiven* (pp. 157–170). Wiesbaden: VS Verlag für Sozialwissenschaften.

Simon, M. (2011). Von der Koalitionsvereinbarung bis Ende 2010: Eine Zwischenbilanz schwarz-gelber Gesundheitspolitik. *Jahrbuch Für Kritische Medizin Und Gesundheitswissenschaften, 47,* 9–28.

Simon, M. (2016). Die ökonomischen und strukturellen Veränderungen des Krankenhausbereichs seit den 1970er Jahren. In I. Bode & W. Vogd (Eds.), *Mutationen des Krankenhauses: Soziologische Diagnosen in organisations- und gesellschaftstheoretischer Perspektive* (pp. 29–45). Wiesbaden: Springer.

Slotala, L. (2011). *Ökonomisierung in der ambulanten Pflege: Eine Analyse der wirtschaftlichen Bedingungen und deren Folgen für die Versorgungspraxis ambulanter Dienste.* Wiesbaden: Springer.

Song, L., Mishel, M., Bensen, J. T., Chen, R. C., Knafl, G. J., Blackard, B., et al. (2012). How does health literacy affect quality of life among men with newly diagnosed clinically localized prostate cancer? Findings from the North Carolina-Louisiana Prostate Cancer Project (PCaP). *Cancer, 118*(15), 3842–3851. https://doi.org/10.1002/cncr.26713.

Sørensen, K., & Brand, H. (2014). Health literacy lost in translations? Introducing the European Health Literacy Glossary. *Health Promotion International, 29*(4), 634–644. https://doi.org/10.1093/heapro/dat013.

Sørensen, K., van den Broucke, S., Fullam, J., Doyle, G., Pelikan, J., Slonska, Z., et al. (2012). Health literacy and public health: A systematic review and integration of definitions and models. *BMC Public Health, 12*, 80. https://doi.org/10.1186/1471-2458-12-80.

Sperlich, S. (2009). *Verringerung gesundheitlicher Ungleichheit durch Empowerment. Empirische Analyse der Gesundheitseffekte für sozial benachteiligte Mütter.* Wiesbaden: VS Verlag für Sozialwissenschaften.

Sperlich, S. (2016). Handlungsorientierte Perspektiven auf Gesundheit und Krankheit. In M. Richter and K. Hurrelmann (Eds.), *Lehrbuch. Soziologie von Gesundheit und Krankheit* (1st ed., pp. 41–54). Wiesbaden: Springer.

Sperlich, S., & Mielck, A. (2003). Sozialepidemiologische Erklärungsansätze im Spannungsfeld zwischen Schicht- und Lebensstilkonzeptionen. *Zeitschrift Für Gesundheitswissenschaften, 11*(2), 165–179.

Statistics Canada & OECD (2005). *Learning a living: First results of the Adult Literacy and Life Skills Survey.* Ottawa, Paris.

Street, B. V. (1984). *Literacy in theory and practice. Digital print.* Cambridge: Cambridge Univ. Pr.

Street, B. (2003). What's 'new' in New Literacy Studies? Critical approach to literacy in theory and practice. *Current Issues in comparative education 5*(2), 7–91.

Sudore, R. L., Yaffe, K., Satterfield, S., Harris, T. B., Mehta, K. M., Simonsick, E., et al. (2006). Limited literacy and mortality in the elderly: The health, aging, and body composition study. *Journal of General Internal Medicine, 21*(8), 806–812. https://doi.org/10.1111/j.1525-1497.2006.00539.x.

Sundmacher, L. (2016). Regionale Variationen in der Gesundheit und Gesundheitsversorgung. In M. Richter and K. Hurrelmann (Eds.), *Lehrbuch. Soziologie von Gesundheit und Krankheit* (1st ed., pp. 197–209). Wiesbaden: Springer VS.

The Scottish Government (2014). *Making it Easier: A Health Literacy Action Plan for Scotland.* The Scottish Government: Edinburgh.

Tiesmeyer, K., Brause, M., Lierse, M., Lukas-Nülle, M., & Hehlmann, T. (Eds.). (2008). *Der blinde Fleck: Ungleichheiten in der Gsundheitsversorgung.* Bern: Huber.

Tokuda, Y., Doba, N., Butler, J. P., & Paasche-Orlow, M. K. (2009). Health literacy and physical and psychological wellbeing in Japanese adults. *Patient Education and Counseling, 75*(3), 411–417. https://doi.org/10.1016/j.pec.2009.03.031.

Tones, K. (2002). Health literacy: new wine in old bottles? *Health Educ Res, 17,* 287–290.

Trout, A. L., Hoffman, S., Epstein, M. H., Nelson, T. D., & Thompson, R. W. (2014). Health Literacy in High-Risk Youth: A Descriptive Study of Children in Residential Care. *Child and Youth Services, 35*(1), 35–45. https://doi.org/10.1080/01459 35X.2014.893744.

Van der Vaart, R., van Deursen, A. J., Drossaert, C. H., Taal, E., van Dijk, J. A., & van de Laar, M. A. (2011). Does the eHealth Literacy Scale (eHEALS) measure what it intends to measure? Validation of a Dutch version of the eHEALS in two adult populations. *Journal of Medical Internet Research, 13*(4), e86. https://doi.org/10.2196/jmir.1840.

Vernon, J. A., Trujillo, A., Rosenbaum, S., & DeBuono, B. (2007). Low health literacy: Implications for national health policy. Retrieved from https://publichealth.gwu.edu/departments/healthpolicy/CHPR/downloads/LowHealthLiteracyReport10_4_07.pdf.

Vester, M. (2009). Milieuspezifische Lebensführung und Gesundheit. *Jahrbuch Für Kritische Medizin Und Gesundheitswissenschaften, 45,* 36–56.

Wallston, K. A., Cawthon, C., McNaughton, C. D., Rothman, R. L., Osborn, C. Y., & Kripalani, S. (2014). Psychometric properties of the brief health literacy screen in clinical practice. *Journal of General Internal Medicine, 29*(1), 119–126. https://doi.org/10.1007/s11606-013-2568-0.

Wångdahl, J., Lytsy, P., Mårtensson, L., & Westerling, R. (2015). Health literacy and refugees' experiences of the health examination for asylum seekers - a Swedish cross-sectional study. *BMC Public Health, 15,* 1162. https://doi.org/10.1186/s12889-015-2513-8.

Wångdahl, J., Lytsy, P., Mårtensson, L., & Westerling, R. (2018). Poor health and refraining from seeking healthcare are associated with comprehensive health literacy among refugees: A Swedish cross-sectional study. *International Journal of Public Health, 63*(3), 409–419. https://doi.org/10.1007/s00038-017-1074-2.

Weiss, B. D. (1999). *20 common problems in primary care.* New York: McGraw-Hill Open University Press.

Weiss, B. D. (2005). The epidemiology of low health literacy. In J. G. Schwartzberg, J. VanGeest, & C. Wang (Eds.), *Understanding health literacy: Implications for medicine and public health* (pp. 65–81). Chicago Ill.: American Medical Association.

Weiss, B. D., Mays, M. Z., Martz, W., Castro, K. M., DeWalt, D. A., Pignone, M., et al. (2005). Quick Assessment of Literacy in Primary Care: The Newest Vital Sign. *Annals of Family Medicine, 3*(6), 514–522. https://doi.org/10.1370/afm.405.

WHO (2009). Nairobi Call to Action - Promoting health and development : closing the implementation gap. Retrieved from https://www.who.int/oral_health/events/2010_seventh_who_global_conference_health_promotion.pdf.

WHO & Europe. (2008). *Closing the Gap in a Generation: Health Equity through Action on the Social Determinants of Health.* Geneva: World Health Organization.

Wilkinson, R. (2005). *The Impact of Inequality: How to Make Sick Societies Healthier.* New York: The New Press. Retrieved from https://ebookcentral.proquest.com/lib/gbv/detail.action?docID=579087.

Wilkinson, R. G. (1996). *Unhealthy Societies: The Affliction of Inequality.* London: Routledge.

Wilkinson, R. G. & Marmot, M. (2003). *Social Determinants of Health: The Solid Facts.* 2nd edition. Retrieved from WHO website: http://www.euro.who.int/__data/assets/pdf_file/0005/98438/e81384.pdf.

Wilkinson, R. G. & Pickett, K. E. (2010). *The spirit level: Why equality is better for everyone* (Publ. with rev). *Pinguin sociology.* London: Penguin Books.

Williams, M. V., Baker, D. W., Parker, R. M., & Nurss, J. R. (1998). Relationship of functional health literacy to patients knowledge of their chronic disease: A study of patients with hypertension and diabetes. *Archives of Internal Medicine, 158,* 166–172. https://doi.org/10.1001/archinte.158.2.166.

Wills, J. (2009). Health literacy: New packaging for health education or radical movement? *International Journal of Public Health, 54*(1), 3–4. https://doi.org/10.1007/s00038-008-8141-7.

Wissenschaftszentrum Berlin für Sozialforschung WZB (Ed.) (1993). *Healthismus: eine Analyse der Präventionspolitik und Gesundheitsförderung in den USA.* Berlin: Edition Sigma.

Wolf, M. S., Davis, T. C., Shrank, W., Rapp, D. N., Bass, P. F., Connor, U. M., et al. (2007). To err is human: Patient misinterpretations of prescription drug label instructions. *Patient Education and Counseling, 67*(3), 293–300. https://doi.org/10.1016/j.pec.2007.03.024.

Wolf, M. S., Wilson, E. A. H., Rapp, D. N., Waite, K. R., Bocchini, M. V., Davis, T. C., et al. (2009). Literacy and learning in health care. *Pediatrics, 124*(Suppl 3), S275–S281. https://doi.org/10.1542/peds.2009-1162C.

World Health Organization. (2016). Shanghai Declaration on promoting health in the 2030 Agenda for Sustainable Development.

Yee, L. M., & Simon, M. A. (2014). The role of health literacy and numeracy in contraceptive decision-making for urban Chicago women. *Journal of Community Health, 39*(2), 394–399. https://doi.org/10.1007/s10900-013-9777-7.

Yin, H. S., Forbis, S. G., & Dreyer, B. P. (2007). Health literacy and pediatric health. *Current Problems in Pediatric and Adolescent Health Care, 37*(7), 258–286. https://doi.org/10.1016/j.cppeds.2007.04.002.

Yin, H. S., Johnson, M., Mendelsohn, A. L., Abrams, M. A., Sanders, L. M., & Dreyer, B. P. (2009). The health literacy of parents in the United States: A nationally representative study. *Pediatrics, 124*(Suppl 3), S289–S298. https://doi.org/10.1542/peds.2009-1162E.

Zarcadoolas, C., Pleasant, A., & Greer, D. S. (2005). Understanding health literacy: An expanded model. *Health Promotion International, 20*(2), 195–203. https://doi.org/10.1093/heapro/dah609.

Zarcadoolas, C., Pleasant, A., & Greer, D. S. (2009). *Advancing health literacy: A framework for understanding and action.* San Francisco: Wiley.

Zhang, N. J., Terry, A., & McHorney, C. A. (2014). Impact of health literacy on medication adherence: A systematic review and meta-analysis. *The Annals of Pharmacotherapy, 48*(6), 741–751. https://doi.org/10.1177/1060028014526562.

Zou, P., & Parry, M. (2012). Strategies for health education in North American immigrant populations. *International Nursing Review, 59*(4), 482–488. https://doi.org/10.1111/j.1466-7657.2012.01021.x.

Health Literacy in Childhood and Adolescence: An Integrative Review

Orkan Okan, Torsten M. Bollweg and Janine Bröder

1   Introduction

Health literacy was introduced as an outcome of school health education in the 1970's in the USA (Simonds 1974). While the 1980s are deemed silent with regard to research, health literacy gained momentum throughout the 1990s and the 2000s, however, the focal population of most studies were adults whereas little research was conducted on the health literacy of children and adolescents during this period (Manganello et al. 2015; Okan et al. 2015; Bröder et al. 2017; Velardo and Drummond 2017). Despite two articles published in 1998 (Nutbeam 1998) and 2000 (Fok and Wong 2002), it was not until 2006 (Davis et al. 2006) that research on the health literacy of children and adolescents began to increase rapidly (Levin-Zamir et al. 2011; Paakkari and Paakkari 2012; Jang and Kim 2015; Okan et al. 2015; Ghanbari et al. 2016; Fairbrother et al. 2016a; Shih et al. 2016; Bröder et al. 2017; Hoffman et al. 2017; Velardo et al. 2017). Especially during the past few years there has been a particular focus on the construction

O. Okan (✉) · T. M. Bollweg
Bielefeld University, Faculty of Educational Sciences, Bielefeld, Germany
e-mail: orkan.okan@uni-bielefeld.de

T. M. Bollweg
e-mail: t.bollweg@uni-bielefeld.de

J. Bröder
Deutsche Gesellschaft für Ernährung e.V., Leipzig, Germany
e-mail: broeder@dge.de

of health literacy concepts and definitions (Levin-Zamir et al. 2011; Paakkari and Paakkari 2012; Bröder et al. 2017; Fairbrother et al. 2016a; Velardo and Drummond 2017), development of measurement tools (Ormshaw et al. 2013; Paakkari 2016; Okan et al. 2018), and the gathering of evidence on health literacy and associated health outcomes (DeWalt and Hink 2009; Sanders et al. 2009; Sansom-Daly et al. 2016). This has also led to the publication of several systematic or scoping reviews related to either one of the aforementioned focal areas (Ormshaw et al. 2013; Okan et al. 2015; Sansom-Daly 2016; Bröder et al. 2017; Okan et al. 2018). Moreover, governmental and non-governmental organisations have made recommendations to improve the health literacy of children and adolescents particularly in schools (Paakkari and Paakkari 2012; Hagell et al. 2015; Kilgour et al. 2015; Okan et al. 2015; McDaid 2016; WHO 2016; Velardo and Drummond 2017). This is closely related to the fact that it is widely acknowledged that the development of health literacy should be addressed from early childhood onwards (Paakkari and Paakkari 2012; Okan et al. 2015; Bröder et al. 2017; Velardo and Drummond 2017) and that the influence of adults, the social environment, and various contexts play a crucial role in health literacy promotion (Nutbeam 2000; Okan et al. 2015; Bröder et al. 2017; Fairbrother et al. 2016b).

The aim of this literature study is to review published material that provides a synthesis of recent evidence regarding the health literacy of children and adolescents in relation to three focus areas: (i) concepts and models, (ii) measurement instruments, and (iii) empirical evidence on the relationship between health literacy and health outcomes.

2   Results

The following section synthesizes the key evidence regarding the health literacy of children and adolescents in three areas: i) concepts and models, ii) measurement instruments, and iii) empirical evidence on the relationship between health literacy and health outcomes.

2.1   Focus Area 1: Conceptual Models and Definitions

The literature provides several approaches to conceptualizing health literacy in children and adolescents. In health care research, early approaches mostly included functional literacy skills (Davis et al. 2006; Chisolm and Buchanan 2007; Driessnack et al. 2014), while newer models take a broader approach by addressing a wide array of dimensions (Massey et al. 2013). In public health, health promotion, and education, health literacy concepts and models have been multidimensional from the beginning, clearly demonstrated by the earliest available model from the mid-nineties reflecting on the "health literate child" and based on the US health education curriculum (Joint Committee on National Health Education Standards 1995). The debates have since evolved with many ties to sociology (Rubene et al. 2015), expanding the concept towards functional, interactive, and critical health literacy (Nutbeam 2000), personal skills (Kickbusch 1997), critical media literacy (Levin-Zamir et al. 2011; Manganello 2008), theoretical/ practical knowledge as well as social responsibility and citizenship (Paakkari and Paakkari 2012), meaning making of health information (Fairbrother and Goyder 2016a), or by including the perspective of multiple literacies as introduced by the paradigm of the New Literacy Studies (NLS) (Papen 2009; Chinn 2011; Okan et al. 2015; Fairbrother and Goyder 2016b). Beyond general health literacy models, over the years, many derivatives and domain-specific health literacies were introduced, such as mental health literacy (Coles et al. 2016), oral health literacy (Naito et al. 2007), diabetes literacy (Black et al. 2017), alcohol related health literacy (Chisolm et al. 2014), or e-health/digital health literacy (Kaufmann et al. 2017), which have since been applied or adopted to younger populations.

A systematic review by Bröder and colleagues (Bröder et al. 2017) identified 12 health literacy definitions and 21 models for children and adolescents. In addition to the sheer number of alternative approaches, the concepts are found to be very heterogeneous, multidimensional, and complex. Within these conceptualisations, health literacy appears to be a variable set of key dimensions related to knowledge, skills, and actions an individual applies in order to understand, use, and evaluate health information. However, available concepts are mainly focused on certain cognitive abilities rather than addressing children's unique attributes or the influence of the social environment on health literacy practices. In addition, most health literacy definitions and concepts were very similar to those for adults and did not consider the target group's unique characteristics, resources and needs. For instance, child development is primarily addressed through a cognitive development perspective, ignoring sociological approaches to development. Specifically, most definitions and concepts focus on older children and adolescents, with little attention being directed towards children younger than ten years old. This may suggest that due to children's early stage of social, emotional, and psychological development, they are perceived as lacking certain formative skills required for health literacy and for processing especially complex health information. However, we argue that health literacy is highly individual. Hence, while there may be common skills – for instance, reading and writing skills, that children typically develop at a certain age, when socialized in the same setting, they do acquire a very unique set of individual skills and experience as they engage with health-related information from an early age onwards. This is supported by a UK based study among 53 children aged 9–10 years (Fairbrother et al. 2016b), which explored how children access and understand health information in relation to food and health. Key results are that children access a wide variety of different food information sources, through their schools, family/parents, or their wider social environment and the media. Family is the most important source of health information, as parents are role models regarding healthy eating and developing values and food practices (Fairbrother et al. 2016b).

The review also concluded that health literacy must be seen as contextually and socially embedded. Hence, the socio-ecological determinants of health literacy as well as its interrelatedness with the social environment and contextual factors need to be closely taken into account. Nevertheless, many conceptual approaches and definitions still strongly emphasise individual attributes. Another conceptual shortcoming that was identified in the systematic review by Bröder and colleagues (Bröder et al. 2017) was that "health information" was often used as a term without specification. We argue that this ignores the complexity of today's information-based society, their multimodality as they 'come in all shapes and sizes' (e.g. digital, written, oral) and the challenges related to actuality, reliability, quality, trustworthiness and credibility of the source.

2.2   Focus Area 2: Measurement Instruments

Currently, two systematic reviews on health literacy instruments for children and adolescents are available, yielding a total of 25 tools published by 2015 (Ormshaw et al. 2013; Okan et al. 2018). The review by Ormshaw et al. (2013) included health literacy as well as mental and oral health literacy tools whereas Okan and colleagues (Okan et al. 2018) focused on generic health literacy tools only. The tools address children and adolescents ranging from 7 to19 years of age. 19 of the tools were novel measures developed for the purposes of the studies, seven were existing tools or adaptations of adult health literacy tools. Regarding the assessment design, 16 tools applied 'objective' measurement (assessing performance), eight 'subjective' measurements (self-report), and one tool used a combination of both measurement types. Six tools used a functional health literacy understanding and 19 applied a multidimensional conceptual underpinning. The tools were applied mostly in school settings and addressed broader health promotion or health education issues. However, eight tools were found to address specific health care related or medical content and two tools mixed health care and health promotion topics. The authors of both reviews found that reporting the quality of evidence and psychometric properties could be improved as could reporting on validation methods. Lastly, the studies did either use a study-specific health literacy concept or did not provide a definition of health literacy at all. This makes it difficult to compare study findings and make general conclusions. An updated search conducted for the purpose of this article found a total of 37 tools published by 2017 (Table 1). Notable new and multidimensional tools that were most recently published are those developed by Paakkari et al. (2016) from Finland or Shih et al. (2016; Liu et al. 2016) from Taiwan.

2.3   Focus Area 3: Review of Empirical Data and Evidence

The earliest systematic review on health literacy in children was published in 2009 (DeWalt and Hink 2009). It focused on parent and child literacy and analysed a total of 24 articles and 11 systematic reviews. One key result was that low literacy in parents was associated with less knowledge and unfavourable health behaviour as well as worse health outcomes in children. Children`s low literacy levels were a predictor for worse health behaviours. Another systematic review (Sanders et al. 2009) analysed 36 studies and discovered that low health literacy in parents/caregivers is wide-spread, associated with limited preventive care behaviours and child-health outcomes, and related to socioeconomic status. Low health literacy was found in one third of all adolescents and young adults. An update on this review published in 2016 included 14 new studies confirming the results (Sansom-Daly 2016). Most studies reported adequate levels of health literacy in more than 60% of the participants. However, only two studies were found to address critical health literacy suggesting that participants had problems in meeting the critical health literacy requirements, despite adequate knowledge and understanding. In addition, findings indicate that the internet is the most common source of health information, which is consistent with another review (Jain and Bickham 2014) on adolescents` online related health information behaviour highlighting the increasing role of the internet for seeking health information. In this context, adolescents experience particular challenges associated with functional, interactive, and critical health literacy in relation to their online health-seeking behaviour. Further results suggest that on the provider level, reliable health information shaped to needs of adolescents is required, and on the individual level,

Table 1 Existing health literacy measures and tools for children and adolescents (source: own depiction)

Study reference/country	Measurement tool	Type	Age group	Health literacy dimensions
Davis et al. (2006)/USA	Rapid Estimate of Adult Literacy in Medicine - Teen (REALM-teen)	Adaptation and modification of the REALM	10–19	Functional health literacy
Burns and Rapee (2006)/ Australia	Adolescent Mental Health Literacy Friend in Need Questionnaire	New tool	15–17	Mental health literacy
Brown et al.(2007)/USA	KidsHealth KidsPoll of Health Literacy	New tool	9–13	Health literacy (understand, access, apply, belief, attitude)
Hubbard and Rainey (2007)/USA	Health Literacy Instrument	New tool	Secondary school	Health literacy (Understand, access, communication, decision-making, goal setting, and self-management)
Chisolm and Buchanan (2007)/USA	Test of Functional Health Literacy in Adolescent population (TOFHLAd)	Adaptation and modification of the TOFHLA	13–17	Functional health literacy
Naito et al.(2007)/ Japan	Oral/ Dental health literacy tool	New tool	11–12	Oral health literacy (seek, understand, interest, health consciousness)
Steckelberg et al.(2009)/ Germany	Critical Health Competence Test (CHC)	New tool	15–42	Health literacy (understand, seek and access, numeracy)
Vardavas et al. (2009)/ Greece	Health Literacy Questionnaire for Children	New tool	12–18	Health literacy (health education, seek and access, satisfaction)
Wharf Higgins et al. (2009)/Canada	Health literacy tool not specified	New tool	11th–12th grade	Health literacy (access, understand, assess, perception)

(continued)

Table 1 (continued)

Study reference/country	Measurement tool	Type	Age group	Health literacy dimensions
Benham Deal et al. (2010)/USA	Health literacy tool	New tool	8–9	Health literacy (knowledge, seek and access)
Primack et al.(2010)/USA	Health literacy tool	New tool	9th grade	Health literacy (mostly knowledge related to chest pain and heart failure)
Chang (2010)/Taiwan	Chinese Short Version Test of Functional Health Literacy in Adolescent population (c-TOF-HLAd)	Translation of the (TOFHLAd)	High school Ø 17	Functional health literacy
Wu et al (2010)/ Canada	Health literacy instrument for high school students	New tool	Secondary school	Health literacy (evaluate, understand)
Olsson and Kennedy (2010)/USA	Mental health problem related case scenarios	New tool	6th–12th grade	Mental health literacy (recognition and identification of health-related problems)
Leighton (2010)/England, UK	Mental and emotional health related case scenarios	New tool	10, 12–15	Mental health literacy (recognise, rate, understand)
Sharif and Blank (2010)/ USA	Short Test of Functional Health Literacy (STOF-HLA)	Modification of the TOFHLA	Ø 11,5	Functional health literacy
Schmidt et al (2010)/ Germany	GeKoKids Health Literacy Questionnaire	New tool	9–13	Health literacy (knowledge, attitudes, communication, behaviour, self-efficacy)

(continued)

Table 1 (continued)

Study reference/country	Measurement tool	Type	Age group	Health literacy dimensions
Levin-Zamir et al.(2011)/ Israel	Media Health Literacy tool	New tool	7th, 9th, 11th grade	Media Health Literacy (identify, critical thinking, evaluate, action)
Paek et al.(2011)/ USA	Health literacy tool	New tool	7th grade	Health literacy (knowledge acquisition, apply)
Wallmann et al. (2012)/ Germany	Health Quiz	New tool	7th grade	Health knowledge (described as functional health literacy)
Yu et al.(2012)/ China	Health Literacy Questionnaire	New tool	Elementary/ Secondary school	Health literacy (knowledge, attitude, practice including health behaviour and lifestyle)
Chinn et al. (2013)/England, UK	All Aspects of Health Literacy Scale (AAHLS)	New tool	15–82	Health literacy (functional, interactive, critical)
Massey et al.(2013)/ USA	Multidimensional health literacy instrument	New tool	13–17	Health literacy related to health care (patient-provider and health care interactions, rights and responsibilities, seek, confidence towards personal and media sources)
Loureiro et al. (2013)/ Portugal	Questionnaire for Assessment of Mental Health Literacy - QuAL-iSMental	Translation, adaptation and modification of the Australian MHL tool	14–24	Mental health literacy (recognition of mental disorders, knowledge, skills, self-help strategies, support disease prevention)
Röthlin et al.(2013)/ Austria	HLS-EU-Q for adolescents	Adaptation of the HLS-EU-Q	15	Health literacy (access, understand, appraise, apply)

(continued)

Table 1 (continued)

Study reference/country	Measurement tool	Type	Age group	Health literacy dimensions
Mulvaney et al. (2013)/ USA	Diabetes Numeracy Test (DNT)	Adapted DNT for the purposes of type 1 diabetes	12–17	Diabetes literacy (self-management, responsibility, reading, and glycaemic control problem solving)
Liu et al.(2016)/ Taiwan	Taiwan Children's Health Literacy Test (TCHL)	New tool	6th grade	Health literacy (functional, interactive, critical, including knowledge)
Driessnack et al.(2014)/ USA	Newest Vital Sign (NVS)	Existing tool	7–12	Functional health literacy
Ueno et al.(2014)/Japan	Oral Health Literacy Instrument	New tool	15–16	Oral health literacy related to evaluation and self-evaluation of tooth related drawings
Naigaga et al. (2015)/ Uganda	Maternal Health Literacy Scale (MaHeLi scale)	Short form of the MaHeLi scale	15–19	Health literacy (appraisal of health information, competence and coping)
Manganello et al. (2015)/ USA	Health Literacy Assessment Scale for Adolescents (HAS-A)	New tool	12–19	Health literacy (functional, communicative, confusion related items, obtain, understand)
Ghanbari et al.(2016)/Iran	Health Literacy Measure for Adolescents (HELMA)	New tool	15–18	Health literacy (access, read, understand, appraise, use, communication, self-efficacy, and numeracy)
Messer et al.(2016)/ Germany	HLS-EU-Q for vulnerable populations	Adaptation and modification of the HLS-EU-Q	15–25	Health literacy (knowledge, functional health literacy, behaviour, health care service use, access, understand, appraise, apply)

(continued)

Table 1 (continued)

Study reference/country	Measurement tool	Type	Age group	Health literacy dimensions
Paakkari et al. (2017)/ Finland	Health Literacy for School-Aged Children (HLSAC)	New tool	7th and 9th grade	Health literacy (theoretical knowledge, practical knowledge, critical thinking, self-awareness, citizenship)
Firnges et al.(2017)/ Germany	MOHLLA questionnaire	Adaptation and modification of the HLS-EU-Q	14–17	Health literacy (access, understand, appraise, apply, knowledge, behaviour)
Okan and Bollweg (2017)/Germany	MoMChild questionnaire	Adaptation and modification of the HLS-EU-Q	9–10	Health literacy (access, understand, appraise, apply, knowledge, behaviour, milieu)

promoting media related health literacy skills might be beneficial in order to better navigate the internet. These findings are supported by 1) an earlier review on teenager's health information behaviour (Kim and Syn 2014), 2) a recent study on adolescent health literacy and credible sources of online health information (Ghaddar et al. 2012), and 3) a review on adolescents' understanding of advertisements which highlights the value of critical media literacy in context of health (Begoray et al. 2013).

2.4   Qualitative Research

2.4.1 Conceptual Research

A UK based study among 53 children aged 9–10 years (Steckelberg et al. 2009; Fairbrother et al. 2016a) explored how children access and understand health information in relation to food and health. Key results are that children access a wide variety of different food information sources, through their schools, family/parents, or their wider social environment and the media. Family is the most important source of health information, as parents are role models regarding healthy eating and developing values and food practices (Steckelberg et al. 2009). This study found particular evidence for children`s engagement with interactive and critical health literacy (Fairbrother et al. 2016a). The findings, however, indicate that critical health literacy goes beyond individual skills and that meaning making of health information is shaped by the social practice of health literacy, which is also embedded within the social context. Similar findings are presented in another study among primary school-aged children (8–11 years old) in Finland (Bhagat et al. 2016). In terms of functional health literacy, the main findings were that meaning making of health information was more relevant than factual understanding. In relation to interactive health literacy, parents were seen as the primary sources of health information, followed by schools and teachers. Critical health literacy was defined in terms of engaging in critical analysis when linking knowledge and facts with personal experience. However, the authors report that the critical health literacy ability in this age group is still under development. Hence, more research and insights are needed for understanding to what extent and how precisely individual health literacy skills are embedded in and influenced by the proximate and distant social context. Among others, this includes if and how children are able to make use of their individual health literacy attributes in a given context, namely considering their potential and actual opportunities in an adult-focused setting to put their health literacy skills into practice.

A Finish study (Parisod et al. 2016) on the determinants of health literacy in the context of tobacco-related health communication was conducted among focus groups of 10–13-year-old early adolescents. The results suggest that health literacy development is mainly influenced by a combination of multidimensional determinants. In addition to determinants of health literacy highlighted earlier, such as age, knowledge, media, social skills, or attitudes, the authors introduce further determinants: (1) personal determinants contain psychosocial factors, such as motives, self-efficacy, and role expectations, whereas (2) external determinants include several social factors such as authorities, idols and random people, and the socio-cultural environment.

2.4.2 Questionnaire Development

In order to develop a child-appropriate health literacy measurement tool, a Taiwanese study (Liao et al. 2016) conducted focus group interviews with sixthsgraders aged 11–12 years old to identify children's practices related to functional, interactive, and critical health literacy. Based on the children`s opinions, the findings resulted in an adaption of the Nutbeam typology for children. The three dimensions were connected to specific school health education goals, such as oral health, healthy diet, mental health, and sex education. The resulting model was used to underpin the Taiwan Children's Health Literacy Scale (Liao et al. 2016; Shih et al. 2016).

An Israeli study aiming to develop a media health literacy questionnaire for adolescents included focus groups of 7th, 9th, and 11th graders (Levin-Zamir et al. 2011). Participants expressed how they conceptualise health, elaborated on their sense for specific determinants of health, their main sources of health information, and the role that media play for their health activities. Based on these findings, different segments were constructed and associated with health promotion topics, such as nutrition, physical activity, tobacco and alcohol consumption, or social behaviour, and finally were used to underpin the media health literacy instrument.

A German study aiming to develop a questionnaire for fourth graders (Okan and Bollweg 2017) was conducted among focus groups of children aged between 8–11 years and found that children have a multidimensional understanding of health, which included notions of well-being as well as mental health. Healthy food, playing games and having fun, physical activity, and the living environment were understood to be closely related to health. While parents were named as the most important source of health information and regarded their primary agents of health communication along with health professionals, doctors were associated with high trustworthiness in the context of health (Okan et al. 2015).

2.5   Quantitative Research

2.5.1 Population-Based Surveys Using Multidimensional Health Literacy Measures

An Austrian study among 15-year-old adolescents, representative for gender, province, and community population, found 58% of the participants to have low health literacy (Röthlin et al. 2013). In contrast, a nationwide Taiwanese study in schoolchildren found that the mean health literacy level was high, while children in the lowest quartile were more likely to be obese than children from the highest quartile (Shih et al. 2016). A German representative study with N=1,000 participants with lower educational background, of which half were aged between 15 and 25, found that 73,5% of adolescents had low levels of health literacy (Messer et al. 2016). When taking into account migration background, 77% had lower levels. In addition, lower parental education, ethnicity, and financial deprivation proved to be determinants of lower health literacy in adolescents. A recently conducted study on health literacy and sports club activities among adolescents (13 and 15 years old) found that self-perceived health literacy was higher when they had regularly participated in sports club activities (Paakkari et al. 2017). While the study found no gender differences, daily physical activity was found to be a factor associated with higher health literacy, but only when children were older and had moderate or high school achievements, whether they were members of a sports club or not.

2.5.2 Functional Health Literacy Studies

A study on health literacy and alcohol use found that 25% of 14-19-year-old adolescents had low health literacy and that lower levels were associated with alcohol consumption and associated problems (Chisolm et al. 2014). Low levels were also associated with low education, belonging to an ethnic minority, or having a migration background. Another study among children and teenagers aged between 10-16 years in Guatemala found that more than two thirds of the participants had inadequate health literacy (Hoffman et al. 2017). Low levels also predicted alcohol and tobacco use, whereas health literacy and parent education were found to be predictors of an increased lifetime alcohol use. Within a parent-child-study on functional health literacy and obesity including children (aged 7–11) and adolescents (aged 12–19), child obesity was mostly associated with parental health literacy or obesity condition. In adolescents, obesity was strongly related to their own health literacy (Chari 2014). Another study found that low child health literacy was negatively correlated with a healthy Body Mass Index in overweight children (Sharif and Blank 2010). A study in Taiwan found that adolescents with low health literacy rated their self-perceived health status worse than adolescents with higher levels. In addition, low levels of health literacy were associated with unhealthy dietary behaviours and interpersonal relations (Chang 2011). A Korean study (Jang and Kim 2015) among fifth and sixths-graders that examined the relationship between health literacy and health behaviour found that 56% of the children had limited health literacy, which was correlated with health behaviour.

2.5.3 Health Literacy and Media

Two studies on health literacy and media found that web-based and other media resources are both significant health socialisation agents and important sources for adolescents to seek health-related information (Levin-Zamir et al. 2011; Paek et al. 2011). The study by Levin-Zamir et al. (2011) conducted in Israel on media health literacy in adolescents found higher levels in girls and that the educational attainment of the mothers had a significant influence on levels. Higher levels were also associated with health empowerment and better health behaviour. An online survey among U.S. high school students aged 14–20 found that health literacy of adolescents was positively associated with self-efficacy and the likelihood of seeking online health information (Ghaddar et al. 2012). This study also found that access to valid online health information can foster health literacy levels. Generally, the internet is of increasing importance in the context of health literacy and health information (Levin-Zamir et al. 2011; Paek et al. 2011; Ghaddar et al. 2012; Begoray et al. 2013; Jain and Bickham 2014; Kim and Syn 2014).

3   Discussion and Conclusion

This literature review provides a brief overview on the current state of health literacy research on children and adolescents with regard to available concepts and models, measurement tools, and evidence-based data. Although there is no health literacy theory that could be adapted to children and adolescents, the conceptual development moves rapidly forward with many models arising out of different contexts and providing several multidimensional concepts based on health promotion, education, or health care principles. However, although there is a lot of overlap, each model incorporates its unique attributes. As there is a difference between health literacy in young children and late adolescents, it seems beneficial to develop tailored concepts for specific target populations. Regarding measurement instruments, tools should be built on specific predefined models or definitions and the assessment should be based on both objective and subjective measurement in order to gather information on health literacy, both perceived and performed. Finally, measures of health literacy should address interactive and critical dimensions as well as components that reflect on the person-environment interplay. Especially qualitative research allows for a better understanding of children`s perspectives on health literacy and highlights the influence of the person-environment interplay. Furthermore, the concept of multi-literacies introduces new possibilities related to health literacy practices and associated social and cultural influences. Deriving meaning from health information is not purely a rational process but is strongly influenced by emotional components and the proximal and distal social context. Health literacy in children seems to be strongly influenced by parental health literacy and further social, cultural, and economic factors, which should be taken into account accordingly. Although the study of health literacy in children and adolescents is rapidly evolving, future research is needed in relation to all focus areas addressed within this review but especially with regard to interactive and critical health literacy as well as media related health literacy and the internet.

References

Begoray D., Higgins J. W., Harrison J., & Collins-Emery A. (2013). Adolescent reading/ viewing of advertisements. *J of Adolescent Adult Literacy. 57*(2), S. 121–130.

Benham Deal T. B., Jenkins J. M., Deal L. O., & Byra A. (2010). The impact of professional development to infuse health and reading in elementary schools. American *Journal of Health Education, 41*(3), 155–166.

Bhagat, K., Howard, D. E., & Aldoory, L. (2016). The relationship between health literacy and health conceptualizations: an exploratory study of elementary school-aged children. *J of Health Communication, 2016,* 1–8.

Black S., Maitland C., Hilbers J., & Orinuela K. (2017). Diabetes literacy and informal social support: a qualitative study of patients at a diabetes centre. *The Journal of Clinical Nursing, 26*(1–2), 248–257.

Bröder J., Okan O., Bauer U., Bruland D., Schlupp S., Bollweg T.M., et al. (2017). Health literacy in childhood and youth: a systematic review of definitions and models. *BMC Public Health, 17*(1), 361.

Brown S. L., Teufel J. A., & Birch D. A. (2007). Early adolescent's perceptions of health and health literacy. *Journal of School Health, 77* (1), 7–15.

Burns, J. R., & Rapee, R. M. (2006). Adolescent mental health literacy: young people's knowledge of depression and help seeking. *Journal of* Adolescent *Health, 29* (2), 225–239.

Chang, L. C. (2011). Health literacy, self-reported status and health promoting behaviours for adolescents in Taiwan. *J of Clinical Nursing,* 20 (1–2), 190–196.

Chari, R, Warsh J., Ketterer T., Hossain J., & Sharif I. (2014). Association between health literacy and child and adolescent obesity. *Patient Education and Counseling,* 94 (1), 61–66.

Chinn, D., & McCarthy, C. (2013). All Aspects of Health Literacy Scale (AAHLS). Developing a tool to measure functional, communicative and critical health literacy in primary healthcare settings. *Patient Education and Counseling,* 90 (2), 247–253.

Chinn, D. (2011). Critical health literacy: A review and critical analysis. *Social Science & Medicine, 2011*(73), 60–67.

Chisolm, D. J., & Buchanan, L. (2007). Measuring adolescent functional health literacy: a pilot validation of the test of functional health literacy in adults. *The Journal of Adolescent Health,* 41 (3), 312–314.

Chisolm D. J., Manganello J. A., Kelleher K. J., & Marshal M. P. (2014). Health literacy, alcohol expectancies, and alcohol use behaviors in teens. *Patient Education and Counseling,* 97 (2), 291–296.

Coles M. E., Ravid A., Gibb B., George-Denn D., Bronstein L. R., & McLeod S. (2016). Adolescent mental health literacy: Young people's knowledge of depression and social anxiety disorder. *The Journal of Adolescent Health,* 58 (1), 57–62.

Davis T. C., Wolf M. S., Arnold C. L., Byrd R. S., Long S. W., Springer T., et al. (2006). Development and validation of the Rapid Estimate of Adolescent Literacy in Medicine (REALM-Teen): A tool to screen adolescents for below-grade reading in health care settings. *Pediatrics,*118 (6), e1707–e1714.

DeWalt D. A. & Hink A. (2009). Health literacy and child health outcomes: a systematic review of the literature. *Pediatrics,* 124 (3 suppl), S265–S274.

Driessnack M., Chung S., Perkhounkova E., & Hein M.(2014). Using the "Newest Vital Sign" to assess health literacy in children. *The Journal of Pediatric Health* Care, 28 (2), 165–171.

Fairbrother, H., Curtis, P., & Goyder, E. (2016a). Making health information meaningful: Children's health literacy practices. *SSM Popul Health., 2016*(2), 476–484.

Fairbrother, H., Curtis, P., & Goyder, E. (2016b). Where are the schools? Children, families and food practices. *Health Place, 2016* (40), 51–57.

Firnges C., Domanska O., Gojdka C., & Jordan S. (2017). Adolescents' health literacy self-reports-insights from the MOHLAA-study. Proceedings. ZPID-Symposium Health Literacy across the Life Span. Papst Science Publishers. 2017: Accepted.

Fok, M. S., & Wong, T. K. (2002). What does health literacy mean to children?.*Contemporary Nurse,*13 (2–3), 249–258.

Ghaddar S. F., Valerio M.A., Garcia C.M., & Hansen L. (2012). Adolescent health literacy: The importance of credible sources for online health information. *Journal of School Health,* 82 (1), 28–36.

Ghanbari S., Ramezankhani A., Montazeri A., Mehrabi Y. (2016). Health Literacy Measure for Adolescents (HELMA): Development and Psychometric Properties. *PloS one,* 11 (2), e0149202.

Hagell A., Rigby E., & Perrow F. (2015). Promoting health literacy in secondary schools: A review. *British Journal of Nursing,* 10 (2).

Hoffman S., Marsiglia F. F., Nevarez L., & Porta M. (2017). Health literacy among youth in Guatemala City. Soc Work Public Health. 2017;(32)1: 30-37.

Hubbard B. & Rainey J. (2007). Health literacy instruction and evaluation among secondary school students. *Journal of Health Education.* 38 (6), 332–337.

Jain A. V. & Bickham D. (2014). Adolescent health literacy and the Internet: challenges and opportunities. *Current Opinion in Pediatrics, 26* (4), 435–439.

Jang B. S. & Kim D. H. (2015). Health literacy and health behavior in late school-age children. *Journal of Korean Academy of Community Health Nursing.* 26 (3), 199–208.

Joint Committee on National Health Education Standards. (1995). *National Health Education Standards – Achieving Health Literacy.* Atlanta: American Cancer Society.

Kaufman D. R., Mirkovic J., & Chan C. (2017). eHealth literacy as a mediator of health behaviors. In *Cognitive Informatics in Health and Biomedicine* (S. 271–297). Springer International Publishing.

Kickbusch I. (1997). Think health: what makes the difference?. *Health Promotion International,* 12 (4), 265–272.

Kilgour L., Matthews N., Christian P., & Shire J. (2015). Health literacy in schools: Prioritising health and well-being issues through the curriculum. *Sport, Education and Society 20* (4), 485–500.

Kim S. U. & Syn S. Y. (2014). Research trends in teens' health information behaviour: A review of the literature. *Health Information & Libraries Journal, 31* (1), 4–19.

Leighton S. (2010). Using a vignette-based questionnaire to explore adolescents' understanding of mental health issues. *Clinical Child Psychology and Psychiatry.* 15 (2), 231–250.

Levin-Zamir D., Lemish D., & Gofin R. (2011). Media Health Literacy (MHL): Development and measurement of the concept among adolescents. *Health Education Research,* 26 (2), 323–335.

Liao L. L., Liu C. H., Cheng C. C., & Chang T. C. (2016). Defining Taiwanese children's health literacy abilities from a health promotion perspective. *Global Health Promotion,* 0 (0), 1–12.

Liu C. H., Liao L. L., Cheng C. C. J., & Chang T. C. (2016). Development and implementation of Taiwan's Child Health Literacy Test. *Global Health Promotion,* 0 (0), 1–13.

Loureiro L. M., Jorm A. F., Mendes A. C., Santos J. C., Ferreira, R. O., & Pedreiro A. T. (2013). Mental health literacy about depression: A survey of Portuguese youth. *BMC Psychiatry,* 13 (1), 129.

Manganello J. A., DeVellis R. F., Davis T. C., & Schottler-Thal C. (2015). Development of the Health Literacy Assessment Scale for Adolescents (HAS-A). *The Journal of Community Health.* 8 (3), 172–184.

Manganello J.A. (2008). Health literacy and adolescents: A framework and agenda for future research. *The Journal of Health Education Research & Development,* 23 (5), 840–847.

Massey, P., Prelip, M., Calimlim, B., Afifi, A., Quiter, E., Nessim, S., et al. (2013). Findings toward a multidimensional measure of adolescent health literacy. *Am J Health Behav., 2013*(37), 342–350.

McDaid, D. (2016). *Investing in health literacy.* European Observatory on Health Systems and Policies: Policy briefs and summaries. World Health Organization.

Messer M., Vogt D., Quenzel G., & Schaeffer D. (2016). Health Literacy bei vulnerablen Zielgruppen. *Präv Gesundheitsf, 11* (2), 110–116.

Mulvaney S. A., Lilley J. S., Cavanaugh K. L., Pittel E. J., & Rothman R. L. (2013). Validation of the diabetes numeracy test with adolescents with type 1 diabetes. *Journal of Health Communication.* 18 (7), 795–804.

Naigaga M. D., Guttersrud Ø., & Pettersen K. S. (2015). Measuring maternal health literacy in adolescents attending antenatal care in a developing country – the impact of selected demographic characteristics. *Journal of Clinical Nursing,* 24 (17–18), 2402–2409.

Naito M., Nakayama T., & Hamajima N. (2007). Health literacy education for children: Acceptability of a school-based program in oral health. *International Journal of Oral Science, 49* (1), 53–59.

Nutbeam D. (2000). Health literacy as a public health goal: A challenge for contemporary health education and communication strategies into the 21st century. *Health Promotion International, 15* (3), 259–267.

Nutbeam, D. (1998). Health promotion glossary. *Health Promot Int., 1998*(13), 349–64.

Okan O. & Bollweg T. M. (2017). Development process of a health literacy measurement instrument for fourth grade schoolchildren: A mixed-method study. In G. Krampen & A.-K. Mayer (Hrsg.), *Health Literacy across the Life Span.* Pabst Science Publishers.

Okan, O., Lopes, E., Bollweg, T. M., Bröder, J., Messer, M., Bruland, D., et al. (2018). Generic health literacy measurement instruments for children and adolescents: a systematic review of the literature. *BMC Public Health, 18*(1), 166.

Okan O., Pinheiro P., Zamora P., & Bauer U. (2015). Health Literacy bei Kindern und Jugendlichen. *Bundesgesundheitsblatt-Gesundheitsforschung-Gesundheitsschutz, 1* 58 (9): 930–941.

Olsson D. P., Kennedy M. G. (2010). Mental health literacy among young people in a small us town: Recognition of disorders and hypothetical helping responses. *Early Interv Psychiatry.* 4(4), 291–298.

Ormshaw M. J., Paakkari L. T., & Kannas L. K. (2013). Measuring child and adolescent health literacy: A systematic review of literature. *The Health Education.* 113 (5), 433–455.

Paakkari, L., Kokko, S., Villberg, J., Paakkari, O., & Tynjälä, J. (2017). Health literacy and participation in sports club activities among adolescents. *Scandinavian Journal of Public Health, 2017,* 1–7.

Paakkari L. & Paakkari O. (2012). Health literacy as a learning outcome in schools. *The Health Education,* 112 (2), 133–152.

Paakkari O., Torppa M., Kannas L., & Paakkari, L. (2016). Subjective health literacy: Development of a brief instrument for school-aged children. *Scand J Public Health. 44* (8), 751–757.

Paek H., Reber B. H., & Lariscy R. W. (2011). Roles of interpersonal and media socialization agents in adolescent self-reported health literacy: A health socialization perspective. *Journal of Health Education Research & Development, 26* (1), 131–149.

Papen U. (2009). Literacy, learning and health – A social practices view of health literacy. *Lit Numer Stud,* 16 (2), 19–34.

Parisod H., Axelin A., Smed J., & Salanterä S. (2016). Determinants of tobacco-related health literacy: A qualitative study with early adolescents. *The International Journal of Nursing Studies,* 62, 71–80.

Primack B. A., Wickett D. J., Kraemer K. L., & Zickmund S.(2010). Teaching health literacy using popular television programming: A qualitative pilot study. *The American Journal of Health Education,* 41 (2), 147–154.

Röthlin F., Pelikan J. M., & Ganahl K. (2013). Die Gesundheitskompetenz der 15-jährigen Jugendlichen in Österreich. http://lbihpr.lbg.ac.at.w8.netz-werk.com/sites/files/lbihpr/attachments/hljugend_bericht.pdf.

Rubene Z., Stars I., & Goba L. (2015). Health literate child: Transforming teaching in school health education. Society, Integration, Education. *Proceedings of the International Scientific Conference, 1,* 331–340.

Sanders L. M., Federico S., Klass P., Abrams M. A., & Dreyer B. (2009). Literacy and child health: A systematic review. *The Archives of* Pediatrics *& Adolescent Medicine,* 163 (2), 131–140.

Sansom-Daly, U. M., Lin M., Robertson E. G., Wakefield C. E., McGill B. C., & Girgis A. (2016). Health literacy in adolescents and young adults: An updated review. *Journal of Adolescent and Young Adult Oncology* 5 (2), 106–118.

Schmidt C. O., Fahland R. A., Franze M., Splieth C., Thyrian J. R., Plachta-Danielzik S., Hoffmann W., et al. (2010). Health-related behaviour, knowledge, attitudes, communication and social status in school children in eastern Germany. *Journal of Health Education Research & Development,* 25 (4), 542–551.

Sharif, I., & Blank, A. E. (2010). Relationship between child health literacy and body mass index in overweight children. *The Patient Education and Counseling,* 79 (1), 43–48.

Shih S. F., Liu C. H., Liao L. L., & Osborne R. H. (2016). Health literacy and the determinants of obesity: A population-based survey of sixth grade school children in Taiwan. *BMC Public Health,* 16(1), 1.

Simonds S.K. (1974). Health education as social policy. Proceedings of the Will Rogers Conf on Health Education. Health Education Monographs. 1974:2(Suppl.1), 1–10.

Steckelberg A., Hulfenhaus C., Kasper J., Rost J., & Muhlhauser I. (2009). How to measure critical health competences: development and validation of the critical health competence test (CHC test). *Advances in Health Sciences Education Theory and Practice.* 14 (1), 11–22.

Ueno M., Takayama A., Adiatman M., Ohnuki M., Zaitsu T., & Kawaguchi Y. (2014). Application of visual oral health literacy instrument in health education for senior high school students. *International Journal of Health Promotion and Education,* 52 (1), 38–46.

Vardavas C.I., Kondilis B.K., Patelarou E., Akrivos P.D., & Falagas M.E. (2009). Health literacy and sources of health education among adolescents in Greece. *The International Journal of Adolescent Medicine* and *Health,* 1, 21 (2), 179–186.

Velardo S. & Drummond M. (2017). Emphasizing the child in child health literacy research. *Journal of Child Health Care,* 21 (1), 5–13.

Wallmann, B., Gierschner, S., & Froböse, I. (2012). Gesundheitskompetenz: was wissen unsere Schüler über Gesundheit. *Präv Gesundheitsf., 2012*(7), 5–10.

Wharf, Higgins J., Begoray, D., & MacDonald, M. (2009). A Social Ecological Conceptual Framework for Understanding Adolescent Health Literacy in the Health Education Classroom. *The American Journal of Community Psychology, 2009*(44), 350–62.

World Health Organisation (WHO) (2016). Shanghai Declaration on promoting health in the 2030 Agenda for Sustainable Development. 9th Global Conference on Health Promotion, Shanghai.

Wu, A. D., Begoray, D. L., MacDonald, M., Higgins, J. W., Frankish J., Kwan B., et al. (2010). Developing and evaluating a relevant and feasible instrument for measuring health literacy of Canadian high school students. *Health Promotion International, 25* (4), 444–452.

Yu, X., Yang, T., Wang, S., & Zhang, X. (2012). Study on student health literacy gained through health education in elementary and middle schools in China. *Health Educ. J., 2012*(71), 452–460.

Health Literacy and Multimodal Adapted Communication

Anja Blechschmidt

1 Introduction

In this paper, I will argue that the 'Multimodal Adapted Communication' (MAC) model of communication can improve health literacy in children. The focus is thus on the adaptation of language, adopting the perspective of linguistics, speech therapy, and special needs education, but simultaneously acknowledging the importance of a multidisciplinary approach.

I will first discuss a broad definition of Health Literacy and maintain that it concerns every member of society. Health-related phenomena should be conceptually accessible by everyone. Language as one fundamental mode of conveying information (e.g. related to health) should therefore be comprehensible by everyone. However, our society is far from a state in which full inclusion is a reality. The MAC model shall be presented as a model that takes into account all aspects of language and that can improve mutual understanding for everyone.

2 Health Literacy

A broad understanding of Health Literacy interweaves the concepts of empowerment, participation, and learning. Health Literacy is further thought to be relevant in every area of life, be it at work or during other everyday activities. According to Theunissen (2002), the target dimension of empowerment is autonomy

A. Blechschmidt (✉)
Pädagogische Hochschule FHNW (ISP), Muttenz, Switzerland
e-mail: anja.blechschmidt@fhnw.ch

© The Editor(s) (if applicable) and The Author(s), under exclusive license to
Springer Fachmedien Wiesbaden GmbH, part of Springer Nature 2021
L. A. Saboga-Nunes et al. (eds.), *New Approaches to Health Literacy*,
Gesundheit und Gesellschaft, https://doi.org/10.1007/978-3-658-30909-1_4

(making independent choices), and it is achieved through a number of aspects of activity orientation; i.e. cooperation (the trust in the other person's potentials and strengths), and the consideration of context (adaptation to different situations and people). Participation is considered to be the "involvement in life situations, which includes being autonomous to some extent or being able to control your own life" (Perenboom and Chorus 2003, p. 578). Thus, participation facilitates joint action, fully utilizing capacity and opportunity through the adaptation of the environment (Nordenfelt 2003). A fundamental type of participation is communicative participation, as it ensures quality of life (Blechschmidt 2008). Finally, 'learning' is a necessary condition for Health Literacy: It awards the possibility of knowledge about the interlocutor's competences at different ages, which can then appropriately be used as a resource for the ability to act.

An extended view of Health Literacy emphasizes (a) competence orientation as the fundament for learning, (b) action orientation to secure the possibility of autonomous action taking, and (c) people orientation (respecting individual competences). It further enables participation under all circumstances and for every member of society, thus expanding the (health) competences of everybody involved.[1] All of these aspects ultimately depend on language competence because they cannot be realized without cooperation[2] and, thus, communication. By focusing on the improvement of interpersonal communication, these aspects can be implemented with high efficiency and promote Health Literacy.

3 Status Quo and Goal

Our society is highly heterogeneous, and the environment has been continually adapted, developed, and refined in order to create multifarious opportunities of participation to a large number of people in various areas of life. Participation is achieved by providing opportunities that align with the competences of a large number of people. For instance, mobility is possible through different means such as cars or public transportation that are adapted to the competences of people.

However, as already implied, there is also a considerable part of society that lack one or more competences attributed to the average citizen (e.g. the ability to

---

[1]The term "health competence" may then be preferable to the term "health literacy".

[2]As stated by Welling (1990), cooperation happens through language action which has a goal, a plan, and is value-based.

walk or to understand complex texts) and thus, the environment fails to warrant equal opportunities to those minority groups (such as children with disabilities), even in everyday activities. This inevitably generates dependence on those who have access to opportunities (due to a match of opportunity-competence), and simultaneously inhibits autonomy for the minority group.

This has substantial consequences in the context of Health Literacy and children: As seen above, Health Literacy ultimately depends extensively on language competence. However, children's language competences differ with regard to syntax, semantics, and pragmatics (Weinert and Grimm 2012). For instance, their language is less complex and consists of a smaller range of vocabulary (Weinert and Grimm 2012). Thus, if opportunities related to Health Literacy require competences that a child does not have, such as the understanding of complex language, children are excluded from an area of life that concerns them personally and is fundamental to their further development (Zamora et al. 2015; Okan et al. 2015; Bröder and Carvalho 2019; Okan 2019).

The goal is to adapt the entire environment to the manifold competences present in our society in order to give every member the opportunity to participate. This especially relates to those areas of life that affect everybody. The adaptation of the environment to the language competences of children is thus a necessary step in order to achieve health literacy.

4   Language as a Means of Communication

According to Strässle (2000), language as one essential means of communication is crucial for participation (and socialization). It is thus indispensable to first examine the phenomenon of language itself. We presume that the communicative function of language is goal-oriented in nature (cf. Blechschmidt 2017), which is why this function is the main focus of this paper. According to Blechschmidt (2015), language acts are regarded in terms of Multimodal Communication, which is defined as the "perspective of oral language with its reference to the situation and context [...], using different modes of communication such as gestures, [etc.]" (p. 145). While oral language is then seen as "context-generating written language [kontextherstellende Schriftlichkeit]" (p. 145), written language is "used for dialogical contextual oral language [dialogisch kontextbezogene Mündlichkeit]" (p. 145). Thus, Multimodal Communication is characterized by a continuous interplay and reciprocal support between the two main domains of language, oral language and written language.

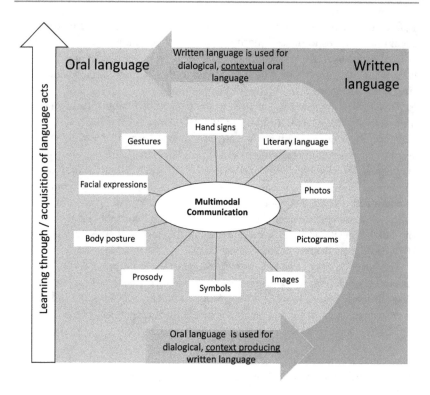

Fig. 1 Multimodal Communication (Blechschmidt 2015)

Figure 1 is based on the entire process of language acquisition. As represented by the white boxes, both oral language and written language can be implemented in a number of modes of communication.[3] Some modes, such as hand signs or symbols, are ambiguous and are therefore assigned to both oral language and written language. There is no communication that does not include at least a range of modes of communication, even when some others are omitted. Choosing which modes of communication are appropriate in a particular interaction

---

[3]Due to the unlimited number of modes of communication and the innumerable possibilities of divisions into subcategories of each mode, the list in the figure does not make a claim for completeness..

depends on the individual competences of the speaker and the hearer. Knowing these appropriate modes that support mutual understanding is a complex and lifelong learning process and is itself seen as a process of adaptation, because it does not only concern a static point in time at the beginning of the conversation, but the communicative event is continuously reassessed in terms of mutual understanding. Thus, a continuous substitution or addition of modes of communication is not only the norm, but necessary in most of the cases. Through this continuous work, then, the competences of the individual interlocutors are merged as common ground is established, and the interdependency can be regarded as a mutual competence. Individual competences are extended and used to develop the mutual competence. This can be illustrated by the example of Management of Understanding [Verstehensmanagement] (Blechschmidt 2017), which is a model of how mutual competences are developed in spoken conversations. It takes into account the dynamic character of interactions and focuses on how interlocutors apply strategies to achieve mutual understanding. It facilitates the process of communication and prevents misunderstandings. Management of Understanding itself is a dynamic process that can only be achieved through joint language action. Interlocutors achieve understanding knowledge (Gerstenkorn 2004) through joint work and mutual evaluation of competences and understanding, for instance through questions, change of subject, but also non-verbal reactions such as eye contact (Blechschmidt 2017). Management of Understanding is defined as a managing activity establishing a mutual code during the language action with the goal of a mutual code, which has the effect of mutual understanding and participation (Blechschmidt et al. 2013b). This managing activity is characterized by strategically targeted, constantly developing organization of procedures towards a mutual code (Blechschmidt 2017).

The spiral of Management of Understanding in Fig. 2 represents the continuous development of processes of understanding in conversations. Deppermann (2010) emphasizes that understanding is indispensable in conversations and considers it a condition of communicative success in professional fields of action. This is relevant for the present argument because it stresses the risk of not being understood, or not making sufficient effort to be understood, when certain modes or complexities of communication (for instance the use of expert definitions and terminology, as is often the case in professional fields) are presupposed. It is also indispensable to create hypotheses of understanding with regard to the meaning of the interlocutor's action, his or her intentions, expectations, and prerequisites of knowledge. Deppermann (2010, p. 8) emphasizes that understanding in communication is highly heterogeneous depending on the professional field of action,

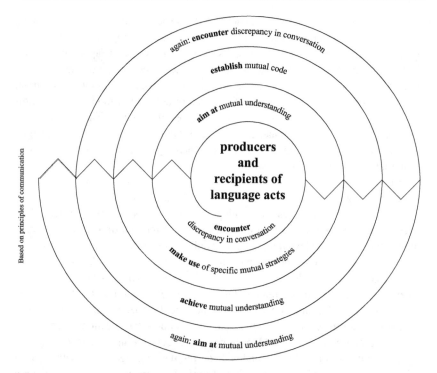

Fig. 2 Spiral of Management of Understanding (Blechschmidt 2017)

and that the specific conditions of interaction and the social structure of different types of interactions are reflected in different types of understanding.

The process of Management of Understanding can be unconscious or conscious, and it is based on an evaluation of the speaker's and the hearer's language competences. Cooperation makes this evaluation possible, and the association Inclusion Europe highlights this aspect with the principle "do not write for us without us" (n.d.). Although this statement refers to people with language disabilities and to written language only, it can be applied to any communicative event due to the reciprocal consideration between the interlocutors elaborated above. In this sense, successful communication (that is, communication which ensures mutual understanding) is achieved through a multimodal and joint process that is continuously adapted. This activity is represented by the Multimodal Adapted Communication model.

5   Multimodal Adapted Communication

As seen in the previous remarks, communication is always multimodal. The Multimodal Adapted Communication (MAC) model elaborates in more detail in which terms communication can and should be adapted by the example of communication with people with language disabilities, as it is usually applied in the context of speech or language impairment of spoken language. This model indicates that the simultaneous consideration of multimodal adapted communication and adapted written language "leads to a close linkage between oral language and written language and dominates language acts in all domains" (Blechschmidt 2015). The benefit of a model that focuses on this linkage is that the individuality of competences is not ignored or even seen as an obstruction but is rather integrated into a dynamic model of communication.

Figure 3 displays the two main domains of language, written language and oral language, and how they can be effectively applied in order to achieve a system of communication in which there is an interconnection between adapted written language and adapted oral language, which ultimately leads to empowerment. Each of the two language domains consists of two types of competence, one regarding the reception of each domain (reading for written language and listening for oral language), and the other regarding the production of each domain (writing for written language and speaking for oral language). Along the objectives of MAC elaborated above, it is essential to link these two domains, or the

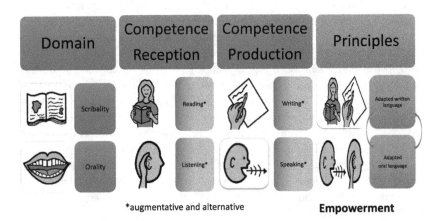

*augmentative and alternative   **Empowerment**

Fig. 3 Three-dimensional thinking about learning and compensation. (Blechschmidt 2015)

four competences respectively, and to communicate in augmentative and alternative terms. This terminology is derived from the concept of AAC (Augmentative and Alternative Communication). AAC has a highly heterogeneous target group of all ages (Erdélyi 2015), and it strongly focuses on those principles of language acts that are indeed essential for every act of communication. This includes communication with children, because similarly to communication in the context of speech or language impairment, it is oftentimes asymmetrical in terms of competences as well (Blechschmidt 2015). MAC then is a basic model of communication in order to manage understanding which draws upon the principles of AAC in order to adapt multimodal communication. In AAC, spoken language is either augmented (when the language user has limited competences of spoken language), or alternated (when spoken language is entirely unavailable to the language user) (Nußbeck 2008). In the context of AAC, it becomes evident that it is not essential for both (or all) interlocutors to have the same competences of production, but it is rather important for both (or all) interlocutors to have the competence of reception of the productive modes of communication involved. The goal of AAC is a maximally effective (Hill 2004) "generalized and functional system of communication, which enables participation in social life" (Nußbeck 2008) and it constitutes the basic model of all communication. The interlocutors aim for a minimization of the communicative asymmetry.

One goal that all models of communication should aim for is to avoid too much generality (i.e. by not considering the numerosity and heterogeneity of subgroups) and too much refinement (statements must still be sufficiently general to be politically reinforceable). Furthermore, the highest applicability, and thus efficiency, of any model is achieved only when it takes into account the most extreme cases of communicative asymmetry, because these are the cases that serve as a basic model for every act of communication (even for the least asymmetrical ones). As elaborated above, it is self-evident that there will be some asymmetry in a conversation between a child and an adult, and thus, the MAC model should be applied in order to achieve mutual understanding. This will ideally empower the child to make autonomous decisions, for instance with regard to health. Even though the child will remain dependent on the adult in some aspects (e.g. advice giving, or putting decisions into practice), he or she will nevertheless gain the experience of being able to make a decision, realizing a decision, and ultimately bearing the consequences of each decision. In the following, I will give some concrete examples of how MAC has already been realized in written language (5.1) and oral language (5.2).

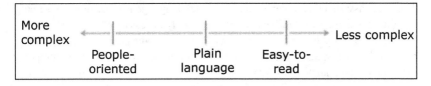

Fig. 4 Continuum of language complexity. (Source: own depiction)

6 Adaptation of Written Language

Besides the various literary modalities which can be used to communicate, written language itself can be adapted to different levels of complexity, which are to be thought of as arranged on a continuum (as seen in Fig. 4). The decision on which level is appropriate should be entirely based on the competences of the target group or target person.

Figure 4 shows this continuum, on which three particular complexities of language are highlighted: People-oriented language, plain language, and easy-to-read language. The first corresponds to a level B1 approximately. It is a text directed towards a specific audience whose language competences (besides the context of the text) should be evaluated before the text is written in order to create mutual understanding. This orientation happens on various levels, the most evident being the choice of language (for instance, if the goal of an academic paper is for it to be read internationally, it is reasonable to write it in English). But it is not only the language itself, but the complexity of language and language style that varies from context to context: For instance, a child may not understand an academic article in terms of its form, but it may well understand its content to a great extent given that the language in which these contents are expressed is simplified. This process of simplification is worth being considered consciously, but it also happens unconsciously in most cases.

The term 'plain language' refers to the simplification of written language following a set of general suggestions, among which are the logical organization of the output, the use of active voice, or the use of everyday words.[4] Plain language does not have a specified target group and its goal is to make public documents understandable and therefore accessible for everyone. It is seen as a service to the reader that can "save time, personnel resources, and money" (Plainlanguage.gov).

---

[4]https://www.plainlanguage.gov/about/definitions/.

Thus, it is asserted that understanding complex language is more time consuming, and that this is ineffective whenever not absolutely necessary.

The term 'easy to read and understand' was introduced by Inclusion Europe and it follows a specific set of standards along which a text must be composed in order to have an 'easy-to-read'-signet (cf. Inclusion Europe 2009). It serves to make written and spoken information understandable. Some examples of standards are the shortness of sentences (the absence of subordinate clauses), the explanation of difficult words as they are mentioned, an overall clear and structured layout, the presence of illustrations, etc. The language level of easy-to-read corresponds to a language level of A1. The aforementioned adaptations are directed at the specified target group of people with language impairments, but it is important to note that the adaptations facilitate the understanding of a text for people without such impairments, too. The idea of plain language that less complex language is more effective in terms of time needed for understanding applies to 'easy-to-read' as well. They can, however, be regarded as more important for people with learning difficulties, non-natives, children, etc., because the difficulty or inability to understand the complex version of the text is much greater for them, and thus, the adaptation is not only a possibility, but a necessity in order to ensure their autonomy.

It can be argued that the simplification of language may reduce not only the form but also the content to a simplicity that does not correspond to the inherent complexity of a certain topic. Or, inversely, a complex content may not be expressible through non-complex language. This is certainly a problem one should be aware of, and it should be reduced through cooperation: in this way, the understanding or misunderstanding of information can be immediately identified and clarified, and the findings of such cooperation can be reutilized as tenets for the writings of future texts. However, it should not be viewed as a reason to suspend the effort of making information accessible for everyone. This becomes especially relevant and noticeable in political contexts: Given that political issues affect and concern every member of society, they should be autonomously accessible by every such member.

One example of political content made accessible to a wide range of people is the United Nations Convention on the Rights of Persons with Disabilities (UNCRPD).[5] In the following, I will discuss three examples by means of an

---

[5]As a matter of fact, it is regulated by law (UNCRPD, article 9) that easy-to-read documents must be available for language impaired people. It should be a matter of future debate whether this law should not be expanded for people with difficulties other than disabilities.

extract of article 4 of the UNCRPD. The first extract is found in the official version, the second is the version composed in plain language with children as the target group, and the third is the version written in easy-to-read, with people language disabilities the target group.

Article 4: General obligations

1. States Parties undertake to ensure and promote the full realization of all human rights and fundamental freedoms for all persons with disabilities without discrimination of any kind on the basis of disability. To this end, States Parties undertake:

   a) To adopt all appropriate legislative, administrative and other measures for the implementation of the rights recognized in the present Convention;

   b) To take all appropriate measures, including legislation, to modify or abolish existing laws, regulations, customs and practices that constitute discrimination against persons with disabilities;

   c) To take into account the protection and promotion of the human rights of persons with disabilities in all policies and programmes.

(UNCRPD 2006)

In this first example, the language style is complicated and the syntax rather convoluted. Moreover, the sentences are long and involve a number of technical terms or designations (understanding this extract presupposes advanced knowledge of legal terms and is thus rather complex for any lay person). Lastly, there are no illustrations included. A second example shows how this extract was adapted to a version understandable by children as it is written in plain language, see Fig. 5.

The language style of this version is likely to be understood by children (less complex and shorter sentences, fewer technical terms, etc.). Furthermore, the design is colorful, the font size is large, and there is an illustration. All of these aspects simplify the text. Reading and understanding this version of the UNCRPD, children have the opportunity to autonomously have insight into a political matter that affects them as well, thus, they have an understanding of their own rights and are empowered to exercise these rights and to participate in discussions about equality. An even more simplified version of the UNCRPD is seen in the Fig. 6, the easy-to-read version.

This document is called the "EasyRead version" of the CRPD. The sentences are simpler than those written in plain language. For instance, there are no subordinate clauses, there are no technical terms, and the sentences are short. The font size is large, and the layout is generally held simpler and plainer that used in the plain language version. There is a lot of free white space, which supports the clear

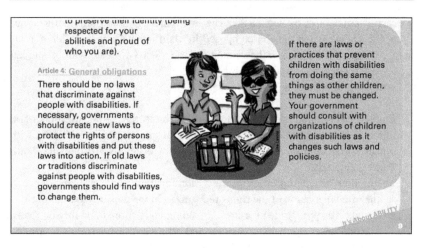

Fig. 5 Plain language example. (Source: UNICEF Victor Santiago Pineda 2008)

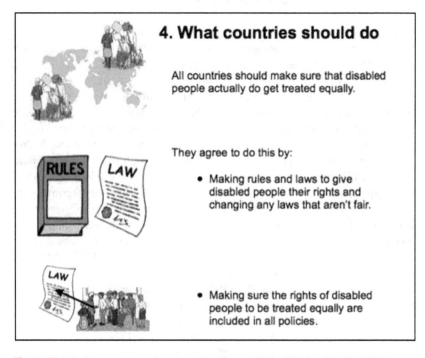

Fig. 6 Plain language easy-reading example. (Source: United Nations Enable 2006)

structure, and illustrations give visual support to the reader. This extract was composed in line with the strict standards of easy-to-read language.

We have seen that this specific document is accessible to people with the most diverse language competences. This is especially important for Health Literacy because not being informed about one's personal rights can lead to political exclusion and even exploitation. This accessibility should now be extended to all contexts that concern a wide range of people, for instance, as this is the special focus of this article, to health contexts.

7 Adaptation of Spoken Language

Regarding the adaptation of oral language, there are three main points to be considered: First, the adaptation has to be a helpful tool for the person's individual progress, and thus, it must be justified in terms of a direct linkage to that person's competence. Second, the process of communication through spoken language must be based on the tenet of cooperation, in order to manage and ensure understanding on both sides. Third, it must be compatible with and usable within the person's environment and circumstances. I will now discuss two types of spoken language adaptation that have already been established: co-construction and modelling.

8 Co-construction

Co-construction is one type of spoken language adaptation which is most commonly used in AAC, and thus, with people who have a disability regarding the use of spoken language. As elaborated earlier in this paper, the positive effects of even the most extreme language adaptation apply to everybody, even though there is no necessity of such an extreme adaptation in terms of the language competences available. Thus, this example can be applied to children as well, even though with children the adaptation of the language through co-construction will have fewer restrictions and will be less intense.

One instance in which co-construction is applied is when one person communicates through a speech-generating computer and has the goal of giving that person the competence of decision-making. There is a variety of uses of such a computer, among which is the control through the eye gaze. In this case, the computer is directed by means of the eye gaze and it can then give language output of the sentence inserted by the user of the computer. The person with the spoken language impairment can then produce spoken language nevertheless and is thus considerably empowered to make decisions in everyday life. Since this person cannot exercise the uttered decisions independently, there is no complete autonomy, but it is radically increased through the computer-based language output. During an interaction, then, there is a process of co-construction between the person with no impairment with regard to language or movement and the person communicating through the speech-generating computer. Co-construction is a cooperative action during which the language impaired person's competences are expanded. This expansion involves language acts such as management of understanding (for instance assuring oneself through questions whether a certain utterance was understood correctly, and receiving an affirmative or negative answer to the question).

9 Modelling

Another established type of spoken language adaptation is modelling, whose most frequent target group are children. Dannenbauer (1994) discusses modelling prevalently in the context of speech, language and communication needs/developmental language disorder and lists communication strategies such as the introduction of the goal structure (and the regular metacommunicative return to this goal structure), parallel speaking (the instructor putting into words the child's intentions), linguistic marking (putting into words something that has caught the child's attention), alternative questions (giving the child two possible answers to choose from), etc. These strategies help the child to understand the contents of a conversation and to produce his or her own expressions of language.

Another context of use of modelling is that of multiple disabilities, as applied and described by Pivit and Hüning-Meier (2011). They state the following general directives have to be considered during the interaction:

a) Contextual communication. E.g.: the instructor says out loud: "I am done, I need more material now" and slowly and articulately says "done" – "need" – "more" in the supported form of communication. Then the instructor asks: "And you? Are you done, too?" and again uses the communicative help in an articulate manner. Finally, where appropriate, the instructor helps the supported child say: "I not done!"

b) Vocalization of structural supporters, that is, saying out loud what needs to be done in order to achieve a specific word. E.g.: The instructor thinks out loud: "What do I want to say? Mmh... Is it about the person on the brown pages? – No! Is it about something one can do? – Yes!! – Then, I have to go see the yellow words (the instructor turns the pages). – Is it on this page? – No! (the instructor keeps turning the pages) – but here!! – I want to go for a ride in the car" (the instructor points at the symbol).

c) Support of utterances, i.e. offering modelled suggestions of answers, e.g. in terms of an opposite pair and/or by leaving out the last word of a phrase.

d) Augmentation of utterances by turning one-word sentences into two- or more-word sentences, augmentation of new words, and offering flexion and synonyms.

All of the aspects along which modelling moves indicate that, like all of the other forms of adapted communication, this one also emphasizes the children's competences. Furthermore, the fact that it can be applied in several contexts, two of which have been mentioned, makes evident that modelling is dynamic by its very nature. The same flexibility should be achieved in any model of communication.

10 Concluding Remarks and Outlook

Health Literacy was viewed as a concept that includes empowerment, participation, and learning. This implies that it affects every member of society, and thus, everybody must be able to understand the messages that are communicated in the context of health. Empowerment, participation, and learning all crucially depend on language because the latter is an essential tool for communication and ultimately greatly influences one's quality of life. However, language competences are as multifarious as our society itself. On the one hand, there are many people who do not have the ability to make productive and/or receptive use of certain modes of communication that a person with average language competences has, e.g. spoken language. On the other hand, the competence of using one such mode may well be given, but the internal complexity of the language may be too high, and thus, the utterance becomes incomprehensible. In many aspects and areas, our society currently does not adapt events of communication (posters, interviews, leaflets, etc.) to non-average language competences. This inevitably leads to a state of society in which some people are not included and thus are not empowered to make autonomous decisions. This can be changed by adapting communicative events, and thus language, in the two areas of competence, reception and production, for instance taking into account MAC as a concept which promotes management of understanding by using people-oriented language, plain language, and easy-to-read language, i.e. models to adapt written language. We then presented co-construction and modelling as examples of the adaptation of spoken language. Choosing a certain form of MAC must be based on the competences of the hearer and of the speaker and must continually be re-evaluated. Through MAC, people who were formerly not able to understand a communicated utterance can understand contents of issues that affect them personally and are thus empowered to make autonomous decisions. Applying Multimodal Adapted Communication with a high frequency in the private and the public sphere will lead to a general increase of Health Literacy in our society.

Future research should be directed towards examining the language competences of different groups of our society in detail. One productive methodological approach would be Conversation Analysis. A possible study design would be the analysis of video recordings of people communicating in a multimodal manner. A special focus on misunderstandings could reveal the acts of adaptation used to deal with such instances (for instance taking into account the Spiral of Management of Understanding). Because this method reveals individual language competences, it could also be a productive means of diagnostics.

References

Blechschmidt, A. (2008). Ich rede mit, Du auch? *Schweizerische Zeitschrift für Heilpädagogik, 11–12*, 32–37.

Blechschmidt, A. (2015). Multimodale Angepasste Kommunikation (MAK) – eine Verbindung von Mündlichkeit und Schriftlichkeit. In A. Blechschmidt & U. Schräpler (Eds.), *Mündliche und schriftliche Texte in Sprachtherapie und Unterricht* (pp. 145–158). Basel: Schwabe Basel.

Blechschmidt, A. (2017). Verstehens-Management in der Multimodalen Angepassten Kommunikation MAK. In Anja Blechschmidt & Ute Schräpler (Eds.), *Unterstützt erzählen – Erzählen unterstützen*. Schwabe: Basel.

Bröder, J. & Carvalho, G. S. (2019). Health literacy of children and adolescents: Conceptual approaches and development considerations. In: O. Okan, U. Bauer, D. Levin-Zamir, P. Pinheiro, & K. Sørensen (Hrsg.): International Handbook of Health Literacy. Research, practice and policy across the lifespan (pp. 39–52). Bristol: POLICY Press.

Dannenbauer, F. M. (1994). Zur Praxis der entwicklungsproximalen Intervention. In: H. Grimm & S. Weinert. Intervention bei sprachgestörten Kinder. Voraussetzungen, Möglichkeiten und Grenzen. Stuttgart: Gustav Fischer Verlag.

Deppermann, A. (2010). Konklusionen: Interaktives Verstehen im Schnittpunkt von Sequenzialität, Kooperation und sozialer Struktur. In: Deppermann, A./ Reitemeier, U./ Schmitt, R./ Spranz-Fogasy, Th.: Verstehen in professionellen Handlungsfeldern (S 363–384). Tübingen: Narr.

'EasyRead' service @ Inspired Services Publishing Ltd. (2007). International agreement on the rights of disabled people. Retrieved from https://www.un.org/development/desa/disabilities/convention-on-the-rights-of-persons-with-disabilities.html

Erdélyi, A. (2015). Unterstützte Kommunikation für Menschen ohne Sprache. Patienteninformation. In: Sprache · Stimme · Gehör 39, 39.

Gerstenkorn, A. (n.d.). (2004). Wissensmanagement Braucht Verstehensmanagement – Konzeption Eines Instrumentariums Zum Verstehen Von Fachtexten Für Experten, Neulinge Und Begrifflich Geschulte Fachfremde. *Wissensorganisation in Kooperativen Lern- Und Arbeitsumgebungen: Proceedings Der 8. Tagung Der Deutschen Sektion Der Internationalen Gesellschaft Für Wissenschaftsorganisation, Regensburg, 9.–11. Oktober 2002*, edited by Gerhard Budin and Peter H. Ohly, Ergon.

Hill, K. (2004). Augmentative and alternative communication and language: Evidence-based practice and language activity monitoring. *Topics in Language Disorders, 24*(1), 18–30.

Inclusion Europe. (n.d.). Do not write for us without us. Involving people with intellectual disabilities in the writing of texts that are easy to read and understand [Brochure].

Nordenfelt, L. (2003). Action theory, disability and ICF. *Disability and Rehabilitation, 25*(18), 1075–1079. https://doi.org/10.1080/0963828031000137748.

Nußbeck, S. (2008). Unterstützte Kommunikation. In: M. Fingerle, & Ellinger, St. (Hrsg.): Sonderpädagogische Förderprogramme im Vergleich. Orientierungshilfen für die Praxis (S. 214–232). Stuttgart: Kohlhammer.

Okan, O. (2019). The importance of early childhood in addressing equity and health literacy development in the life-course. *Public Health Panorama, 5*(2–3), 170–176.

Okan, O., Pinheiro, P., Zamora, P., & Bauer, U. (2015). Health Literacy bei Kindern und Jugendlichen. In: Bundesgesundheitsblatt – Gesundheitsforschung – Gesundheitsschutz 58 (9), 930–941. https://doi.org/10.1007/s00103-015-2199-1.

Perenboom, R. J., & Chorus, A. M. (2003). Measuring participation according to the International Classification of Functioning, Disability and Health (ICF). *Disability and Rehabilitation, 25*(11–12), 577–587. https://doi.org/10.1080/0963828031000137081.

Pineda, V. S. (2008). It's About Ability. An explanation of the Convention on the Rights of Persons with Disabilities. New York, NY: United Nations Children's Fund (UNICEF).

Pivit, C., & Hüning-Meier, M. (2011). Wie lernt ein Kind unterstützt zu kommunizieren? – Allgemeine Prinzipien der Förderung und Prinzipien des Modellings. *Handbuch der Unterstützten Kommunikation, Karlsruhe, 01*(32), 001.

Strässle, J. (2000). *Wortlos Erwachsen Werden*. Edition SZH/SPC: Zur Kommunikativen Situation Junger Erwachsener Mit Cerebralen Bewegungsstörungen.

Theunissen, G. (2002). *Handbuch Empowerment und Heilpädagogik*. Freiburg im Breisgau: Lambertus.

UN Enable - Text of the Convention on the Rights of Persons with Disabilities. (2006, December 6). Retrieved from: http://www.un.org/esa/socdev/enable/rights/convtexte.htm.

Weinert, S. & Grimm, H. (2012). Sprachentwicklung. In: Schneider, W.; Lindenberger, U. (eds.): Entwicklungspsychologie. 7th Edn. (pp. 433–456), Weinheim, Basel: Beltz.
What is Plain Language? (o.J.). Retrieved from: https://www.plainlanguage.gov/about/definitions/.
Zamora, P., Pinheiro, P., Okan, O., Bitzer, E.-M., Jordan, S., Bittlingmayer, U. H., et al. (2015). „Health Literacy" im Kindes- und Jugendalter. *Prävention und Gesundheitsförderung, 10*(2), 167–172. https://doi.org/10.1007/s11553-015-0492-3.

The Significance of Health Literacy for Public Health and Health Promotion

Eva Maria Bitzer and Hanna E. Schwendemann

1 Introduction

To achieve public health goals such social and health outcomes, it is not sufficient to focus on individual health literacy only. It might be more effective to improve environmental, social and economic conditions, and to strengthen patient-centredness of the health system. This chapter first looks at current definitions, strategies and practices of public health. We then refer to the idea of health literacy as a public health goal (Nutbeam 2000) and briefly describe the current understanding of health literacy. We examine the role of individual health literacy as proximal outcome of health education compared to public health practices on the macro- and meso-levels in three case studies: (1) fighting infectious diseases, (2) participation in population-based cancer screening, and (3) management of chronic diseases. In the discussion we introduce the concept of health literacy responsiveness and argue that in many situations increasing the health literacy responsiveness of the system is of equal, if not of more importance than attempts to increase individual health literacy.

E. M. Bitzer (✉) · H. E. Schwendemann
Departement of Public Health and Health Education, University of Education Freiburg (Germany), Freiburg, Germany
e-mail: evamaria.bitzer@ph-freiburg.de

H. E. Schwendemann
e-mail: hanna.schwendemann@ph-freiburg.de

2 Public Health

From a public health perspective, health is a human right and maintaining or promoting health is not merely a task of the health system or of the individual person, it is a task of the society (Resnik 2007). Public health as the science and practice of preventing disease, prolonging life and promoting health through the organized efforts of society (Acheson 1988) includes the equitable and efficient allocation of resources as well (Gerhardus et al. 2012). Activities to strengthen public health capacities and services aim to provide conditions under which people can aim to be healthy, improve their health and wellbeing and furthermore prevent the deterioration of their health. To achieve this vision, the public health approach involves collaboration with other sectors to address the wider determinants of health. A unifying principle of public health is its essentially "public" nature and the fact that it is mainly focused on the health of the whole population.

3 How to Maintain and Promote Health?

More than 30 years ago, the Ottawa Charter provided a framework on how to maintain and promote health. The Charter defined health promotion as a public health action, directed towards improving people's control over all modifiable determinants of health (World Health Organization Europe 1986). What are we doing when we try to promote and maintain health? We, society, political leaders, public health practitioners and researchers, intervene. Intervention can take place on the macro, meso, and micro levels and include public policy, addressing living and working conditions, as well as education to influence individual behaviour directly and indirectly. Public health interventions aim ultimately to improve health and social outcomes, i.e. morbidity and mortality, functional independence, disability and (health-related) quality of life. Changing determinants of health and social outcomes is part of the theoretical model on how interventions might work, and such determinants of health and social outcomes are regarded as intermediate outcomes of public health efforts. The immediate targets of public health actions are those individual, social and structural factors that can be modified to improve determinants of health, the so-called proximal outcomes. How can we be sure that public health and health promotion interventions achieve those goals? We measure direct, mostly short term (proximal) outcomes that lead to indirect outcomes in the mid-term, and finally improve health and social outcomes.

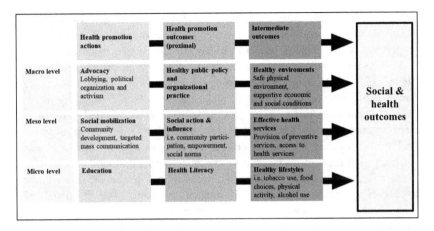

Fig. 1 Maintain and promote health on individual, community and population level (Figure adapted using (Nutbeam 2000; Walter et al. 2012))

Figure 1 describes common public health and health promotion actions on the micro, meso, and macro levels and their proximal, intermediate and health outcomes.

On the macro level it is advocacy, i.e. lobbying and activism that encourages a healthy public policy and organizational practice that will finally lead to improved health outcomes. On the meso-level we think of social mobilization and community development, as well as targeted mass communication with proximal outcomes such as community participation or the shaping of cultural and social norms, leading to effective health (care) services, i.e. the provision of preventive services, and access to health services (intermediate outcomes). Public health and health promotion action on the micro level comprises health education. Modern health education supports public health interventions and aims to increase health outcome by fostering healthy lifestyles (intermediate outcome) via increasing health literacy (proximal outcome).

4   What do we mean when we refer to Health Literacy?

Health literacy was introduced nearly 50 years ago and is gaining importance in public health. The wealth of models and definitions of health literacy has been synthesized to a comprehensive model (Sørensen et al. 2012) health literacy is linked to literacy and entails people's knowledge, motivation and competences to access, understand, appraise, and apply health information in order to make judgements and take decisions in everyday life concerning heath care, disease prevention and health promotion to maintain or improve quality of life during the life course. To be health literate means placing one's own health and that of one's family and community into context, understanding which factors are influencing it, and knowing how to address them. At the heart of the model are the four steps accessing, understanding, appraising and applying information relevant for health. The first step encompasses the ability to know how and where to search for health information, to be able to recognize health information (i.e. instead of advertisement) and get hold of the information. The second step addresses the ability to comprehend health information, including basic functional skills such as reading, calculating and writing, whereas the third step looks for more advanced judgement skills that help to answer questions like "Is this information credible and relevant for my health problem?". Step four addresses the issue of applying health information for one's own health, i.e. taking decisions to act health consciously in order to maintain and promote health (Sørensen et al. 2012).

When you ask lay people and experts in the field of health promotion, or health professionals "What constitutes health literacy", a more personal model evolves. From their point of view, basic abilities like literacy and numeracy, and knowledge about health as well as the health care system are "supplemented" by a third facet, namely the motivation to take responsibility for one's personal health. Basic abilities, knowledge, and motivation are the prerequisites for the main domain of health literacy, namely agency, the ability to act on behalf of one's own health, including the facets navigation and action in the health system, communication & co-operation, information retrieval, appraisal, and self perception & self regulation (Osborne et al. 2013; Soellner et al. 2010).

Health literacy is context specific. Each specific health decision situation defines the amount and type of health literacy a patient needs to cope with the situation. The level and type of the health literacy required depends largely on the type of health decision, the situation, and environmental factors. A person may exhibit high levels of health literacy when it comes to interacting with healthcare providers dealing with a common condition, but exhibit low health literacy when confronting an unfamiliar condition in a different setting (Kickbusch 2013). Individual health behaviour is always an expression of the interaction between individual skills or abilities and the demands or complexity of the social and natural environment. In a health care situation, the individual interacts in the structural and organisational framework of the health care system. Acting in a health literate way is thus the ability to deal with the available information, the health care system, one's resources and possible support. Individuals, patients and citizens differ regarding their health literacy, their abilities and skills. The health system, health care institutions and health care professionals must acknowledge that it is not a "one size fits all". Institutions must respond to the health literacy needs of their clients appropriately. Apart from that, improving individual health literacy might be of varying significance on the way to good health and social outcomes.

In accordance with what has been said previously, we will now focus on three case studies. The first of these studies, entitled "Fighting Infectious Diseases" addresses actions to improve health literacy, as compared with macro-level actions. The second example explores the role of health literate health professionals and the health literacy of the population when faced with the decision of whether to participate in population-based cancer screening. The third case study links health literacy as an important resource to managing chronic conditions.

5   Where does Individual Health Literacy Matter? Three Case Studies

Case 1: Fighting infectious diseases

Efforts to fight infectious diseases encompass three strategies that can be linked to the micro and macro levels. Micro level individual strategies focus on medical therapy (i.e. antibiotics, quarantine) and prevention via fostering protective individual behaviour like personal hygiene, food preparation, and housekeeping. Macro level interventions are linked to environmental measures aiming at safe food and water, infection and vector control, both based on sound legislation.

Cholera is an acute enteric infection caused by the ingestion of bacterium Vibrio Cholerae present in faecal contaminated water or food. Primarily linked to insufficient access to safe water and proper sanitation, its impact can be even more dramatic in areas where basic environmental infrastructures are disrupted or have been destroyed. Cholera causes a lot of watery diarrhoea and vomiting and can lead to death from dehydration (the loss of water and salts from the body) within hours if not treated (Lamond and Kinyanjui 2012). First line therapy of cholera consists in oral rehydration with simple sugar-salt-solution (Glass and Stoll 2018). Current recommendations to prevent cholera consist of drinking bottled water with unbroken seals, washing hands with soap and safe water, cooking food hot and eating it hot, and peeling fruits and vegetables (World Health Organisation 2018). Clearly, a person that happens to be informed and educated about these measures and is willing to act according to those recommendations should be regarded as health literate—meaning: individual health literacy matters in infection control and prevention!

However, interventions on the macro level might be of even more importance—as in the case of the cholera epidemic in 1892 in Hamburg. Between 15th of August and 15th of October 1892 cholera accounted for more than 17.000 cases and more than half of those infected died from the disease. Epidemics of diseases like cholera struck big cities time and again in the nineteenth century; the spread over continents, across country borders, and from city to city was an unfortunate side-effect of the expansion of commerce and trade routes. These epidemics ultimately led to increased cooperation between the state and scientific institutions to improve public hygiene in cities (German Historical Institute 2018). The City of Hamburg consulted Robert Koch from Berlin, who discovered the cholera pathogen. He was appalled by the state of public hygiene, particularly in the city's slum quarters. The cholera epidemic in Hamburg led to the foundation of the Hygiene Institute in the September of 1892, the city's first waste incinerator, a sewage system, and a filtering plant for drinking water (all in 1893), the rebuilding of a complete quarter, strong legislation to prohibit unsafe and unsanitary buildings, and changes in the city constitution to increase political participation of larger parts of the population (Winkle 1983, 1984).

The permanent eradication of cholera in Germany was not a matter of individual health literacy. Political decisions and organized efforts of the society to improve community hygiene led to safe and sanitary buildings, clean water and better hygienic conditions. The fighting of infections is an example showing that not only individual health literacy but also health literacy of the system matters in prolonging life and improving quality of life. Individual health literacy is necessary, but to maintain and promote health on population level advocacy (i.e. lobbying, political organizations and activism), as well as good governance is needed (United Nations Economic and Social Commission for Asia and the Pacific 2009). On the macro level it is necessary to create healthy public policies and organisational practices to provide a safe and healthy physical environment, supportive economic and social conditions, thus to achieve, in the longer term, lower mortality (see fig. 2).

Case 2: Individual decision to participate in screening for prostate cancer and health professionals

To be able to judge whether to participate in a screening or not, one has to ponder the benefits and harms of screening. Knowledge about these facts concerning cancer screening is essential for healthy individuals to make informed decisions as well as for physicians supporting informed decisions. But only five in a hundred

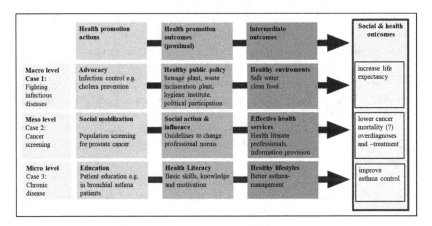

Fig. 2 Maintain and promote health on population level, practical examples

healthy individuals correctly estimate the benefits of screening, many overestimate the benefits or cannot name them. Some persons rely on the physicians' judgment alone when they have to decide about screening (Gigerenzer and Wegwarth 2008). Not only lay persons but also physicians have difficulties in understanding the meaning of statistical information on screening effectiveness, i.e. they are statistical illiterate (Gaissmaier and Gigerenzer 2008). From that point of view, to allow citizens to act in a health literate manner regarding the decision on whether to participate in cancer screening, a sound public health intervention would have to change cultural and professional norms in that it would first enable health care professionals to provide risk communication, non-directive counselling and shared-decision-making—as part of being a health literate health care organization (Bitzer and Sørensen 2018). The case of PSA-testing for early detection of prostate cancer illustrates some of the difficulties with such an approach.

Prostate cancer is a common male cancer and the second leading cause of cancer death in Germany and in the USA. More than 60% of all prostate cancers are diagnosed in men older than 65 (Robert Koch-Institut 2014b; The american cancer society 2018). Early detection of prostate cancer is possible with a blood test (PSA). But does early detection of prostate cancer with PSA increase live expectancy and quality of life?

The benefits of PSA-screening for prostate cancer have been reported to be one death of cancer of the prostate prevented per 1000 screened men for 11 years (four in 1000 non-screened men and three in 1000 screened men die because of prostate cancer, this is an absolute risk reduction of 1 per 1000 and a relative risk reduction of 25%) Screening for prostate cancer has no effect on overall mortality (Keller et al. 2018). PSA-screening for prostate cancer leads to overdiagnosis and overtreatment, the diagnosis and treatment of carcinomas that would not have bothered men during their lifetime in a situation without screening. Treating cancer of the prostate is often accompanied by complications and persisting side effects (urinary incontinence, impotence (Henninger et al. 2014)). The harms of PSA-screening for prostate cancer include 160 of 1000 men screened experience a biopsy of the prostate with a benign result (false positive PSA-test), 20 of 1000 men screened are affected by overtreatment—eight to ten of those men are affected by urinary incontinence, and impotence (Ilic et al. 2013; Keller et al. 2018).

Against this background it is difficult to justify the fact that annual screening for cancer of the prostate in men 50 years of age and older has been recommended by many doctors and professional organisations. Only recently several organisations have begun to caution against routine population screening (Grossman et al. 2018; Moyer 2012). In a difficult process, supported by public health researchers and independent public health agencies, professional guidelines at least acknowledge that men who are considering PSA-screening have the right to be informed in detail about the potential harms and benefits in advance (Pickles et al. 2015) using absolute rather than relative numbers (Keller et al. 2018). As mentioned above, to implement this recommendation into usual health care, health care institutions and professionals engaged with prostate cancer screening would have to offer risk communication, non-directive counselling and shared-decision-making—as part of being a health literate health care organization (Bitzer and Sørensen 2018). However, physicians of various backgrounds happen to be unable, unwilling or reluctant to offer such counselling and the majority still recommends PSA-screening (Hall et al. 2017; Pickles et al. 2015; Stiftung Warentest 2015). And, more disturbingly from a public health perspective, at least in the U.S. patient-provider communication on the benefits and harms of prostate cancer screening increases (!) PSA-screening uptake (Haider et al. 2017). This raises concern on how physicians provide such information on benefits and harms of PSA-testing for prostate cancer (easy to understand, non-threatening and non-directive?). Obviously, it is more than the level of evidence or (un)certainty that guides professional behaviour. Other determinants are the history of the prostate screening policy in a respective country, the health system's organisational structures and funding models and the extent to which professional decisions reflect a consistent, organisationally embedded approach based on local evidence-based recommendations to discourage screening (Pickles et al. 2015).

The case of PSA-screening for prostate cancer illustrates the significance of health literate health care organizations and professionals for improving health care utilization and sound individual decisions on (not) taking up preventive services. It highlights the importance of public health actions directed at changing cultural and professional norms on the meso level, and to improve health outcomes, apart from increasing individual health literacy.

Case 3: Individual asthma control
The third case study examines the significance of health literacy as an individual resource to manage chronic conditions in everyday life, and health education as the means to increase health literacy on the micro level. Health education is a key component in the management of chronic diseases and aims to promote health literacy and self-management (Bitzer et al. 2009; Chodosh et al. 2005; Faller et al. 2005; Weingarten et al. 2002). Modern health education does not only consist in knowledge transfer but also enables patients to control and manage their symptoms, fosters the adequate adaption of therapies and the integration of new behavioural habits in a patient's daily life (Bäuerle et al. 2017). We use bronchial asthma in adults as an example, and asthma patient education as the public health action to increase health literacy.

Bronchial asthma is a chronic inflammatory disease of the lower respiratory tract. It leads to a reversible constriction of the bronchi with inflammatory swollen bronchial mucosa and an increased production of viscous secretions. The main symptom is seizure-related breathlessness with whistling exhalation (Robert Koch-Institut 2014a). With current anti-asthmatics management, the prognosis of asthma has greatly improved, however, even in industrialized countries there are still people dying from asthma. Two in three deaths from asthma could be prevented by better management of the condition including personal asthma plans for patients, timely reviews of asthma care, and the prescription of more appropriate drugs (Crellin et al. 2018). Health professionals are responsible not only for prescribing appropriate drugs but also for fostering health literacy in asthma patients by health education to fully exploit the merits of asthma therapy.

This kind of health education is an important component of modern asthma management (Bundesärztekammer (BÄK), Kassenärztliche Bundesvereinigung (KBV), Arbeitsgemeinschaft der Wissenschaftlichen Medizinischen Fachgesellschaften 2018; National Heart Lung and Blood Institute 2007) and improves asthma control (Gibson et al. 2003), the main health outcome in asthma care (Gibson et al. 2003; Nathan et al. 2004; Schatz et al. 2009). Better asthma control is associated with a substantial, clinically relevant und sustainable reduction of asthma-related disabilities (Jones 2002).

In Germany, four in ten asthma patients entering medical rehabilitation attended some sort of patient education prior to rehabilitation. However, all of these patients are in need of patient education, since only five in a hundred arrive with controlled asthma, 35% of patients have a sufficiently controlled asthma, the majority (60%) arrives with inadequately controlled asthma (Bitzer and Steurer-Stey 2019). Asthma patient education in German inpatient rehabilitation addresses skills (i.e. how to measure peak flow correctly), offers knowledge to support individual asthma management (i.e. why monitoring peak flow on a daily bases matters and what to learn from peak flow charts), and strives to enable asthma patients to take responsibility for their own health, trains adequate self-perception of asthma symptoms and teaches patients to take appropriate (medical and non-medical) steps to manage their asthma (Bäuerle et al. 2017). One year after discharge from such an inpatient rehabilitation scheme the proportion of patients with controlled asthma more than doubles (from 5% to 12%) and the proportion of patients with poorly controlled asthma decreases markedly (from 60% to 45%) (Bäuerle et al. 2017). With reference to fig. 1, health literacy is a proximal outcome of health education, and modern asthma health education increases patients' asthma-specific health literacy and leads to improved health outcomes, such as asthma control (see fig. 2).

6   Discussion and Conclusion

From a public health and health promotion perspective, health literacy matters on every level of the system. On the macro level, in public health strategies, on the meso level via health professionals and on the micro-level through health literate individuals. In this chapter we illustrated that to achieve public health goals it is not sufficient to focus on individual health literacy only, and that it might be more effective to improve environmental, social and economic conditions and to strengthen the patient-centeredness of the health system using three case studies.

On the micro level of public health interventions, we examined the individual health literacy as a proximal outcome of health education using the case study of patient education in asthma patients. Central abilities of patients are knowing when and where to seek for information, verbal communication, assertiveness, literacy, retaining and processing information and the application of the acquired skills (Jordan et al. 2010). Limited health literacy affects individual health significantly, it is associated with riskier health choices, poor adherence to medication, more hospitalization and increased morbidity. Building personal health literacy skills is a lifelong process that includes informal and formal education. From a public health perspective it is important to facilitate and support these learning processes, to enable patients to judge health information, to make decisions in health care, disease prevention and health promotion (Bitzer et al. 2009; Kickbusch 2013; Quaglio et al. 2017).

However, regarding health and social outcomes, public health strategies should not only focus on improving individual health literacy. Health literacy is an added value to current strategies within healthcare, disease prevention and health promotion if it focuses on making a more coherent match between the needs of people and the services of our health system in order to reduce waste and barriers. Actions that aim to fix people's low health literacy by educating them to match the demands of the health system's complexity are of much less significance compared to actions focusing on the health system's skills to meet the complex demands of people (Sørensen 2018). This might be called *health literacy responsiveness*, the extent to which a health system is responsive to its users' needs (Dodson et al. 2018). To increase the health literacy responsiveness of the (health) system and to improve citizens health literacy, systematic efforts are needed. Optimising health literacy to improve health and equity would be an important public health goal. Such an approach would support the identification of community health literacy needs, and the development and testing of potential solutions. It would ask "what strategies are appropriate and effective, for what organisations and individuals?" (Batterham et al. 2014, p. 2) and would rely on eight principles: focussing on improving health and wellbeing, increasing equity among people with different health literacy needs, prioritising, responding to local and changing needs, engaging with stakeholders, focussing on all levels of the health system and creating sustainability (Dodson et al. 2017).

In such an environment, individual health literacy would not be that important in order to lead a long and healthy life. To achieve public health goals, it might be more effective to intervene on the macro and meso levels, which means improving environmental, social and economic conditions and creating health literate responsive (health care) systems.

References

Acheson. (1988). *Public health in England: The report of the committee of inquiry into the future development of the public health function.* London.

The american cancer society. (2018). Cancer Facts & Figures. https://www.cancer.org.

Batterham, R. W., Buchbinder, R., Beauchamp, A., Dodson, S., Elsworth, G. R., & Osborne, R. H. (2014). The OPtimising HEalth LIterAcy (Ophelia) process: Study protocol for using health literacy profiling and community engagement to create and implement health reform. *BMC Public Health, 14*, 694. https://doi.org/10.1186/1471-2458-14-694.

Bäuerle, K., Feicke, J., Scherer, W., Spörhase, U., & Bitzer, E.-M. (2017). Evaluation of a standardized patient education program for inpatient asthma rehabilitation: Impact on patient-reported health outcomes up to one year. *Patient Education and Counseling, 100*(5), 957–965. https://doi.org/10.1016/j.pec.2016.11.023.

Bitzer, E. M., Dierks, M. L., Heine, W., Becker, P., Vogel, H., Beckmann, U., et al. (2009). Teilhabebefähigung und Gesundheitskompetenz in der medizinischen Rehabilitation – Empfehlungen zur Stärkung von Patientenschulungen [Empowerment and health literacy in medical rehabilitation – recommendations for strengthening patient education]. *Die Rehabilitation, 48*(4), 202–210. https://doi.org/10.1055/s-0029-1231060.

Bitzer, E. M., & Sørensen, K. (2018). Gesundheitskompetenz – Health Literacy [Health Literacy]. *Gesundheitswesen, 80*(8–09), 754–766. https://doi.org/10.1055/a-0664-0395.

Bitzer, E. M., & Steurer-Stey, C. (2019). Patientenschulung und Selbstmanagement im Rahmen der Rehabilitation von Erwachsenen mit Asthma. In K. Schultz, H. Buhr-Schinner, K. Vonbank, R. H. Zwick, M. Frey, & M. Puhan (Eds.), *Pneumologische Rehabilitation: Ein Lehr- und Lernbuch für das Reha-Team*. Oberhaching: Dustri-Verlag Dr. Karl Feistle GmbH & Co. KG.

Bundesärztekammer (BÄK), Kassenärztliche Bundesvereinigung (KBV), Arbeitsgemeinschaft der Wissenschaftlichen Medizinischen Fachgesellschaften. (2018). Nationale VersorgungsLeitlinie Asthma – Langfassung. www.asthma.versorgungsleitlinien.de.

Chodosh, J., Morton, S. C., Mojica, W., Maglione, M., Suttorp, M. J., Hilton, L., et al. (2005). Meta-analysis: Chronic disease self-management programs for older adults. *Annals of Internal Medicine, 143*(6), 427. https://doi.org/10.7326/0003-4819-143-6-200509200-00007.

Crellin, E., Mansfield, K. E., Leyrat, C., Nitsch, D., Douglas, I. J., Root, A., et al. (2018). Trimethoprim use for urinary tract infection and risk of adverse outcomes in older patients: Cohort study. *BMJ, 360*, k341. https://doi.org/10.1136/bmj.k341.

Dodson, S., Beauchamp, A., Batterham, R. W., & Osborne, R. H. (2017). Ophelia Toolkit: A step-by-step guide for identifying and responding to health literacy needs within local communities. www.ophelia.net.au.

Dodson, S., Beauchamp, A., Batterham, R. W., & Osborne, R. H. (2018). Informationsheet 1: What is health literacy? Ophelia Toolkit: A step-by-step guide for identifying and responding to health literacy needs within local communities. www.ophelia.net.au.

Faller, H., Reusch, A., Vogel, H., Ehlebracht-König, I., & Petermann, F. (2005). Patientenschulung [Patient education]. *Die Rehabilitation, 44*(5), 277–286. https://doi.org/10.1055/s-2005-866954.

Gaissmaier, W., & Gigerenzer, G. (2008). Statistical illiteracy undermines informed shared decision making. *Zeitschrift Für Evidenz, Fortbildung Und Qualität Im Gesundheitswesen, 102*(7), 411–413. https://doi.org/10.1016/j.zefq.2008.08.013.

Gerhardus, A., Blättner, B., Babitsch, B., Bolte, G., Dierks, Marie Luise, Gusy, B. et al. (2012). Situation und Perspektiven von Public Health in Deutschland – Forschung und Lehre. http://www.deutsche-gesellschaft-public-health.de/fileadmin/user_upload/_temp_/DGPH_-_Public_Health_in_Deutschland.pdf.

German Historical Institute. (2018). Cholera Epidemic in Hamburg (1892). http://ghdi.ghidc.org/sub_image.cfm?image_id=1608.

Gibson, P., Powell, H., Coughlan, J., Wilson, A., Abramson, M., Haywood, A., Walters, E. et al.(2003). Self-management education and regular practitioner review for adults with asthma. *Cochrane Database Syst. Rev.*, CD001117.

Gigerenzer, G., & Wegwarth, O. (2008). Risikoabschätzung in der Medizin am Beispiel der Krebsfrüherkennung. *Zeitschrift Für Evidenz, Fortbildung Und Qualität Im Gesundheitswesen, 102*(9), 513–519. https://doi.org/10.1016/j.zefq.2008.09.008.

Glass, R. I., & Stoll, B. J. (2018). Oral Rehydration Therapy for Diarrheal Diseases: A 50-Year Perspective. *JAMA, 320*(9), 865–866. https://doi.org/10.1001/jama.2018.10963.

Grossman, D. C., Curry, S. J., Owens, D. K., Bibbins-Domingo, K., Caughey, A. B., Davidson, K. W., et al. (2018). Screening for prostate cancer: US preventive services task force recommendation statement. *JAMA, 319*(18), 1901–1913. https://doi.org/10.1001/jama.2018.3710.

Haider, M. R., Qureshi, Z. P., Horner, R., Friedman, D. B., & Bennett, C. (2017). What have patients been hearing from providers since the 2012 USPSTF recommendation against routine prostate cancer screening? *Clinical Genitourinary Cancer, 15*(6), e977–e985. https://doi.org/10.1016/j.clgc.2017.05.002.

Hall, I. J., Rim, S. H., Massetti, G. M., Thomas, C. C., Li, J., & Richardson, L. C. (2017). Prostate-specific antigen screening: An update of physician beliefs and practices. *Preventive Medicine, 103*, 66–69. https://doi.org/10.1016/j.ypmed.2017.08.004.

Henninger, S., Neusser, S., Lorenz, C., & Bitzer, E. M. (2014). Prostatakarzinom in der Routineversorgung: Gesundheitsbezogene Lebensqualität nach stationärer Behandlung [Prostate cancer in routine healthcare: health-related quality of life after inpatient treatment]. *Der Urologe. Ausg. A, 53*(12), 1793–1799. https://doi.org/10.1007/s00120-014-3615-0.

Ilic, D., Neuberger, M. M., Djulbegovic, M., & Dahm, P. (2013). Screening for prostate cancer. *The Cochrane Database of Systematic Reviews.* (1), CD004720. https://doi.org/10.1002/14651858.CD004720.pub3.

Jones, P. W. (2002). Interpreting thresholds for a clinically significant change in health status in asthma and COPD. *European Respiratory Journal, 19*, 398–404.

Jordan, J. E., Buchbinder, R., & Osborne, R. H. (2010). Conceptualising health literacy from the patient perspective. *Patient Education and Counseling, 79*(1), 36–42. https://doi.org/10.1016/j.pec.2009.10.001.

Keller, N., Jenny, M. A., Gigerenzer, G., & Ablin, R. J. (2018). PSA-Screening: Möglicher Nutzen und Schaden. *Deutsches Ärzteblatt, 115*(13), A583–A587.

Kickbusch, I. (2013). *Health Literacy. The Solid Facts.* Geneva: World Health Organization. http://gbv.eblib.com/patron/FullRecord.aspx?p=1582975.

Lamond, E., & Kinyanjui, J. (2012). Cholera outbreak guidelines. https://www.unicef.org/cholera/Annexes/Supporting_Resources/Annex_6B/OXFAM_Cholera_guidelines.pdf.

Moyer, V. A. (2012). Screening for prostate cancer: U.S. Preventive Services Task Force recommendation statement. *Annals of Internal Medicine, 157*(2), 120–134. https://doi.org/10.7326/0003-4819-157-2-201207170-00459.

Nathan, R. A., Sorkness, C. A., Kosinski, M., Schatz, M., Li, J. T., Marcus, P., et al. (2004). Development of the asthma control test: A survey for assessing asthma control. *The Journal of Allergy and Clinical Immunology, 113*(1), 59–65. https://doi.org/10.1016/j. jaci.2003.09.008.

National Heart Lung and Blood Institute (2007). Expert Panel Report 3: Guidelines for the Diagnosis and Management of Asthma Clinical Practice Guidelines National Asthma Education and Prevention Program, Third Expert Panel on the Diagnosis and Management of Asthma. http://www.nhlbi.nih.gov/guidelines/asthma/asthgdln.htm.

Nutbeam, D. (2000). Health literacy as a public health goal: a challenge for contemporary health education and communication strategies into the 21st century. *Health Promotion International, 15*(3), 259–267. https://doi.org/10.1093/heapro/15.3.259.

Osborne, R. H., Batterham, R. W., Elsworth, G. R., Hawkins, M., & Buchbinder, R. (2013). The grounded psychometric development and initial validation of the Health Literacy Questionnaire (HLQ). *BMC Public Health, 13*(1), 658. https://doi.org/10.1186/1471-2458-13-658.

Pickles, K., Carter, S. M., & Rychetnik, L. (2015). Doctors' approaches to PSA testing and overdiagnosis in primary healthcare: A qualitative study. *British Medical Journal Open, 5*(3), e006367. https://doi.org/10.1136/bmjopen-2014-006367.

Quaglio, G., Sørensen, K., Rübig, P., Bertinato, L., Brand, H., Karapiperis, T., et al. (2017). Accelerating the health literacy agenda in Europe. *Health Promotion International, 32*(6), 1074–1080. https://doi.org/10.1093/heapro/daw028.

Resnik, D. B. (2007). Responsibility for health: Personal, social, and environmental. *Journal of Medical Ethics, 33*(8), 444–445. https://doi.org/10.1136/jme.2006.017574.

Robert Koch-Institut (2014a). Asthma bronchiale. Faktenblatt zu GEDA 2012: Ergebnisse der Studie »Gesundheit in Deutschland aktuell 2012«. www.rki.de/geda.

Robert Koch-Institut (2014b). Prostatakrebs (Prostatakarzinom). www.krebsdaten.de.

Schatz, M., Kosinski, M., Yarlas, A., Hanlon, J., Watson, J., & Jhingran, P. (2009). The minimally important difference of the Asthma Control Test. *J. Allergy Clin. Immunol., 124,* 719.

Soellner, R., Huber, S., Lenartz, N., & Rundiger, G. (2010). Facetten der Gesundheitskompetenz – eine Expertenbefragung. Projekt Gesundheitskompetenz. In E. Klieme, D. Leutner, & M. Kenk (Eds.), *Kompetenzmodellierung. Zwischenbilanz des DFG-Schwerpunktprogramms und Perspektiven des Forschungsansatzes* (pp. 104–114). Weinheim: Beltz.

Sørensen, K. (2018). Shifting the Health Literacy Mindset to Enhance People-Centred Health Services. https://health.gov/news/blog/2018/07/shifting-the-health-literacy-mindset-to-enhance-people-centred-health-services.

Sørensen, K., Van den Broucke, Stephan, Fullam, J., Doyle, G., Pelikan, J. M., Slonska, Z., & Brand, H. (2012). Health literacy and public health: A systematic review and integration of definitions and models. *BMC Public Health, 12*(1), 80. https://doi. org/10.1186/1471-2458-12-80.

Warentest, Stiftung. (2015). Mann muss abwägen. *Test, 49*(4), 88–91.

United Nations Economic and Social Commission for Asia and the Pacific (2009). What is Good Governance? https://www.unescap.org/sites/default/files/good-governance.pdf.

Walter, U., Robra, B.-P., & Schwartz, F. W. (2012). Prävention. In F. W. Schwartz, U. Walter, J. Siegrist, P. Kolip, R. Leidl, M. L. Dierks,··· N. Schneider (Eds.), *Public Health* (pp. 196–222). Elsevier. https://doi.org/10.1016/B978-3-437-22261-0.00010-1.

Weingarten, S., Henning, J., Badamgarav, K., Knight, K., & Hasselblad, V. (2002). Interventions used in disease management programmes for patients with chronic illness which one works? Meta-analysis of published reports. *Brit. Med J, 325,* 1–8.

Winkle, S. (1983). Chronologie und Konsequenzen der Hamburger Cholera von 1892. *Hamburger Ärzteblatt, 12.* http://www.collasius.org/WINKLE/04-HTML/hhcholera.htm.

Winkle, S. (1984). Chronologie und Konsequenzen der Hamburger Cholera von 1892. *Hamburger Ärzteblatt, 1.*

World Health Organisation (2018). cholera prevention and control. http://www.who.int/water_sanitation_health/emergencies/cholera-prevention/en/.

World Health Organization Europe (1986). Ottawa Charter of Health Promotion. http://www.euro.who.int/__data/assets/pdf_file/0004/129532/Ottawa_Charter.pdf?ua=1.

Renewing the Conceptual Framework for Health Literacy: The Contribution of Salutogenesis to Tapered the Health Gap

Luis A. Saboga-Nunes, Didier Jourdain and Uwe H. Bittlingmayer

1 Introduction

Health and Health Literacy (HL) have been mostly discussed from the bio-medical pathogenic paradigm. This has had as a consequence serious hindrances to sustainability which is a critical component to human wellbeing. Breaking apart from traditional bio-medical approaches to health, the salutogenic approach was introduced by Aaron Antonovsky (1984). The main contribution of this perspective is that it considers health to be a part of a disease-ease continuum and to be a resource that is dependent on other resources. HL is one of these other resources that has drawn attention, being today considered a valuable standing reserve to humanity. From the stand point of the Sense of Coherence theory, HL is regarded as a Macro Social General Resistance Resource.

L. A. Saboga-Nunes (✉)
Institute of Sociology, Public Health Research Centre, University of Education Freiburg (Germany), Freiburg, Germany
e-mail: luis.saboga-nunes@ph-freiburg.de

D. Jourdain
UNESCO Chair Global Health & Education—WHO Collaborating Centre for Research in Education & Health, Université Clermont Auvergne, Clermont-Ferrand, France
e-mail: didier.jourdan@uca.fr

U. H. Bittlingmayer
Institute of Sociology, University of Education Freiburg (Germany), Freiburg, Germany
e-mail: uwe.bittlingmayer@ph-freiburg.de

2   Health, a Concept in Motion

We consider Health as a concept in motion. After establishing the starting moment for this motion, it is our aim to re-visit the frames of reference and enhance the diversity and richness of human experience. We argue that instead of competition of the fittest (and their natural predatory activity against the less fit), we would have the shared knowledge of the unique human experience in the pursuit of health.

2.1   Health and the Pursuit of Life

Health has been called a basic human right: "The enjoyment of the highest attainable standard of health is one of the fundamental rights of every human being without distinction of race, religion, political belief, economic or social condition". This statement of the *Constitution of the World Health Organization*, stands today as a beacon to the actions that thrive human existence.[1]

During these 70 years a lot has been written and said about what this statement means and its consequences. Although it will not be discussed here in all details, some minutiae of this declaration need to be revisited, as they may constitute prejudice against humans. Without proper consideration, some of these details can set the tone to much entropic (e.g. chaotic) situations of individuals and countries because of the social representations they can embrace.

For instance, the idea of the "right to health" does not imply the right to be protected from diseases (absence of disease or infirmity) and to be in a state of complete physical, mental and social well-being, since this is not achievable. Health depends on many determinants and some of them are not dependent on social interventions or personal choices (see below). Therefore what is at stake is the right for somebody to benefit of the conditions to reach the best possible health (Jourdan 2012). As stated by the UN it is "the right to a standard of living adequate for the health and well-being of himself and of his family, including food, clothing, and housing and medical care and necessary social services." (UN 1948). At the foot of these, are social representations that with a persistent grip can hinder the very basic goals established at the foundation of these organizations.

---

[1]The first meeting of the World Health Assembly took place on 22 July 1946 and on the 7 April 1948, WHO was formed.

2.2   "Without Distinction of Race" and the Persistence Categorization of Racism

Besides the "right to health" (see before) the concept "race" inserted in the previous statement needs to be highlighted in this discussion since it is structural to the health field. The statement quoted above was made at a time when racist views—although commonly accepted—where already under severe scrutiny (UNESCO 1945).[2]

In the discussion about the use of the race concept, we need to go back to the sixteenth century to find the word race connected to the aprioristic division of anatomically modern humans (Homo Sapiens). The modern meaning of this concept emerges with physical anthropology in the mid-nineteenth century, when measuring skulls was supposed to entail different races in the quest for the superior race. Charles Darwin[3] gave this a strong impulse and not that long after, we have (again) extermination of "inferior races" as a civilizational goal for several nations (Darwin, 1871). Slavery, apartheid, the extermination of Abyssinians, Ovaherero and Nama, Armenians, Jews, Tutsis or Yazidis (to name a few) are the land marks of how racism can bring increased levels of entropy (e.g. chaos) to individuals or communities, i.e., to humanity.

We need to wait until the XX century to find a number of scientists, philosophers and humanists to dismantle the long heritage of the sociobiological construction of race. One of them, Claude Lévi-Strauss in his "Race and History" argues in favor of cultural relativism. The prioritization of values, ideas, ways of living, tastes or any other human dispositions, were to be relativized since

---

[2]More than two years before WHO was founded, at the foundation of UNESCO, November 16, 1945, it's constitution already declared that "The great and terrible war which now has ended was made possible by the denial of the democratic principles of the dignity, equality and mutual respect of men, and by the propagation, in their place, through ignorance and prejudice, of the doctrine of the inequality of men and races." (UNESCO 11/16/1945).

[3]In the "The Descent of Man", Darwin wrote: "Man has been studied more carefully than any other animal, and yet there is the greatest possible diversity amongst capable judges whether he should be classed as a single species or race, or as two (Virey), as three (Jacquinot), as four (Kant), five (Blumenbach), six (Buffon), seven (Hunter), eight (Agassiz), eleven (Pickering), fifteen (Bory St. Vincent), sixteen (Desmoulins), twenty-two (Morton), sixty (Crawfurd), or as sixty-three, according to Burke. This diversity of judgment does not prove that the races ought not to be ranked as species, but it shews that they graduate into each other, and that it is hardly possible to discover clear distinctive characters between them" (Darwin 1871).

the culture of the person performing the ranking of cultures/humans would inevitably advocate for his/her own values and ideas.

The concept of frame of reference used by Claude Lévi-Strauss, was a word of caution at a time when each observer had the inclination to use their own culture as a fixed frame of reference, passing over all others cultures (Lévi-Strauss 1952).

Lévi-Strauss proposed that looking at the context of different human expressions not only would relativize those static frames of reference but enhance the diversity and richness of human experience. Instead of competition of the fittest (and their natural predatory activity against the less fit), we would have the shared knowledge of the unique human experience.

Nevertheless, one of the consequences of racism was that the superiority of the technologically most advanced Western societies, increasingly took the lead in the health field also, eliminating elementary forms of answering the needs of humans from the perspective of the origins of health, and replacing this perspective with the origins of disease (pathogenesis). A natural ecology of knowledge (Sousa Santos 2008) distributed among all humans in different settings and latitudes, was smashed by totalitarian views on what is "superior knowledge" that were most of the times concerned with disease and with the utopian perspective of the definition of health proposed at the meeting of WHO (quoted above). Moreover, the association between racism (where certain human groups would consider themselves in a superior condition) and technology, produced a combination that—as a result—is at the basis, with many other negative consequences, of the health gap we have in humanity today. Alienation, ethnocentrism or hyperspecialization are all consequences that indicate what could be the result of this destruction of humanity's health knowledge, made up, as it is, of experiences considered to be obsolete by the superior social trend (to guarantee the survival of the fittest).

As a result, not only most of human social groups saw their frames of references in terms of health, being replaced by dominant monolithic views, but also initiated a process of acculturation and assimilation to the predominant culture, considered to be the most advanced and reliable, this way losing their own frames of reference and rich heritage. This process saw the widening of the health gap. For some this is the natural consequence of the selection of the fittest. For others it is the ground where the battle for human dignity is fought, reviving the vision of establishing the principles and rights of all humans.

Having established this, it is relevant to retrace the line of history and explore the question: *unde venis* (where do we come from), before establishing the vision of *quo vadis* (where are we going from here) regarding the health gap.

2.3   Relativizing the Western Positivist and Negative Construct of Health

What did the founders of WHO have in mind when they defined a human right all its own, called "health"? For the WHO founders health was "not only ... the absence of disease and infirmity, but the state of complete physical, mental and social wellbeing" (WHO 1946).

During the thirty years following the establishment of WHO, the pursuit of the perfect state of health aimed at worldwide expansion. Nevertheless, results fell short of expectations and in 1978, WHO organized the first conference after its foundation, gathering representatives of most nations of the world in Alma Ata (WHO and UNICEF 1978). At this convention, it was stated again that health is a fundamental right. Policy changes, along with the involvement of ordinary people, were considered basic strategies for the safeguarding of this right. Primary health care, as a way of strategic thinking was launched. In the same year, Dr. Halfdan Mahler (Mahler 2010), Director-General of the World Health Organization from 1973–1988, lead the introduction of a fourth dimension (spirituality) to the three previously defined in 1948 (physical, mental and social), concerning the well-being of individuals (WHO 1983). At the same time, he opened the way to other scientific perspectives. Dynamic ideas from different fields led scientists working in various fields to explore new theories and models (see below). New approaches allowed further discoveries about what cures a person or prevents that individual from experiencing disease. In a reaction to the prevailing, biomedical model, George Engel, a medical scientist, proposed a *bio-psychological model* (Engel 1977). This perspective considers relevant psychosocial, not only somatic, factors. The expanded bio-psychological model introduced other pertinent dimensions. Besides the body (*soma*), these dimensions need to be considered with regard to the emergence and development of a disease.

From Alma Ata a snowball of developments has evolved through ten major events that are known today by reference to where they took place: Ottawa (WHO 1986), Adelaide (WHO 1988), Sundsvall (WHO 1991b), Rio de Janeiro (UNCED 1992), Jakarta (WHO 1997), Mexico (WHO 2000), Bangkok (WHO 2005), Nairobi (WHO 2009), Helsinki (WHO 2013) and Shang Hai (WHO 2016). Each of these WHO conferences contributed to the development of public health as a whole, with special emphasis on health promotion. New ideas were proposed in connection with extending the right to health to all inhabitants of the planet. But beneath each of them a prevailing question was persistently lurking: why aren't we getting the "absence of disease and infirmity, (and) the state of complete physical, mental and social well-being", despite all of our best intentions?

2.4   Toward Empowerment

In 1986, a few years after Alma Ata, an international conference promoted by the WHO took place in Ottawa (WHO 1986). It was the First International Conference on Health Promotion. In the Ottawa Charter the focus was given to health, instead of disease, and more specifically to health promotion, which was considered to be "*The process of enabling people to increase control over, and to improve, their health*" (WHO 1986, p. 1).

The Charter set the course for a move towards this new public health dimension by reaffirming social justice and equity as prerequisites for health, and advocacy and mediation as the processes needed for their achievement. With the health promotion proposal, key foundations were laid in the form of the lifestyle concepts. The novelty was that measures to prevent disease were seen as a partnership between specialists (the health practitioners—HPs) and members of the public.

The promotion of health was not a goal, but a means to benefiting from life; and in this context the *socio-ecological model* emerged (Kothari et al. 2007; Bauer et al. 2003). The empowerment concept (Labonte 1993, 1994), was introduced as one of the principles of health promotion but also as a synonym for health promotion itself (Rappaport 1987; Stark 1996). *Empowerment* became the new point of reference in the process of strengthening the competence, responsibility and resourcefulness of persons or groups. Health was considered in a multidimensional way.

2.5   The Public-Health call to fill the Health Gap

In 1988, two years after this conference in Ottawa, the WHO organized a second world conference on health promotion, in Adelaide. The declaration drawn up in Australia considered the value of health and emphasized equity, establishing as a goal that "*by the year 2000 the actual differences in health status between countries and between groups within countries should be reduced by at least 25% by improving the level of health of disadvantaged nations and groups*" (WHO 1991a). Four areas were underlined, involving: 1) support for women's health; 2) working on issues related to food and nutrition; 3) decreasing the use of tobacco and alcohol 4) creating supportive environments. Particularly relevant is the assumption of the relationship between health and socio-economic conditions. For example, those who were poorer also tended to smoke more than those who were well off. Therefore, decreasing this gap by 25% (at least) by the turn of last century, seemed a feasible and appropriate goal in the context of the aims of the WHO.

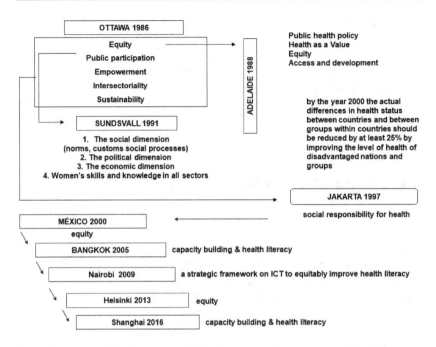

Fig. 1 International Conferences on Health Promotion. (Source: own depiction)

2.6   The Social Dimension of Health

At the Third International Conference on Health Promotion, which took place in Sundsvall, Sweden, in 1991, under the auspices of WHO, specialists looked at four aspects of supportive environments (see fig. 1). The first of these was the social dimension of health; conference delegates considered ways in which norms, customs and social processes affect health (WHO 1991a).

2.7   Health for all

The importance of these environments was emphasized one year after that, in 1992, in Rio de Janeiro (3). The Rio Agenda XXI reads: *"Health ultimately depends on the ability to manage successfully the interaction between the physical, spiritual, biological and economic/social environment"* (UNCED 1992), and established in particular that *"health is for all"* and thus that every person must be involved in the process of achieving it. The ultimate goal is to extend a healthy reality to every human being. Among the objectives, it was proposed that the health and well-being of all urban dwellers must be improved so that they could contribute to economic and social development. The global objective was to *"achieve a 10 to 40 per cent improvement in health indicators by the year 2000"* (UNCED 1992). Once again, the last years of the twentieth century offered a special opportunity for the realization of a better world as far as human health was concerned.

2.8   Health and Social Responsibility

The Fourth International Conference on Health Promotion, entitled *New Players for a New Era*, was held in Jakarta in 1997, focused on promoting social responsibility for health. The conference declaration states, *"Decision-makers must be firmly committed to social responsibility. Both the public and private sectors should promote health by pursuing policies and practices that avoid harming the health of individuals, protect the environment and ensure sustainable use of resources, restrict production of and trade in inherently harmful goods and substances..."* (WHO 1997).

Health promotion is carried out *by* and *with* people, not *on* or *to* people. It improves both the ability of individuals to take action and the capacity of groups, organizations or communities to influence the determinants of health. Improving the capacity of communities to undertake health promotion requires practical education and means empowering individuals' demands by assisting them with more consistent, reliable access to the decision-making process and the skills and knowledge essential to effect change. Both traditional communication and the new information media can support this process.

2.9   Bridging the Equity Gap

In June 2000 the Fifth International Conference on Health Promotion took place in Mexico. It stressed *"Bridging the Equity Gap"*. It also emphasized the view that information and communications technologies (ICT) should play a major role (in terms of efficiency and productivity) in the development of education, information and knowledge (WHO 2000).

2.10   The Call for Capacity Building

The Sixth International Conference on Health Promotion took place in Bangkok in 2005. Among the five required actions for improving the health of individuals, the third emphasized *"building capacity for policy development, leadership, health promotion practice, knowledge transfer and research, and health literacy"* (WHO 2005).

The emphasis on "health literacy" (HL) becomes a critical issue in related health considerations. It is the first time this expression emerges in WHO declarations. According to the WHO, HL *"represents the cognitive and social skills which determine the motivation and ability of individuals to gain access to, understand and use information in ways which promote and maintain good health"*. The definition implies the *"achievement of a level of knowledge, personal skills and confidence to take action to improve personal and community health by changing personal lifestyles and living conditions"* (WHO 1998).

2.11   The Role of Information and Communication Technologies

The seventh Global Conference on Health Promotion organized by the WHO in Africa was held in 2009, in Nairobi. This conference had the motto, *"Call to Action for Closing the Implementation Gap in Health Promotion"*. Its aims were focused on *"...putting people at the centre of care; assure universal access by guaranteeing that health systems provide accessible, appropriate and comprehensive health services for all...that are culturally, linguistically, age, gender and ability appropriate"* (WHO 2009). In order to achieve this, the need to implement innovative approaches is outlined in five conference working documents. In one of them, the conference working document entitled *Health Literacy and Health Promotion: Definitions, Concepts and Examples in the Eastern Mediterranean Region—Individual Empowerment*, Health Literacy is closely linked with health promotion (WHO 2009).

One issue considered in Nairobi is related to the need to implement innovative approaches because of inadequate financial and other resource. One of the suggested innovations is the use of *"information and communication technologies (ICT) by formulating a strategic framework on ICT to equitably improve*

Health Literacy, ... *by building the ICT capacity of health professionals and communities, and maximize* (sic. maximizing) *the use of available ICT tools"* (WHO 2009).

2.12   The Highest Attainable Standard of Health

Interestingly, the first words of the Helsinki declaration (of the 8th Global Conference on Health Promotion, Helsinki, Finland, 10–14 June 2013 (WHO 2013)) under the title *"Building on our heritage, looking to our future"* are *"Affirm our commitment to equity in health"*, followed by exactly the same words that were used at the foundation of the WHO *"(Affirm our commitment to equity in health) and recognize that the enjoyment of the highest attainable standard of health is one of the fundamental rights of every human being without distinction of race, religion, political belief, economic or social condition."*

The emphasis on equity, as the fundamental principle of health promotion, is given a special place when the declaration adds that *"We recognize that governments have a responsibility for the health of their people and that equity in health is an expression of social justice... Likewise, action aimed at promoting equity significantly contributes to health, poverty reduction, social inclusion and security. Health inequities between and within countries are politically, socially and economically unacceptable, as well as unfair and avoidable"* (WHO 2013).

It is extremely relevant today to bring up this topic of the government's responsibility for the health of their people. The state has all resources, but often it is the best-manager of the "best fit" interests, in a power relationship that retrieves resources from the "inferior humans" (those who don't have) to maximize those who have, those whose voices are listen (and who will get even more). Some states become the worst enemy of basic human rights (e.g. to live anywhere). Also, many governments have fallen short of taking the responsibility for the health of their people, and this has been the embryo of the public health problem of re-enforcing state action, that punishes the poor, widening social inequalities. The movements of human and civil rights needed to take into their own hands (e.g. handicapped children) what public health in many circumstances failed to do, i.e., promote inclusive systems. This expresses the tension that persists until today since the Ottawa charter and was again emphasized here in Helsinki.

The Helsinki declaration ends up by "(We) *commit to health and health equity as a political priority by adopting the principles of health in all policies and taking action on the social determinants of health, include communities, social movements and civil society in the development, implementation and monitoring of health in all policies, building Health Literacy in the population*"(WHO 2013). Here, HL is again highlighted shedding the relevance of its principle.

2.13 Health Literacy and Sustainable Development Goals

The last WHO conference to date, was held in Shanghai in 2016 (WHO 2016). Here HL assumes a central role in the overall achievement of the Sustainable Development Goals:

> *"we recognize Health Literacy as a critical determinant of health and invest in its development; develop, implement and monitor intersectoral national and local strategies for strengthening HL in all populations and in all educational settings; increase citizens' control of their own health and its determinants, through harnessing the potential of digital technology; ensure that consumer environments support healthy choices through pricing policies, transparent information and clear labelling. We will promote health through action on all the SDGs"* (WHO 2016).

After WWII, and following the lead taken at Alma Ata, WHO conferences on health promotion have drawn up guidance principles about what the focus ought to be, so that every nation can promote the health of its citizens. Citizen centeredness, primary health care, policy implementation, and the use of ICT are just some of the many areas that have received international consensus.

Since population health is influenced by a complex interplay of determinants (biological, sociocultural, environmental and behavioral factors, and those linked to the healthcare system), this renewed vision of health is not limited to the physical or medical dimensions. One can have an influence on health in two ways:

- Action on the living settings and conditions that influence health (e.g. the physical or social environments, access to appropriate health, social or educational services).
- Individual and population HL in order to give everyone the means (knowledge, attitudes, behaviors and skills) to manage their own health in an autonomous and responsible way, i.e. *conscientização* (Freire 1980), (Jourdan et al. 2020).

3   A Renewed Framework for Health

In this second section we consider the building blocks for a renewed framework for health today. A personal journey of the first author into salutogenesis, as one possible theoretical backbone, is recalled with the intention to make this framework more tangible.

3.1   For a whole Society we need a Sound Theory

One question that needs then to be asked is, why have we not achieved *"not only the absence of disease and infirmity, but the state of complete physical, mental and social wellbeing"*? Two possible answers might emerge: first because we have not followed the correct map (e.g., theoretical approaches that will lead to best practices and results). Another possible answer deals with the very nature of the goal set in 1948, and that is the substance of the definition of *health*.

When considering the broad approach to public health set out in the Ottawa charter, a good theory, which would maximize its potential, was missing. For the *healthy* society there is a need for a theory (Kickbusch 2006). Also, as stated earlier, at conference after conference organized by WHO, there was a sense of goals having been missed. The noble objective of extending health to every single human being was far from being achieved. Health promotion, basically a dynamic process that focuses on peoples' empowerment, in order to facilitate their control over their health (WHO 1986), has been declared a missed opportunity for most of the inhabitants of the world.

But efforts have been put into it and countless researchers have been on the quest for the ways in which health is procured, looking for answers. To exemplify this quest, during these years, theories emerged such as the *locus of control* (Rotter 1966), *self-esteem* (Crandall 1979), Kobasa's *personality hardiness* (Kobasa 1982), *self direction* (Kohn 1983), *stamina* (Thomas 1981), *social interest* (Crandall 1984), Ben-Sira's *potency* (Ben-Sira 1985), *optimism* (Scheier and Carver 1985), *sense of humour* (Lefcourt and Martin 1986), *sense of coherence* (*Antonovsky* 1987), Rosenbaum's *learned resourcefulness* (Rosenbaum 1988), *self-efficacy and human agency* (Bandura 1977) or *resiliency* (Mccubbin et al. 1994).

3.2 Moving on with Theoretical Foundations in Different Disciplines

Super distinguished hygiology and psychopathology (Super 1955). Theories like Maslow's *personality* of third strength (Maslow 1954) or Rogers' concept of *personality of total functioning (Rogers* 1959), Rotter's *social learning* (Rotter 1973), or White's idea of *competence-motivation* (White 1959) later elaborated by (Deci 1975), are just some examples that gave new emphasis to the need to consider a new perspective when searching for "ease/health", pointing out that a new perspective was needed (besides the pathological/pathogenesis paradigm), focusing on health promotion in context.

Khun (1970), used the word *paradigm* to characterize a change in basic assumptions regarding a scientific field (p. 24). It could be said that, in the domain of health, the prevailing paradigm (pathogenesis) was more and more revealing it shortness perspective in the search for health. Along with the pathogenic paradigm that influenced the concept of *disease,* a set of constructs emerged, regarding the *promotion* of *health,* as a major target and not simply as a cure for *disease* or prevention of illness. It was Aaron Antonovsky (of whom more will be said shortly) who would name such a new emerging perspective *salutogenesis,* a composite of two words: *salus* (Latin for "health") and *genesis* (Greek for "origins") (Antonovsky 1979). Various scientific areas contributed to the emergence of this model (including theories from the fields of medicine, sociology and psychology). All these authors do not say the same thing but they share the same theoretical bases of research (Gholson and Barker 1985).

3.3 Racism, Prejudice and Health Creation: Theoretical Framework to Move Forward

This is where the prejudice of racism becomes the starting point for looking deeper into the human condition and health creation. Antonovsky wondered why, after the carnage of concentration camps, the ultimate expression of the survival of the fittest dogma, some were able to get out and re-capture life consistence, while others were not.[4] This view led him to research various deprived groups in

---

[4]It is a closed box the dimension of the arbitrary killings performed during WWII concentration camps, and the rationale behind them. Indeed many of those killed could have had a high sense of coherence but nevertheless were not accounted for, in the carnage that took them away. Research was never able to fully grasp their strength to face such a foe destiny.

society, affected by poverty and marginalization (Antonovsky 1979): Afro-Americans or women who survived Nazi concentration camps (p. 77) during WWII (Antonovsky et al. 1971) (Datan et al. 1981). It was particularly relevant to him that 29% of the women in his study who survived the camps were doing well and considered their health to be in good shape. Despite extreme conditions and terrible stressors, certain individuals could recover and live normal lives as *"stressors are omnipresent in human existence, in fact, the human condition is stressful... given the ubiquity of pathogens—microbiological, chemical, physical, psychological, social and cultural—it seems to me self-evident that everyone should succumb to this bombardment and constantly be dying"* (Antonovsky 1979) (9–13). Organisms have been able to survive in the midst of stressful situations that occur all the time. They are equipped to manage the impact of stressors, defined as *"... a demand made by the internal or external environment of an organism that upsets its homeostasis, restoration of which depends on a non-automatic and not readily available energy-expending action"* (Antonovsky 1979) (72).

The question that Antonovsky poses was, so to speak, born from the prejudice inherent in the race concept. With this source of input Antonovsky set out to design a totally new perspective regarding the prevailing pathogenic paradigm. "How can the human being survive despite these stressors?" Instead of the declaration of the inevitability of the extinction of the "less fit" Antonovsky is another voice that joins the call to consider the inevitability of the human condition, where altruism set the tone for sustainability. The answer lies in the process that is at the heart of the origin of health. Proceeding from here he introduced a new theory of health that led the way to a new perspective (Antonovsky 1984).

3.4 The Quest for a Theory of Health Promotion

Antonovsky was born in the United States in 1923. After serving in the U.S. army in WW II, he obtained his PhD in sociology from Yale University. Aaron Antonovsky became a professor and investigator working with Louis Gutman at the Israel Institute of Applied Social Research, where he immigrated in 1960. He settled in Jerusalem and worked at this Institute in the programme leading to the Master's degree in Public Health, and in the Department of Social Medicine at the Hebrew University of Jerusalem-Hadassah. One of the founders of the medical school at the Ben-Gurion University of the Negev, in 1974, he became Head of the Department of Sociology of Health of the Faculty of Health Sciences. His work was focused on the sociological aspects of health and medicine.

By the end of the 1960's, Antonovsky's role as a leading figure in medical sociology was established when he published several articles on the impact of social class differences in relation to morbidity and mortality. His first major paper, published in 1967 and reprinted countless times throughout the world, emphasizes the important role that social stratification plays in the context of public health (Antonovsky 1967).

He started his quest by posing an unusual research question: *"Why do certain persons suffer less than others?"* From this starting point he caught worldwide attention. From Russia to Scandinavia, he taught frequently at universities, such as the Nordic School of Public Health (where he was awarded an honorary doctorate in 1993) and as a visiting professor in Sweden at the Institute of Child Psychiatry. He also had a permanent influence in Switzerland and in Finland at the department of Social Policy of Turku. As a visiting professor at Berkeley for a year, he started to write his newsletters that linked researchers all over the world and kept them updated about improvements in the new research. Invited to speak in Australia and New Zealand, he had a definitive impact on the WHO Europe meeting organised by Kathyn Dean (Kickbusch 1996).

His very last trip was to Lisbon (Portugal) (Saboga-Nunes 2017), where he was the special guest at the post-graduation series of conferences held at the auditorium of the Faculdade de Medicina de Lisboa, in Santa Maria. That is where the first author heard him for the first time. After the conference, for more than an hour, Prof. Antonovsky took time to personally clarify many of the questions introduced to him.

A special request was answered a few days after Aaron Antonovsky left Lisbon; he sent the first author all his newsletters, among other materials. Most of the details of the progress of his research were discussed. To continue this exchange and go more deeply into the new perspective, a second letter was sent to Aaron Antonovsky with new questions. But in the middle of that year (1994), only a few weeks after the Lisbon conference, he succumbed to myeloid leukaemia.

His sudden departure led to a void. To compensate for this, the first author created the first web site dedicated to salutogenesis, where the ten newsletters were made accessible to researchers, along with the first electronic database on salutogenesis. Special permission from Prof. Antonovsky's wife Helena, who the first author continued to correspond with and receive materials from, helped the first author to establish the seed left Aaron Antonovsky by for the quest for a theory on health promotion.

4 A Renewed Vision of Heath for All

In this third and last section, HL is considered the very core of this renewed vision of heath for ALL. Taking the sense of coherence theoretical foundation, Salutogenesis not only provides a structural answer to the question "why we have not been able to decrease the health gap and health inequalities", but it incorporates the HL perspective in this discussion.

4.1 The Sense of Coherence Construct

For Antonovsky (Saboga-Nunes et al. 2019), looking at *health* (*ease*) and it's the lack of it (*dis-ease*) is not focused on building the perfect health condition (*ease*). While Antonovsky was not looking for a state of total or perfect health (besides the absence of *dis-ease*), he noted that the natural condition of every human being is fighting the chaos of everyday life, managing stressors in a healthy (*ease*) way (Saboga-Nunes 2019).

Life is a negentropic asset; every breath, action and move catalysis order from the chaotic circumstances of everyday life. The basic question is then, "*Why do some people do this better than others?*"

Thus, the point of departure is not the search for what is pathological, with a consequent focus on eliminating that particular "*disease*" from the affected body; it is not the elimination of all states of *diseases* until perfect health is attained. Instead it is the direction towards life (salus), the teleonomic perspective that every being has inscribed in their most basic actions and aspirations.

Antonovsky's salutogenesis perspective (Antonovsky 1979) is built upon the key concept of the *sense of coherence* (SOC) as the center of life control (Antonovsky 1987). This construct proposes answers to the *salutogenesis question*—and is considered to be the motivational basis of any action enacted and attitude held by an individual or a group. The SOC, as a global orientation within the world, perceives it as *comprehensible, manageable* and *meaningful*. It is a central dispositional orientation in the lives of all human beings.

It is in constructing the health dis-ease/ease continuum (Antonovsky 1987) (3) of the Sense of Coherence, that HL emerges as a foundation to what are referred to as the Macro Social General Resistance Resources (Saboga-Nunes 2019).

Antonovsky compared life to a river which he called the river of life. Resources are needed to be in that river. From a pathogenic perspective a bunch of resources are outside the reach of those in the river, making it mandatory to rescue people from the river, whatever the cost. In terms of the salutogenic perspective, it is necessary to learn how to swim (e.g. HL), since people jump into the river of their own free will, and nothing can deter them from doing so. He then referred to the salutogenic approach, writing that

> *"my fundamental philosophical assumption is that the river is the stream of life. No-one walks the shore safely. Moreover, it is clear to me that much of the river is polluted, literally and figuratively. There are forks in the river that lead to gentle streams or to dangerous rapids and whirlpools. My work has been devoted to confronting the question: "Wherever one is in the stream – whose nature is determined by historical, social-cultural, and physical environmental conditions – what shapes one's ability to swim well?"* (Antonovsky 1987) (90).

Today, HL is recognized as one component of the answer to this question, and it is in the context of the Sense of Coherence theory that HL fits in a comprehensive approach, emphatically establishing the holistic perspective.

4.2 From Ethnocentrism to People Centeredness: Dismantling Racism and Launching Health Creation

This brings us to the second component: breaking away from the racist perspective will do much good to the wellbeing of every simple human being, and more particularly, to humanity as a unique entity.

The racist perspective, being ethnocentric, judges all other forms of knowledge as inferior. Nevertheless, taking into account people centeredness (so well highlighted by the WHO declarations above referred), every human being carries a parcel of the puzzle of wellbeing and ease. HL would thus mean the strategic approach to become literate about health and to get the "whole picture". Therefore, the sum of all individual and group HL bits in every latitude—a global integrative scale of learning—will contribute to filling the gaps of the puzzle, towards the completion of patterns of health creation (salutogenesis) (Bauer et al. 2019). That will give us "humanity HL", which by the three dimensions (of the Sense of Coherence), i.e. comprehensibility, manageability and meaningfulness, will embed "ease" as a fundamental right of every human being.

Salutogenesis not only provides a structural answer to the question "why we have not been able to decrease the health gap and health inequalities", but it incorporates the HL perspective that can only thrive and bring good results in a world where no one is above any other one. Finally, this was already foreseen by the WHO. The importance of this perspective is shown by the inclusion of this perspective in the WHO *Health for All* guidelines:

> *Proposed strategies: A **sense of coherence**, where life is experienced as **comprehensible**, **manageable** and **meaningful**, is a great health resource for all people. Health is created if people are confident that life makes sense emotionally, and that they have adequate resources (mental, physical, emotional, social and material) to meet whatever demands are placed on them. As outlined above, this **sense of coherence** must be built up from infancy and childhood through a range of family, kindergarten and health care experiences. Policies that have an immediate effect on young people, as well as on the settings in which they learn, work, live or spend leisure time, should be oriented towards strengthening this sense of coherence (WHO 1999) (28–29).*

5   Conclusion

The aim of this chapter was to define a renewed comprehensive framework for health literacy. The question that was ahead of this exploration was: how to bridge the health gap that is today pervasive? Salutogenesis as a framework for Health Literacy, is considered worthy an investment in this endeavor.

The bio-medical pathogenic perspective has narrowed our views of Health and HL. This has affected sustainability and wellbeing. Aaron Antonovsky helped us break apart from traditional bio-medical approaches with salutogenesis. The disease-ease continuum has drawn attention, and the Sense of Coherence theory, assembles today health literacy as a Macro Social General Resistance Resource.

We may move now from the utopia of the WHO to the utopia of salutogenesis, by the hand of WHO itself. As to the first WHO health utopia definition (in 1948), we know now that it is a dead end, a pit where scores of resources are dumped, but are never enough. This insatiability to achieve "not only the absence of disease and infirmity, …" is surely an eroding utopia. On the other hand, opening up the possibility that the quest for the origins and the creation of health will be leading the way to utopia with the acumen of bits of HL, will make us look at every single human being as a perfect match towards the completion of the puzzle of human wellbeing.

References

Antonovsky, A. (1967). Social class, life expectancy and overall mortality. *The Milbank Memorial Fund Quarterly, 45*(2), 31–73.
Antonovsky, A. (1979). *Health, stress and coping: New perspectives on mental and physical well-being*. Jossey-Bass.

Antonovsky, A. (1984). A call for a new question – salutogenesis - and a proposed answer: the sense of coherence. *Journal of Preventive Psychiatry., 2,* 1–13.

Antonovsky, A. (1987). *Unraveling the mystery of health: How people manage stress and stay well* (1st ed.). The Jossey-Bass health series: Jossey-Bass.

Antonovsky, A., Maoz, B., Dowty, N., & Wijsenbeek, H. (1971). Twenty-five years later: A limited study of the sequelae of the concentration camp experience. *Social Psychiatry and Psychiatric Epidemiology, 6*(4), 186–193.

Bandura, A. (1977). Self-efficacy: Toward a unifying theory of behavioral change. *Psychological Review, 84*(2), 191–215. https://doi.org/10.1037/0033-295X.84.2.191.

Bauer, G. F., Roy, M., Bakibinga, P., Contu, P., Downe, S., Eriksson, M., Espnes, G. A., Jensen, B. B., Juvinya Canal, D., Lindström, B., Mana, A., Mittelmark, M. B., Morgan, A. R., Pelikan, J. M., Saboga-Nunes, L., Sagy, S., Shorey, S., Vaandrager, L., & Vinje, H. F. (2019). Future directions for the concept of salutogenesis: A position article. *Health Promotion International.* Advance online publication. https://doi.org/10.1093/heapro/daz057.

Bauer, G., Davies, J. K., Pelikan, J., Noack, H., Broesskamp, U., & Hill, C. (2003). Advancing a theoretical model for public health and health promotion indicator development: Proposal from the EUHPID consortium. *European Journal of Public Health, 13*(3 Suppl), 107–113. https://doi.org/10.1093/eurpub/13.suppl_1.107.

Ben-Sira, Z. (1985). Potency: A stress-buffering link in the coping-stress-disease relationship. *Social Science and Medicine, 21*(4), 397–406. https://doi.org/10.1016/0277-9536(85)90220-5.

Crandall, J. E. (1984). Social interest as a moderator of life stress. *Journal of Personality and Social Psychology, 47*(1), 164–174. https://doi.org/10.1037/0022-3514.47.1.164.

Crandall, R. (1979). The measurement of self-esteem and related constructs. In J. P. Robinson and P. R. Shaver. Measures of Social Psychological Attitudes. (Rev. ed.) Ann Arbor, MI: Institute for Social Research, The University of Michigan, 1973. 750 pp. *Group and Organization Studies, 4*(1), 122. https://doi.org/10.1177/105960117900400115.

Darwin, C. (1871). *The Descent of Man: And Selection in Relation to Sex.* J. Murray.

Datan, N., Antonovsky, A. & Maoz, B. (1981). *A time to reap: the middle age of women in five Israeli sub-cultures.* John Hopkins University Press.

de Sousa Santos, B. (2008). Volume III: Another Knowledge is Possible: Beyond Northern Epistemologies. *Capital and Class, 32*(2), 166–177. https://doi.org/10.1177/030981680809500117.

Deci, E. L. (1975). *Intrinsic Motivation.* Springer US. https://doi.org/10.1007/978-1-4613-4446-9.

Engel, G. L. (1977). The need for a new medical model: A challenge for biomedicine. *Science, 196*(4286), 129–136. https://doi.org/10.1126/science.847460.

Freire, P. (1980). *Conscientização: teoria e prática da libertação – uma introdução ao pensamento de Paulo Freire* (3. ed). Cortez and Moraes.

Gholson, B., & Barker, P. (1985). Kuhn, Lakatos, and Laudan: Applications in the history of physics and psychology. *The American Psychologist, 40*(7), 755–769. https://doi.org/10.1037/0003-066X.40.7.755.

Jourdan, D., Faucher, C., Cury, P., Lamarre, M.-C., Mebtoul, M., Matelot, D., Diagne, F., & Damus, O. (2020). *Plurality of knowledge to meet the challenges of tomorrow in Humanistic futures of learning. Perspectives from UNESCO Chairs and UNITWIN Network* (UNESCO).

Jourdan, D. (2012). *La santé pubique au service du bien commun?* (Editions de Santé).

Kickbusch, I. (1996). Tribute to Aaron Antonovsky – 'What creates health'. *Health Promotion International, 11*(1), 5–6. https://doi.org/10.1093/heapro/11.1.5.

Kickbusch, I. (2006). The health society: The need for a theory. *Journal of Epidemiology and Community Health, 60*(7), 561.

Kobasa, S. C. (1982). The hardy personality: toward a social psychology of stress and health. *Social Psychology of Health and Illness.*, 3–32.

Kohn, M. L. (1983). *Work and personality*. Modern Sociology: Ablex.

Kothari, A., Edwards, N., Yanicki, S., Hansen-Ketchum, P., & Kennedy, M. A. (2007). Socioecological models: strengthening intervention research in tobacco control. *Drogues, Santé Et Société.*, 6(1 Supplément 3), 1–24. http://www.drogues-sante-societe. org/vol6no1/DSS_v6n1_art11_ang.pdf.

Kuhn, T. S. (1970). *The structure of scientific revolutions* (2nd ed.). University of Chicago Press.

Labonte, R. (1993). Health promotion and empowerment: Practice Framework. *Issues in Health Promotion Series HP-10-0102.* https://www.researchgate.net/publication/246362374_ Health_Promotion_and_Empowerment_Practice_Frameworks.

Labonte, R. (1994). Health promotion and empowerment: Reflections on professional practice. *Health Education Quarterly, 21*(2), 253–268. https://doi. org/10.1177/109019819402100209.

Lefcourt, H. M. & Martin, R. A. (1986). *Humor and Life Stress*. Springer New York. https://doi.org/10.1007/978-1-4612-4900-9.

Lévi-Strauss, C. (1952). *Race and history*. UNESCO. https://archive.org/details/racehistory00levi/page/n63/mode/2up.

Maslow, A. H. (1954). *Motivation and personality*. Harper and Row.

Mccubbin, H. I., Thompson E. A., Thompson, A. I. & Fromer, J. E. (Eds.). (1994). *Sense of coherence and resiliency: Stress, coping and health*. University of Wisconsin Press.

Rappaport, J. (1987). Terms of empowerment/exemplars of prevention: Toward a theory for community psychology. *American Journal of Community Psychology, 15*(2), 121–148. https://doi.org/10.1007/BF00919275.

Rogers, C. R. (1959). *A theory of therapy, personality, and interpersonal relationships, as developed in the client-centered framework. In Koch, S. ed lit. – Psychology: a study of a science.* Mc Graw-Hill.

Rosenbaum, M. (1988). *Learned resourcefulness, stress and self-regulation. In Fisher, S.; Reason, J. ed lit. Handbook of life-stress, cognition and health.* Wiley.

Rotter, J. B. (1966). Generalized expectancies for internal versus external control of reinforcement. *Psychological Monographs: General and Applied, 80*(1), 1–28. https://doi. org/10.1037/h0092976.

Rotter, J. B. (1973). *Social learning and clinical psychology, by Julian B. Rotter. Englewood Cliffs, N.J., Prentice-Hall, 1954.* Johnson Reprint Corp.

Saboga-Nunes, L. (2017). The handbook of salutogenesis: Perspectives on salutogenesis of scholars writing in Portuguese. In M. B. Mittelmark, S. Sagy, M. Eriksson, G. F. Bauer, J. M. Pelikan, B. Lindström, and G. A. Espnes (Eds.), *The Handbook of Salutogenesis: Introduction to the Handbook of Salutogenesis.* https://doi.org/10.1007/978-3-319-04600-6_46.

Saboga-Nunes, L., Bittlingmayer, U. H., & Okan, O. (2019). Salutogenesis and health literacy: The health promotion simplex! In O. Okan, U. Bauer, D. Levin-Zamir, P. Pinheiro, and K. Sørensen (Eds.), *International Handbook of Health Literacy: Research, practice and policy across the lifespan* (pp. 649–664). POLICY Press.

Scheier, M. F., & Carver, C. S. (1985). Optimism, coping, and health: Assessment and implications of generalized outcome expectancies. *Health Psychology, 4*(3), 219–247. https://doi.org/10.1037/0278-6133.4.3.219.

Stark, W. (1996). *Empowerment: Neue Handlungskompetenzen in der psychosozialen Praxis*. Lambertus.

Super, D. E. (1955). Transition: From vocational guidance to counseling psychology. *Journal of Counseling Psychology, 2*(1), 3–9. https://doi.org/10.1037/h0041630.

Thomas, C. B. (1981). Stamina: The thread of human life. *Journal of Chronic Diseases, 34*(2–3), 41–44. https://doi.org/10.1016/0021-9681(81)90049-7.

UNCED. (1992). *Rio Declaration on Environment and Development (1992)*. In London: Graham and Trotman/Martinus Nijhoff.

UNESCO. (1945, November 16). UN Educational, Scientific and Cultural Organisation (UNESCO) - Constitution of the United Nations Educational, Scientific and Cultural Organisation (UNESCO). https://www.refworld.org/docid/3ddb73094.html.

White, R. W. (1959). Motivation reconsidered: The concept of competence. *Psychological Review, 66*, 297–333. https://doi.org/10.1037/h0040934.

WHO. (1946). Constitution of the World Health Organization: International Health Conference, New York 19 June – 22 July 1946. *American Journal of Public Health and the Nations Health, 36*(11), 1315–1323. https://doi.org/10.2105/AJPH.36.11.1315.

WHO (1983). Thirty-sixth World Health Assembly (2-16 May, 1983). In *WHA36/1983/REC/1. WHA 36/1983/REC/2 and WHA 36/1983/REC/3*. 224.

WHO. (1986). Ottawa Charter For Health Promotion. *Health Promotion International, 1*(4), 405. https://doi.org/10.1093/heapro/1.4.405.

WHO (1988). Adelaide recommendations on healthy public policy1988.

WHO (1991a). *Sundsvall statement on supportive environments for health*. World Health Organization. https://apps.who.int/iris/handle/10665/59965.

WHO (1991b). Sundsvall statement on supportive environments for health. https://www.who.int/healthpromotion/conferences/previous/sundsvall/en/.

WHO (1997). *The Jakarta Declaration: On leading health promotion into the 21st century*. World Health Organization. https://apps.who.int/iris/handle/10665/63698.

WHO (1998). *The WHO Health Promotion Glossary* (WHO/HPR/HEP/98.1). https://www.who.int/healthpromotion/about/HPR%20Glossary%201998.pdf?ua=1.

WHO (1999). *Health 21: The health for all policy framework for the WHO European Region. European health for all series, 1012–7356: no. 6*. World Health Organization.

WHO (2000). *Mexico Fifth Global Conference on Health Promotion, Health Promotion: Bridging the Equity Gap*. World Health Organization. www.who.int/healthpromotion/conferences/mexico.pdf.

WHO (2005). *The Bangkok statement on supportive environments for promoting health*. World Health Organization. https://apps.who.int/iris/handle/10665/61542.

WHO (2009). *Nairobi Call to Action - Promoting health and development: closing the implementation gap*. https://www.who.int/oral_health/events/2010_seventh_who_global_conference_health_promotion.pdf.

WHO (2013). The Helsinki statement on Health in All Policies: Framework for Country Action. https://www.who.int/healthpromotion/conferences/8gchp/frameworkandstatement/en/.

WHO (2016). Shanghai declaration on promoting health in the 2030 Agenda for Sustainable Development, Article WHO/NMH/PND/17.5. https://apps.who.int/iris/rest/bitstreams/1090104/retrieve.

WHO & UNICEF (1978). *International Conference on Primary Health Care; World Health Organization; United Nations Children's Fund (UNICEF): Primary health care: Report of the International Conference on Primary Health Care, Alma-Ata, USSR, 6–12 September 1978/ jointly sponsored by the World Health Organization and the United Nations Children's Fund* (Health for all series). World Health Organization, *no. 1.* https://apps.who.int/iris/handle/10665/39228.

Health Literacy in the Education Setting

Implementing Complex Interventions in Childcare Settings: Potentials and Challenges of Creating Screen Media Sensitive Environments for a Healthier Childhood

Hanna E. Schwendemann, Simone Flaig, Lea Kuntz, Anja Stiller, Paula Bleckmann, Thomas Mößle and Eva Maria Bitzer

H. E. Schwendemann (✉) · S. Flaig · L. Kuntz · A. Stiller · E. M. Bitzer
Department of Public Health and Health Education, University of Education Freiburg
(Germany), Freiburg, Germany
e-mail: hanna.schwendemann@ph-freiburg.de

S. Flaig
e-mail: simone.flaig@ph-freiburg.de

L. Kuntz
e-mail: lea.kuntz@ph-freiburg.de

E. M. Bitzer
e-mail: evamaria.bitzer@ph-freiburg.de

P. Bleckmann
Institute of School Pedagogy and Teacher Education, Alanus University of Applied
Science, Alfter, Germany
e-mail: paula.bleckmann@alanus.edu

T. Mößle
Vice Director of the Criminological Research Institute of Lower Saxony,
Hannover, Germany
e-mail: thomas.moessle@kfn.de

1   Introduction

1.1   Growing up in the Digital World

Screen media devices, like television sets, DVD players, video games, computers, smartphones and tablets are omnipresent in children's lives today. Nearly all children grow up in a household with a TV and some type of mobile device (common sense media 2017). International studies report an increase in the amount of time children spent with screen media (Vaala and Hornik 2014). Mobile electronic devices play an increasing role in children's lives, but television is still the dominant medium in families (Paudel et al. 2017). Over 40% of the two to five-year-old children watch on average 43 min television every day (Feierabend et al. 2015). Another study shows that children aged two to four years and five to eight years watch television for more than one hour a day on average. Nearly half of American children watch TV before bedtime, with 42% the TV is "always" or "most of the time" turned on in their home (common sense media 2017). One third of children six years of age and younger have a television in their bedroom (Maniccia et al. 2011). In Germany, nearly every household owns at least one screen media device, but only 5% of the children between two to five years of age have a television in their bedroom. Daily usage times and bedroom screen media equipment increase substantially during the kindergarten and elementary school years (Feierabend et al. 2013; Mößle 2012).

Screen media usage results in an enormous amount of sedentary behaviour and is related to health and developmental risks (Reid Chassiakos et al. 2016). Population based studies show associations between early childhood viewing and cognitive, language and social/emotional delays (Reid Chassiakos et al. 2016), like poor school performance (Acevedo-Polakovich et al. 2007; Ferguson 2011; Mößle et al. 2010; Nunez-Smith et al. 2008), antisocial behaviour (Robertson et al. 2013), attention problems (Christakis and Zimmerman 2007; Gentile et al. 2012; Nunez-Smith et al. 2008) and further neurological changes (Sigman 2017). Higher use of screen media results in an increased risk for obesity/adiposity (Bener et al. 2011; Nunez-Smith et al. 2008; Staiano et al. 2013), low sleep quality (Cain and Gradisar 2010; Marino et al. 2016) and addictive use (Rehbein et al. 2013). In addition, studies have shown that low socio-economic status is related to higher and, in the long run, more problematic screen media use, which in turn leads to an increase of negative outcomes (Coombs et al. 2013; Schmidt et al. 2012). Children from lower income households spend more time with screen media than children in higher income families (common sense media 2017).

Problematic screen media use is described as a major public health issue and requires primary prevention efforts (Christakis et al. 2013; Sigman 2017). Health departments, practitioners and experts recommend that children under the age of three should not be using screen media at all, for children in kindergarten a maximum of half an hour per day is recommended (Bitzer et al. 2014; Strasburger 2010; Vaala and Hornik 2014).

2 Guiding Children in the Digital World

Children learn and master health literacy related skills through their social environment (Borzekowski 2009). In the family as the primary social environment parents are central mediators of children's media use with an influence on bedroom screen media equipment, usage times and exposure to age-inadequate media content (Bleckmann and Mößle 2014; Mößle 2012; Vandewater et al. 2005). Parental media education attitudes influence the home environment and media education of the child, e.g. positive parental attitudes towards media are a significant predictor of the time children watch TV. If the parents believe that using screen media has a positive effect on their children's development, they may further encourage their use (Lauricella et al. 2015).

Besides the family, child care settings, such as kindergartens and grade schools, are also important bases of socialization and play an important role in limiting screen time, because nearly every child at the age of three years and older, independent of their background, is enrolled there. They spend many hours in care and the institutions provide the opportunities for pre-schoolers to learn and adopt healthy behaviours (Kobel et al. 2017; Vanderloo 2014; Yilmaz et al. 2015). Research indicates that a negative association exists between screen-viewing in children and levels of staff education; that is, children in day care with higher educated teachers watch less TV than children in day care with lower educated staff (Vanderloo 2014).

Current models of eHealth literacy focus on skills to master digital media to support health (Kayser et al. 2015; Norman and Skinner 2006). However, they are too narrow to serve as a theoretical model in designing and evaluating an intervention to prevent problematic screen media use in children. We consider an age-appropriate use of digital media to be a special case of general health literacy and propose the term Digital Balance Literacy for children in settings. On the first level Digital Balance Literacy addresses informed decision-making, where eHealth chances and eHealth risks are carefully weighed depending on the age of the user and other situational variables. On the second level, it incorporates both use-oriented and reduction-oriented eHealth Literacy skills.

To guide children in the digital world and help them grow up healthy, parents and teachers must acquire the skills needed for this demanding task. Preventive programs addressing problematic screen media use may be helpful to teach these skills. There are only a few evaluated prevention programs addressing the prevention of problematic screen media use and most of these programs aim specifically at screen time reduction as a measure for increasing physical activity (Altenburg, Kist-van Holthe and Chinapaw 2016; Friedrich et al. 2014; Marsh et al. 2014). In general, there are only a few interventions in Germany regarding screen media that are scientifically monitored. These programs are either school-based (Möller et al. 2012; Schultze-Krumbholz et al. 2014); or combine different settings (Fachstelle für Suchtprävention der Drogenhilfe Köln 2014; Müller et al. 2012). Regarding other countries most of the preventive programs are school-based as well (Friedrich et al. 2014; Maniccia et al. 2011; Schmidt et al. 2012). Only some programs combine different settings and then most frequently parents are involved (Altenburg et al. 2016; Wahi et al. 2011). There are fewer studies on the effects in younger age groups (Friedrich et al. 2014; Maniccia et al. 2011; Schmidt et al. 2012; Wahi et al. 2011), despite ever younger age groups devoting increasingly more portions of their time to screen media (Feierabend et al. 2013; Feierabend and Klingler 2000; Njoroge et al. 2013). But, in line with the Digital Balance Literacy model, it is necessary to involve not only the children in the intervention, but also the parents and educational institutions. Thus, a multi-setting approach provides the opportunity to sustainably learn and adopt healthy behaviours in childhood.

MEDIA PROTECT aims to support screen media sensitive environments in the home and the childcare setting. It was renamed in 2017 as "ECHT DABEI— gesund groß werden im digitalen Zeitalter/REALLY PRESENT—growing up healthy in the digital age" (BKK Dachverband e. V. 2017)). It is a program to sustainably prevent children's problematic and, in the long run, addictive use of screen media in a multi-setting approach through targeting parents, children and teachers (Bleckmann et al. 2014; Stiller et al. 2018). At the core of the intervention are MEDIA PROTECT coaches, specially trained professionals of pedagogical and therapeutic fields. The overall objective is to empower teachers to prevent unhealthy screen media use and promote active, age-adequate and accompanied media use in the family and the childcare setting through their daily work with parents and children. Apart from information about problematic screen media use and strategies to guide parents, the staff develops a "screen-free leisure time map" of locations addressing the parents and their children (e.g., playgrounds).

Furthermore, there is an optional program component with hands-on support for installing child protection software for limiting online time and content (technical support evening). For the children, an interactive stage play is part of the intervention. Pedagogical staff can refer to the play afterwards and use parts of it like the songs and the movement games in their daily work with the children (for more details see Stiller et al. 2018).

The aim of this this chapter is to describe practical experiences gained while implementing MEDIA PROTECT in child care settings. We analyse the structural prerequisites of child care settings for the willingness to participate in an evaluation study to evaluate the MEDIA PROTECT intervention on guiding children in the digital world. Furthermore, we describe the sociodemographic characteristics of the target group reached. One part of this description addresses the children's bedroom screen media equipment and screen time. We examine the parents' perceived need for media education support to analyse a need for prevention in the target group. Based on Prochaska's transtheoretical model of behavioural change (Prochaska and Velicer 1997), we assume that parents are a heterogeneous group in different stages of behavioural change. Some of the parents might not feel that something must be changed (precontemplation, purposelessness), other parents might perceive a need to change their behaviour and some have possibly already been trying to change it (contemplation, preparation). We therefore describe the different stages of the target group reached. We conclude afterwards whether we were able reach the planned target group.

3 Methods

3.1 Design and Recruitment Process

In a cluster-controlled trial to analyse the effectiveness of MEDIA PROTECT, we recruited child care settings in two regions of Germany, namely Hanover (Lower Saxony) and Lörrach (Baden-Württemberg). We recruited parents of four-to-seven-year-old children attending child day care (kindergarten) or elementary school located in areas with a special need in the social field (e.g. low income, high percentage of ethnic minorities). Between August and November 2015, kindergartens and schools were contacted by telephone to motivate them to participate in the study. We gained a positive ethical approval by the Ethic Commission of the State Chamber of Physicians Baden-Württemberg (No. F2015-107). The study is registered in the German Clinical Trial Register (DRKS00010608).

3.2   Data Collection

3.2.1 Childcare Settings

During the recruiting process, we asked the kindergarten managers who refused participation in the intervention study for their reasons. We documented the answers of the kindergarten managers in a short description for both regions, Hanover and Lörrach. These text documents are the basis for the analysis of the reasons for non-participation in the study.

We documented the structural characteristics of every childcare setting in both regions as to their location, sponsorship, the migration background of the children in care, total number of children and group size.

3.2.2 Parents

In the evaluation study carried out in the successfully recruited educational institutions, a written questionnaire for parents was used. To assess children's screen time we used items from the study on health of children and adolescents in Germany (KiGGS) that record screen time during the week and on weekends (Robert Koch-Institut 2003). *Sample question: "How long does your child watch TV/ DVD during the week?"*. The answers ranged on a Likert-Scale from 1 = "never", 2 = "30 min per day", 3 = "1 to 2 h per day", 4 = "3 to 4 h per day", to 5 = "more than 4 h per day". We calculated a weekly screen media time index (WSMTI) (separate for TV and PC) with weighted averages as follows: The screen time during the week was multiplied by five and the screen time on weekend was multiplied by two. Afterwards the two products were added up and divided by seven (Mößle 2012).[1] The WSMTI ranges from 1 = "never" to 5 = "more than 4 h per day", values lower than or equal to two correspond to expert recommended maximum daily screen time (Bitzer et al. 2014). We dichotomized screen media usage time into 1 = "recommended daily screen media use time" and 2 = "more than the recommended screen media use time".

Children's bedroom screen equipment, parental media education and perceived need for support was measured via the parent questionnaire, developed and validated in the Berlin longitudinal study of media (Mößle 2012) and adapted through ideas of (Knop et al. 2015; Wagner and Eggert 2013). It assesses the use of media, media equipment, parental educational and media educational

---

[1]Example: 30 min per day during the week (=2) and 1 to 2 h per day on weekends (=3)=((5 x 2)+(2 x 3))/ 7=2,3. This corresponds to 3 (1 to 2 h per day).

behaviour. *Sample question: "Does your child have one of the following electronic devices in its room?"*.

We documented the parental satisfaction with their own media education with the item *"If you look at your children's media education, how satisfied are you with your parenting?"*. The answers ranged on a Likert Scale from 1 = "strongly satisfied" to 4 = "not satisfied at all". Furthermore, we asked the parents for their intention to change their media education throughout the next weeks or months and they could answer from 0 = "I don't have this intention at all" to 5 = "I strongly intend to do so."

We asked for the parental willingness to change their own media education with a single item: *"Do you want to change something about your media parenting style?"*. The answers ranged from 1 = "I am content and don't need to change s.th.", 2 = "I suppose I have my weaknesses, but there is nothing that I need to change"; 3 = "I thought about making changes before but I never went through with it", 4 = "I am working on changing my media education" to 5 = "I have changed my media education already and I want to stick to it".

Furthermore, we asked the parents about topics on which they would like to learn more with a multiple answers kit of 10 items (a. o. screen media effects on the development of children, filter and time limiting software, recommendations concerning TV programs).

3.3   Statistical Analysis

3.3.1 Child Care Settings

We modelled the propensity to participate in the study and to participate in the intervention on kindergarten level, using logistic regression models, regarding structural characteristics (location, sponsorship, migration background, total number of children and group size).

For the analysis of the non-participation by the kindergarten management, categories were developed inductively, as the answers were analysed by one rater. To ensure coherence, an independent rater coded all answers using the given categories. Cohen's Kappa was determined and used to denote consistency with a rating of >0.6 being considered substantial (Viera and Garrett 2005). Interrater agreement ranged from moderate ($\kappa = .573$ for Hanover) to almost perfect ($\kappa = .881$ for Lörrach) prior to correcting discrepant items. Every unmatched category was discussed among the independent raters until common agreement was achieved.

3.3.2 Parents

We calculated frequencies and descriptive statistics for screen time and bedroom screen media equipment separately for the IG and CG and the parents' perceived need for support. We tested the children's screen media equipment and the usage time between IG and CG by calculating chi-square tests. We used SPSS (version 24) for the analysis.

4   Results

4.1   The Willingness to Participate in the Study from the Child Care Settings

4.1.1 Structural Characteristics

Overall n = 254 child care settings in both regions were identified based on our inclusion criteria. We contacted n = 169 kindergartens and n = 39 elementary schools after institutional approval. Of the total contacted child care settings, n = 49 kindergartens and n = 9 elementary schools (with a total of n = 140 groups/ classes) agreed to participate (see Table 1). More kindergartens in Hanover agreed to participate in the study (recruitment rate in Hanover was 42.4% and in Lörrach 21.8%). For elementary schools, the recruitment rate was 10.3% for Hanover and 38.5% for Lörrach (Table 1).

The participating kindergartens are 30.6% church-run, 34.7% municipal and 34.7% independently operated. In Hanover most of the kindergartens are independent (56,0%) while in Lörrach they are predominantly church-run (45,8%) or municipal (41,7%; p = .004). The elementary schools are all in public

Table 1 Identification und recruitment of institutions. (Source: own depiction)

Region	Institutions identified (n)	Organisations approving (n)	Kindergartens contacted (n)	Schools contacted (n)	Kindergartens recruited (n)	Schools recruited (n)
Hanover	105	66	59	26	25 11 (CG) 14 (IG)	4 3 (CG) 1 (IG)
Lörrach	149	93	110	13	24 13 (CG) 11 (IG)	5 1 (CG) 4 (IG)

CG = control group; IG = intervention group

sponsorship. In nearly 50% of the participating kindergartens and one third of the participating elementary schools more than 35% of the children have a migration background. However, in Hanover significantly more institutions have a high percentage of children with a migration background (more than 35%) in their care: 65.0% in Hanover as compared to 24.1% in Lörrach (p = .002). The average number of children per kindergarten was n = 64, organized in three age groups. The elementary schools are attended by an average of n = 243 children within ten forms. There is no further significant difference between both regions in the structural characteristics except for the migration background and the sponsorship in kindergartens (see Table 2).

1) From 3 of the recruited schools there are no data about the migration background of the children.
2) From 2 of the recruited schools of the IG there are no data about the migration background of the children.

From a multivariate perspective, the location Lörrach reduces the kindergartens' willingness to participate by OR = 0.35 (95% CI 0.18 to 0.70; p = 0.003).

Table 2 Structural characteristics of kindergartens and elementary schools (n = 58). (Source: own depiction)

Characteristic	Forms	Recruited kindergartens (n = 49)	IG kindergartens (n = 25)	Recruited schools (n = 9)	IG schools (n = 5)
Region	Hanover	25 (51.0%)	11 (45.8%)	4 (44.4%)	1 (20.0%)
	Lörrach	24 (49.0%)	13 (54.2%)	5 (55.6%)	4 (80.0%)
Operated by	Church	15 (30.6%)	8 (33.3%)		
	Municipality	17 (34.7%)	9 (37.5%)		
	Independent	17 (34.7%)	7 (29.2%)		
	Public			9 (100.0%)	5 (100.0%)
Migration background	≥35%	23 (46.9%)	11 (45.8%)	3 (33.3%)1	1 (20.0%)[2]
Number of children	M (SD)	63.5 (21.9)	62.7 (23.5)	242.8 (71.6)	213.0 (66.1)
Number of groups/classes	M (SD)	3.0 (1.1)	3.0 (1.0)	11.3 (3.4)	9.6 (2.9)

M = mean; SD = standard deviation

None of the other structural characteristics considered are significant predictors of the willingness to participate in the study (see Table 3). The institutions decided whether to take part in the control or intervention group. N = 25 (51%) kindergartens preferred to participate in the intervention group (see Table 1). The structural characteristics of the kindergartens in both groups are very similar (see Table 2). We found no evidence for confounding, none of the available structural variables (region, sponsorship, migration background, number of children and number of groups) proved to be an independent statistically significant predictor on the decision to participate in the intervention.

4.1.2 Reasons for Non-Participation

Overall, 63 kindergarten managers out of 120 (52.5%) provided information on their reasons for not participating in the study.

In total, four categories for non-participation of the kindergartens were identified: lack of time, staff shortage, no interest in the subject and difficult cooperation with parents. The most common reason for non-participation in the study was "lack of time" (46.0%; Table 4) but with substantial differences by region. Nearly two thirds of the kindergarten managers in Hanover mentioned

Table 3 Willingness to participate in the study (logistic regression, kindergartens only n = 169). (Source: own depiction)

Variable	ß	OR	95% CI		P
Location Lörrach (reference Hanover)	−1.04	0.35	0.18	0.70	.003
Constant	−0.24	0.79			.36
Model statistic		AUC	.62	Nagelkerke R^2	.07	

ß = regression coefficient; OR = Odds Ratio; 95% CI = 95% confidence interval; p < .05; AUC = Area under the curve

Table 4 Generated categories and their frequency of occurrence. (Source: own depiction)

	Hanover (n = 27)	Lörrach (n = 36)	Total (n = 63)
	% (n)	% (n)	% (n)
Lack of time	63.0 (17)	33.3 (12)	46.0 (29)
Staff shortage	14.8 (4)	33.3 (12)	25.4 (16)
No interest in the subject	7.4 (2)	27.8 (10)	19.1 (12)
Difficult cooperation with parents	14.8 (4)	5.6 (2)	9.5 (6)

"lack of time" compared to only one third of the kindergarten managers in Lörrach (63.0% vs. 33.3%). Overall, a quarter mentioned "staff shortage" as the main reason for non-participation in the study, more pronounced in Lörrach than in Hanover (33,3% vs. 14.8%). Every fifth institution was not interested in the subject "prevention of problematic screen media use" (19.1%) with large differences between Hanover and Lörrach, with kindergarten managers in Lörrach being far less interested in this topic than their colleagues in Hanover (7.4% vs. 27,8%), Only one in ten kindergarten managers felt difficulties in cooperation with parents to be the main reason for not participating in the study.

4.2   Parents

4.2.1 Who Participates in the Parental Survey?
We distributed n = 2.241 questionnaires in the participating institutions in both regions, with n = 395 parents in the IG and n = 361 parents in the CG participating in the baseline survey (response rate of 33,7%.) We excluded a total of n = 64 children due to age: n = 10 children due to missing age information, n = 5 children who were three years and younger and n = 49 children who were older than seven years.

Table 5 shows the sociodemographic characteristics of IG and CG in the baseline survey. The participating parents in the IG were 1.4 years older than the parents of the CG (38.1 vs. 36.7 years; p = .002). In addition, children in the IG were a slightly older than children in the CG (M_{IG} = 6.0 vs. M_{CG} = 5.7; p = .00). Compared to the CG, we see fewer single parents in the IG (13.6% vs. 5.6%; p = .015). There were no statistically significant differences between IG and CG regarding the children's or the respondent parents' sexes, length of day care (full-day or half-day), parental occupational status, or migration background.

4.2.2 Screen Media Equipment and Use Times
At baseline, 42.7% of the children in the target group owned or had access to at least one screen media tool, with tablet computers (37.0%) the most important and game consoles (5.6%) the least important devices. 56.6% of the children in our sample watched TV more than 30 min per day and 15.4% of the children used the computer more than 30 min daily.

Table 6 shows the number of our survey participants complying with the recommendations on screen media usage time ($\leq$ 30 min/day), and the screen media equipment rate, by study group and by children's age. There was a significant difference regarding daily TV time, with more children in the IG than

Table 5 Sociodemographic characteristics of study participants at baseline (n = 756). (Source: own depiction)

	IG (n = 395)			CG (n = 361)			
	N	Mean	SD	N	Mean	SD	p
Parental age	388	38.1	6.4	353	36.7	5.9	.002
Children's age	395	6.0	0.8	361	5.7	0.9	.000
	N valid	n	%	N valid	n	%	
Parental sex = female	390	334	85.6	356	311	87.4	n.s.
Children's sex = female	395	199	50.5	360	164	45.6	n.s.
Children in full-day care	393	149	37.9	354	138	39.0	n.s.
Parental occupational status[a]	395			361			n.s.
Employed		385	97.5		350	97.0	
Unemployed		8	2.0		8	2.2	
Not employed		2	0.5		3	0.8	
Migration background[b]	387	91	23.0	348	95	26.3	n.s.
Single parent	374	21	5.6	337	46	13.6	.000

[a] Employed = at least one parent was employed; unemployed = one parent was unemployed and one parent was not employed or unemployed, too; not employed = both parents were not employed, [b](Schenk et al. 2006), IG = intervention group, CG = control group

in the CG complying with daily TV-screen time recommendations (45.7% vs. 38.0%, p = 0.035). There were no substantial or statistically significant differences between IG and CG in daily PC usage time, screen media equipment ownership or screen media access.

In both groups, we see a statistically significant association between the children's age and the number of electronic devices. Older children owned or had access to at least one screen media device more frequently compared with younger children. Older age is associated with lower rates of children watching less than 30 min TV or computer per day, however, this is not consistently seen in both groups.

Table 6 Usage times and screen media equipment in MEDIA PROTECT study partici-pants (n = 756). (Source: own depiction)

		Total		Age groups (%)				
		N	%	4 years	5 years	6 years	7 years	p
Daily TV time	IG	175	45.7	21,4	50,0	49,4	40.5	n.s.
(≤30 min)	CG	135	38.0	48.6	39.8	41.6	22.5	.019
Daily computer time	IG	322	84.5	78.6	82.6	90.7	78.3	.032
(≤30 min)	CG	295	84.8	86.5	90.1	83.2	77.5	n.s.
Owns or has access to at least one	IG	184	46.6	28.6	50.0	40.2	54.8	.039
Electronic device	CG	139	38.5	21.6	34.4	42.1	47.9	.033

IG = intervention group, CG = control group

Screen media ownership and access was higher in children with migration background (p = .00), as were the reported TV and computer times (p = .00, results not presented) compared to children without migration background.

4.2.3 Parents' Perceived Need for Media Education Support

At baseline more than one third of the parents (38.9%) are satisfied with their media education and 39.4% of the parents did not want to change their media education principles during the next few weeks. Dissatisfaction was low (5.6%) and about a fifth of the participating parents (21.4%) wanted to or were about to change their media education behaviour at baseline. These differences are statistically significant (see Table 7). Satisfaction with media education behaviour and the perceived need to change media education is significantly associated with the actual media exposition of the children. Nearly every second parent whose child owns no screen media feels no need to change media education behaviour (45.0%) compared to only one in four parents whose children own two or more screen media devices (27.7%; p = .005; see Table 7). More parents whose children own two or more screen media devices think about changing something, but never did so, compared to parents whose children have less than two screen media devices.

We asked the parents what interests they had regarding media education (see Fig. 1). The parents were most interested to learn about how to prevent exposure of their child to problematic screen media content. The parents expressed a slightly lower interest in screen media equipment, and screen media usage time was considered less important, but still 75% of the parents are interested in this topic.

Table 7 Parental satisfaction with media education and willingness of the parents to change media education in relation to bedroom screen media equipment. (Source: own depiction)

	Total Sample	Screen media equipment			
		0	1	≥ 2	p
Parental satisfaction with media education	(n = 737)	(n = 423)	(n = 209)	(n = 105)	**.001**
Satisfied	38.9%	43.7%	33.0%	31.4%	
Rather satisfied	55.5%	53.2%	59.3%	57.1%	
(Rather) dissatisfied	5.6%	3.1%	7.7%	11.4%	
Parental willingness to change media education	(n = 724)	(n = 416)	(n = 207)	(n = 101)	**.005**
I do not need to change	39.4%	45.0%	33.8%	27.7%	
There are weaknesses, But I feel no need to change	36.9%	33.9%	40.6%	41.6%	
I thought about changing something, but never did	12.7%	12.7%	10.9%	16.8%	
I'm working on changes	8.7%	6.0%	12.1%	12.9%	
I have changed something	2.3%	2.4%	2.9%	1.0%	

5   Discussion

MEDIA PROTECT is an intervention for children between four and seven years of age to both prevent problematic screen media use and promote age-adequate, active and accompanied media use. The intervention pursues a multi-setting approach and addresses teachers in kindergartens and elementary schools as well as parents and their children (Bleckmann et al. 2014; Stiller et al. 2018). It is a setting-oriented intervention to change kindergartens and elementary schools into screen media-sensitive environments. The intervention shows teachers ways to

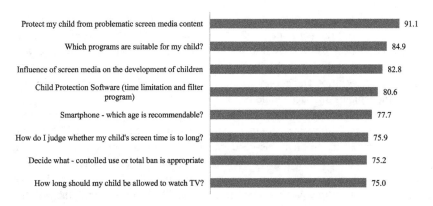

Fig. 1 Parental interests in media education (N = 762, % important, multiple answers possible). (Source: own depiction)

promote an age-adequate use of screen media in the family, provides direct guidance for parents and fosters healthy leisure time activities for children.

In this chapter, we analysed structural characteristics of the participating kindergartens and elementary schools to identify prerequisites for a nationwide implementation of MEDIA PROTECT. Despite the lack of randomisation, the influence of structural characteristics on the decision to participate in the study is small. Only the rural location has an influence on the willingness to participate. There is no significant influence on the decision to participate in the intervention group. The kindergartens and schools did or did not decide to participate in the intervention because of their individual schedules. But the recruitment of kindergartens was challenging and hindered by institutional lack of time and staff shortages. Other studies report these challenges as well. Kobel et al. (2017) suspects the reason might be that kindergartens in Germany already take part in some programmes, like health promotion, language support or dental prevention. They had the same experiences when recruiting kindergartens, that constant staff shortages make it difficult for the institutions to take part in interventions and are reluctant to agree to any further work (Kobel et al. 2017). During the recruitment process of the MEDIA PROTECT intervention, additionally the kindergartens were experiencing challenges because of the high proportion of refugee children who had to be integrated into the kindergartens, and therefore lack of staff was very common (UNHCR - The UN Refugee Agency 2016). However, it was still possible to recruit 49 kindergartens to participate in the study. For a nationwide implementation we must ensure that even rural areas are reached and the importance of the topic "problematic screen media use" has to be stressed. Moreover, an open communication with the participants about what they have to expect is essential, e.g. the teachers need to be fully informed beforehand how much time the intervention will take (Kobel et al. 2017). We informed the childcare managers about the time the intervention and survey would take by mail and in the telephone contact. In further studies this fact should be more stressed.

Considering the response rate of just under 30% among participating parents, it wasn't easy to motivate parents to participate in the MEDIA PROTECT evaluation study. This problem has been much discussed in connection with health promotion strategies. Especially socially disadvantaged parents are difficult to motivate to participate in health promotion strategies. The setting approach is the best practice to attract parents (Hurrelmann et al. 2013). In this light, the MEDIA PROTECT components which empower kindergarten staff to integrate media education issues in their regular meetings with individual parents seem promising and could be strengthened in an improved future version of the program.

Nearly half of the children owned or had access to at least one screen media device in the target group reached. The increased number of children who had access to tablet PCs, while most of them did not personally own the device shows that the established risk factor "screen media bedroom equipment" will soon no longer be suitable for assessing children's access to screen media. Especially portable screen media devices like smartphones and tablet PCs are gaining in importance (Paudel et al. 2017; Statistisches Bundesamt [Destatis] 2017). They are replacing stationary devices, which is supported by the low number of game consoles owned by the children in our sample. In our sample more than half of the children watched TV more than the recommended half an hour per day. We found only minor statistically significant differences in the sociodemographic characteristics and in the screen media usage times between IG and CG.

Parents are central mediators of children's media use with an influence on bedroom media equipment and screen usage time. Nearly four in ten parents in our sample were satisfied with their media education. Only a fifth of the parents wanted to or were about to change their media education behaviour at baseline. The parents whose children owned or had access to two or more screen media devices were more likely to be dissatisfied with their media education behaviour but less likely to perceive a need for change. This is a very encouraging finding. According to research in "parental mediation of children's media use", there might also have been a group of parents whose children display a mildly or highly problematic screen media use while the parents show hardly any problem awareness. This combination could have been expected for the "social co-viewing" (Valkenburg et al. 1999) or the "laissez-faire/unlimited use" (Barkin et al. 2006) style of parental mediation. There is a small group of parents in the German sample who fit into this problematic pattern: Their children have access to screen media and they did not state any dissatisfaction with their media education behaviour or perceive a need for change. So possibly, the prevalence of the different parental mediation styles differs between Germany and the countries the classifications were derived from. For achieving changes in behaviour, the higher problem awareness among parents with more problematic media education in the family is of course very good news. We assume that apart from the small group of "laissez-faire" parents, other parents whose children had high screen media use time, and diverse items of screen media equipment, were aware of the problems, but they need and ask for support in their media education.

Parents stated a high interest in providing appropriate media content for children and avoiding inappropriate content, whereas screen media bedroom equipment and recommended screen media usage times were less relevant. This might be explained by the hypothesis that parents who tend to use screen media for "babysitting" purposes would need to have their children spend a substantial amount of TIME with screen media. Or parents might not be able or willing to enforce time limits. In order not to feel guilty about either of these practices, the claim that "I make sure my child uses only age-adequate or even educationally valuable content" would serve as a functional rationalization strategy. This has been identified as a common pattern among parents of elementary school children in Germany. Media education is often not so much based on knowledge and theory but evolves in the practice of (stressful) daily family life. Parents find it helpful to justify the practice ex post (Seidel 2013). However, we want to emphasise that three quarter of the participating parents judge that all media education items are important and want to learn more about these contents. These findings stress the need for prevention in the target group.

To implement complex health-related interventions in child care settings it is necessary to inform the participating institutions about the urgency of addressing the issue at hand in their daily work, in this case the topic of media education. Furthermore, it is relevant to focus on the important issues in the intervention for educational staff and to inform all educational staff, and not just the kindergarten and school managers, about the effort required for participating in the intervention well beforehand. A multi-setting approach, though, as we have pointed out, it is not without its obstacles, still appears to be the best way to an environment where children and their parents learn eHealth Literacy skills.

References

Acevedo-Polakovich, I. D., Lorch, E. P., & Milich, R. (2007). Comparing television use and reading in children with ADHD and non-referred children across two age groups. *Media Psychology, 9*(2), 447–472.

Altenburg, T. M., Kist-van Holthe, J., & Chinapaw, M. J. M. (2016). Effectiveness of intervention strategies exclusively targeting reductions in children's sedentary time: A systematic review of the literature. *The International Journal of Behavioral Nutrition & Physical Activity, 13*, 65. https://doi.org/10.1186/s12966-016-0387-5.

Barkin, S., Ip, E., Richardson, I., Klinepeter, S., Finch, S., & Krcmar, M. (2006). Parental media mediation styles for children aged 2 to 11 years. *Archives of Pediatrics and Adolescent Medicine, 160*(4), 395–401. https://doi.org/10.1001/archpedi.160.4.395.

Bener, A., Al-Mahdi, H. S., Ali, A. I., Al-Nufal, M., Vachhani, P. J., & Tewfik, I. (2011). Obesity and low vision as a result of excessive Internet use and television viewing. *International Journal of Food Sciences and Nutrition, 62*(1), 60–62. https://doi.org/10.3109/09637486.2010.495711.

Bitzer, E. M., Bleckmann, P., & Mößle, T. (2014). *Prävention problematischer und suchtartiger Bildschirmmediennutzung: Eine deutschlandweite Befragung von Praxiseinrichtungen und Experten. Forschungsbericht Nr. 125*. Hannover: Kriminologisches Forschungsinstitut Niedersachsen.

BKK Dachverband e.V. (2017). ECHT DABEI-gesund groß werden im digitalen Zeitalter. Really present-growing up healthy in the digital age. Retrieved from http://www.echt-dabei.de.

Bleckmann, P., & Mößle, T. (2014). Position zu Problemdimensionen und Präventionsstrategien der Bildschirmnutzung. *Sucht, 60*(4), 235–247. https://doi.org/10.1024/0939-5911.a000313.

Bleckmann, P., Rehbein, F., Seidel, M., & Mößle, T. (2014). MEDIA PROTECT—a programme targeting parents to prevent children's problematic use of screen media. *Journal of Children's Services, 9*(3), 207–219. https://doi.org/10.1108/JCS-10-2013-0036.

Borzekowski, D. L. (2009). Considering children and Health Literacy: a theoretical approach. *Pediatrics, 124*, 282–288. https://doi.org/10.1542/peds.2009-1162D.

Cain, N., & Gradisar, M. (2010). Electronic media use and sleep in school-aged children and adolescents: A review. *Sleep Medicine, 11*(8), 735–742. https://doi.org/10.1016/j.sleep.2010.02.006.

Christakis, D. A., Frintner, M. P., Mulligan, D. A., Fuld, G. L., & Olson, L. M. (2013). Media education in pediatric residencies: A national survey. *Academic Pediatrics, 13*(1), 55–58. https://doi.org/10.1016/j.acap.2012.10.003.

Christakis, D. A., & Zimmerman, F. J. (2007). Violent television viewing during preschool is associated with antisocial behavior during school age. *Pediatrics, 120*(5), 993–999. https://doi.org/10.1542/peds.2006-3244.

Common sense media (2017). The common sense census: media use by kids age zero to eight. Retrieved from https://www.commonsensemedia.org/research/the-common-sense-census-media-use-by-kids-age-zero-to-eight-2017.

Coombs, N., Shelton, N., Rowlands, A., & Stamatakis, E. (2013). Children's and adolescents' sedentary behaviour in relation to socioeconomic position. *Journal of Epidemiology and Community Health, 67*(10), 868–874. https://doi.org/10.1136/jech-2013-202609.

Fachstelle für Suchtprävention der Drogenhilfe Köln (2014). *Abschlussbericht ESCapade.* final report ESCapade. Retrieved from http://www.escapade-projekt.de/fileadmin/user_upload/Abschlussbericht_ESCapade_final.pdf.

Feierabend, S., Karg, U. & Rathgeb, T. (2013). *miniKIM 2012 Kleinkinder und Medien: Basisuntersuchung zum Medienumgang 2- bis 5-Jähriger in Deutschland.* miniKIM 2012-small children and the media. Basic examination on media use of 2 to 5 year olds in Germany: Stuttgart.

Feierabend, S. & Klingler, W. (2000). *KIM-Studie 2000. Kinder und Medien, Computer und Internet. Basisuntersuchung zum Medienumgang 6- bis 13-Jähriger.* children and the media, computer and internet. Basic examination on media use of 6 to 13 year olds ((Keine Angabe)). Baden-Baden.

Feierabend, S., Plankenhorn, T., & Rathgeb, T. (2015). *miniKIM 2014 Kleinkinder und Medien: Basisuntersuchung zum Medienumgang 2- bis 5-Jähriger in Deutschland.* Stuttgart.

Ferguson, C. J. (2011). The influence of television and video game use on attention and school problems: A multivariate analysis with other risk factors controlled. *Journal of Psychiatric Research, 45*(6), 808–813. https://doi.org/10.1016/j.jpsychires.2010.11.010.

Friedrich, R. R., Polet, J. P., Schuch, I., & Wagner, M. B. (2014). Effect of intervention programs in schools to reduce screen time: A meta-analysis. *Jornal De Pediatria, 90*(3), 232–241. https://doi.org/10.1016/j.jped.2014.01.003.

Gentile, D. A., Swing, E. L., Lim, C. G., & Khoo, A. (2012). Video game playing, attention problems, and impulsiveness: Evidence of bidirectional causality. *Psychology of Popular Media Culture, 1*(1), 62–70. https://doi.org/10.1037/a0026969.

Hurrelmann, K., Hartung, S., Kluwe, S., & Sahrai, D. (2013). Gesundheitsförderung durch Elternbildung in „Settings". *Prävention Und Gesundheitsförderung, 8*(4), 267–275. https://doi.org/10.1007/s11553-013-0402-5.

Kayser, L., Kushniruk, A., Osborne, R. H., Norgaard, O., & Turner, P. (2015). Enhancing the effectiveness of consumer-focused health information technology systems through eHealth Literacy: A Framework for Understanding Users' Needs. *JMIR Human Factors, 2*(1), e9. https://doi.org/10.2196/humanfactors.3696.

Knop, K., Hefner, D. & Schmitt, S. (2015). *Mediatisierung mobil: Handy- und mobile Internetnutzung von Kindern und Jugendlichen.* mobil media-smartphone and mobile internet consumption of children and adolescents. *Schriftenreihe Medienforschung der Landesanstalt für Medien Nordrhein-Westfalen: Vol. 77.* Leipzig: Vistas.

Kobel, S., Wartha, O., Wirt, T., Dreyhaupt, J., Lämmle, C., Friedemann, E.-M., et al. (2017). Design, implementation, and study protocol of a kindergarten-based health promotion intervention. *BioMed Research International, 2017,* 4347675. https://doi.org/10.1155/2017/4347675.

Lauricella, A. R., Wartella, E., & Rideout, V. J. (2015). Young children's screen time: The complex role of parent and child factors. *Journal of Applied Developmental Psychology, 36,* 11–17. https://doi.org/10.1016/j.appdev.2014.12.001.

Maniccia, D. M., Davison, K. K., Marshall, S., Manganello, J. A., & Dennison, B. A. (2011). A meta-analysis of interventions that target children's screen time for reduction. *Pediatrics, 128*(1), 193–2010. https://doi.org/10.1542/peds.2010-2353.

Marino, C., Vieno, A., Lenzi, M., Borraccino, A., Lazzeri, G., & Lemma, P. (2016). Computer use, sleep difficulties, and psychological symptoms among school-aged children: The mediating role of sleep difficulties. *International Journal of School Health, 4*(1), 50–58. https://doi.org/10.17795/intjsh-32921.

Marsh, S., Foley, L. S., Wilks, D. C., & Maddison, R. (2014). Family-based interventions for reducing sedentary time in youth: A systematic review of randomized controlled trials. *Obesity Reviews: An Official Journal of the International Association for the Study of Obesity, 15*(2), 117–133. https://doi.org/10.1111/obr.12105.

Möller, I., Krahé, B., Busching, R., & Krause, C. (2012). Efficacy of an intervention to reduce the use of media violence and aggression: An experimental evaluation with adolescents in Germany. *Journal of Youth and Adolescence, 41*(2), 105–120. https://doi.org/10.1007/s10964-011-9654-6.

Mößle, T. (2012). *"dick, dumm, abhängig, gewalttätig?": Problematische Mediennutzungsmuster und ihre Folgen im Kindesalter. Ergebnisse des Berliner Längsschnitt Medien* (1. Aufl.). *Interdisziplinäre Beiträge zur kriminologischen Forschung: Vol. 42.* Baden-Baden: Nomos.

Mößle, T., Kleimann, M., Rehbein, F., & Pfeiffer, C. (2010). Media use and school achievement-boys at risk? *British Journal of Developmental Psychology, 28*(3), 699–725. https://doi.org/10.1348/026151009X475307.

Müller, A., Marci-Boehncke, G., & Rath, M. (2012). KidSmart - Medienkompetent zum Schulübergang. *Medienimpulse-Online, 1*, 1–11. Retrieved from http://www.medienimpulse.at/articles/view/393.

Njoroge, W. F. M., Elenbaas, L. M., Garrison, M. M., Myaing, M., & Christakis, D. A. (2013). Parental cultural attitudes and beliefs regarding young children and television. *JAMA Pediatrics, 167*(8), 739–745. https://doi.org/10.1001/jamapediatrics.2013.75.

Norman, C. D., & Skinner, H. A. (2006). eHealth Literacy: essential skills for consumer health in a networked world. *Journal of Medical Internet Research, 8*(2), e9. https://doi.org/10.2196/jmir.8.2.e9.

Nunez-Smith, M., Wolf, E., Huang, H. M., Emanuel, E. & Gross, C. P. (2008). *Media + child and adolescent health: A Systematic Review.* Retrieved from http://ipsdweb.ipsd.org/uploads/IPPC/CSM%20Media%20Health%20Report.pdf.

Paudel, S., Jancey, J., Subedi, N., & Leavy, J. (2017). Correlates of mobile screen media use among children aged 0-8: A systematic review. *British Medical Journal Open, 7*(10), e014585. https://doi.org/10.1136/bmjopen-2016-014585.

Prochaska, J. O., & Velicer, W. F. (1997). The transtheoretical model of health behavior change. *American Journal of Health Promotion, 12*(1), 38–48. https://doi.org/10.4278/0890-1171-12.1.38.

Rehbein, F., Mößle, T., Arnaud, N. & Rumpf, H.-J. (2013). Computerspiel- und Internetsucht: Der aktuelle Forschungsstand. *Nervenarzt, 84*, 569–575. https://doi.org/10.1007/s00115-012-3721-4.

Reid Chassiakos, Y. L., Radesky, J., Christakis, D., Moreno, M. A., & Cross, C. (2016). Children and adolescents and digital media. *Pediatrics, 138*(5). https://doi.org/10.1542/peds.2016-2593.

Robert Koch-Institut (2003). KiGGS-Basiserhebung: Erhebungsinstrumente. KiGGS basic survey: measurement instruments. Retrieved from https://www.kiggs-studie.de/deutsch/studie/kiggs-basiserhebung/instrumente.html.

Robertson, L. A., McAnally, H. M., & Hancox, R. J. (2013). Childhood and adolescent television viewing and antisocial behavior in early adulthood. *Pediatrics, 131*(3), 439–446. https://doi.org/10.1542/peds.2012-1582.

Schenk, L., Bau, A.- M., Borde, T., Butler, J., Lampert, T., Neuhauser, H., Weilandt, C, et al. (2006). Mindestindikatorensatz zur Erfassung des Migrationsstatus. Empfehlungen für die epidemiologische Praxis [A basic set of indicators for mapping migrant status. Recommendations for epidemiological practice]. *Bundesgesundheitsblatt, Gesundheitsforschung, Gesundheitsschutz, 49*(9), 853–860. https://doi.org/10.1007/s00103-006-0018-4.

Schmidt, M. E., Haines, J., O'brien, A., McDonald, J., Price, S., Sherry, B. and Taveras, E. M. (2012). Systematic review of effective strategies for reducing screen time among young children. *Obesity (Silver Spring), 20*(7), 1338–1354. https://doi.org/10.1038/oby.2011.348.

Schultze-Krumbholz, A., Zagorscak, P., Wölfer, R., & Scheithauer, H. (2014). Das Medienhelden Programm zur Förderung von Medienkompetenz und Prävention von Cybermobbing: Konzept und Ergebnisse der Evaluation. *Praxis Der Kinderpsychologie Und Kinderpsychiatrie, 63*(5), 379–394. https://doi.org/10.1007/978-3-662-48199-8_6.

Seidel, M. [M.] (2013, November). *Supporting parents to limit children's problematic media use. Results and lessons learned from MEDIA PROTECT.* European Society for Prevention Research. Understanding differences in prevention outcomes, Paris. Retrieved from http://euspr.org/wp-content/uploads/2013/04/EUSPR_Conference2013_booklet.pdf.

Sigman, A. (2017). Screen dependency disorders: a new challenge for child neurology. *Journal of the International Child Neurology Association., 17,* 119.

Staiano, A. E., Harrington, D. M., Broyles, S. T., Gupta, A. K., & Katzmarzyk, P. T. (2013). Television, adiposity, and cardiometabolic risk in children and adolescents. *American Journal of Preventive Medicine, 44*(1), 40–47. https://doi.org/10.1016/j.amepre.2012.09.049.

Statistisches Bundesamt (2017). *Laufende Wirtschaftsrechnungen – Ausstattung privater Haushalte mit ausgewählten Gebrauchsgütern – Fachserie 15 Reihe 2 – 2017. Fachserie 15: Vol. 2.*

Stiller, A., Schwendemann, H., Bleckmann, P., Bitzer, E. M., & Mößle, T. (2018). Involving teachers in reducing children's media risks. *Journal of Health Education, 118*(1), 31–47.

Strasburger, V. C. (2010). Media education. *Pediatrics, 126*(5), 1012–1017. https://doi.org/10.1542/peds.2010-1636.

UNHCR-The UN Refugee Agency (2016). Global Trends: Forced displacement in 2015. Retrieved from http://www.unhcr.org/statistics/unhcrstats/576408cd7/unhcr-global-trends-2015.html.

Vaala, S. E., & Hornik, R. C. (2014). Predicting US infants' and toddlers' TV/video viewing rates: Mothers' cognitions and structural life circumstances. *Journal of Children and Media, 8*(2), 163–182. https://doi.org/10.1080/17482798.2013.824494.

Valkenburg, P. M., Krcmar, M., Peeters, A. L., & Marseille, N. M. (1999). Developing a scale to assess three styles of television mediation: „Instructive mediation", „restrictive mediation", and „social coviewing". *Journal of Broadcasting & Electronic Media, 43,* 52–66.

Vanderloo, L. M. (2014). Screen-viewing among preschoolers in childcare: A systematic review. *BMC Pediatrics, 14,* 205. https://doi.org/10.1186/1471-2431-14-205.

Vandewater, E. A., Park, S.-E., Huang, X., & Wartella, E. A. (2005). "No - you can't watch that": parental rules and young children's media use. *American Behavioral Scientist, 48*(5), 608–623. https://doi.org/10.1177/0002764204271497.

Viera, A. J. and Garrett, J. M. (2005). Understanding interobserver agreement: the kappa statistic. *Family Medicine, 37*(5), 360–363. Retrieved from http://www.stfm.org/fmhub/fm2005/May/Anthony360.pdf.

Wagner, U., & Eggert, S. (Eds.) (2013). *Schriftenreihe Medienforschung der Landesanstalt für Medien Nordrhein-Westfalen: Vol. 72. Zwischen Anspruch und Alltagsbewältigung: Medienerziehung in der Familie.* Berlin: Vistas-Verl. Retrieved from http://www.lfm-nrw.de/forschung/schriftenreihe-medienforschung/band-72.html#c18828.

Wahi, G., Parkin, P. C., Beyene, J., Uleryk, E. M., & Birken, C. S. (2011). Effectiveness of interventions aimed at reducing screen time in children: A systematic review and meta-analysis of randomized controlled trials. *Archives of Pediatrics and Adolescent Medicine, 165*(11), 979–986. https://doi.org/10.1001/archpediatrics.2011.122.

Yilmaz, G., Demirli Caylan, N., & Karacan, C. D. (2015). An intervention to preschool children for reducing screen time: A randomized controlled trial. *Child: Care, Health and Development, 41*(3), 443–449. https://doi.org/10.1111/cch.12133.

Towards New Perspectives on Health Literacy for Children: From 'Health Information' to Recognizing Young Citizens' Capacities for Meaning-Making (Debate from a 'Liquid Network')

Paulo Pinheiro, Shanti George, Orkan Okan, Elise Sijthoff, Uwe H. Bittlingmayer, Rahel Kahlert, Almas Merchant, Dirk Bruland, Janine Bröder and Ullrich Bauer

P. Pinheiro (✉) · O. Okan · U. Bauer
Faculty of Educational Sciences, Bielefeld University, Bielefeld, Germany
e-mail: paulo.pinheiro@uni-bielefeld.de

O. Okan
e-mail: orkan.okan@uni-bielefeld.de

U. Bauer
e-mail: ullrich.bauer@uni-bielefeld.de

S. George
Independent Researcher and Learning for Well-Being Foundation (the Netherlands), The Hague, The Netherlands

E. Sijthoff
Founder ChildPress.Org, Publishing House Fysio Educatief Amsterdam, Amsterdam, The Netherlands
e-mail: elise@sijthoff.nl

U. H. Bittlingmayer
Institute of Sociology, University of Education Freiburg (Germany), Freiburg, Germany
e-mail: uwe.bittlingmayer@ph-freiburg.de

R. Kahlert · A. Merchant
Ludwig Boltzmann Institute, Health Promotion Research Vienna, Vienna, Austria
e-mail: rahel.kahlert@lbihpr.lbg.ac.at

© The Editor(s) (if applicable) and The Author(s), under exclusive license to Springer Fachmedien Wiesbaden GmbH, part of Springer Nature 2021
L. A. Saboga-Nunes et al. (eds.), *New Approaches to Health Literacy*, Gesundheit und Gesellschaft, https://doi.org/10.1007/978-3-658-30909-1_8

1 Introduction

Unusual amongst the chapters in this volume—many of which represent formal academic products of the Health Literacy in Childhood and Adolescence (HLCA) project—what follows below provides a glimpse of insights that were generated by the project in the course of wider exchange with researchers from elsewhere, notably those within the Working together Internationally on Social development and Health in Every School and family (WISHES) network.

This chapter depicts what is not often captured on paper, the vibrant exchanges (usually spoken) between researchers working in allied areas, notably at more open and fluid gatherings than those which assemble members of a single entity. In this particular case, WISHES and HCLA were invited to co-host a pre-conference on 'Recognizing Children and Young People as Active Citizens within Health Literacy: Theory and practice across Europe', at the Third European Health Literacy Conference held in Brussels in November 2015.

During this pre-conference, and through the different presentations that were given (largely by the co-authors of this chapter), the researchers concerned and many other participants felt and expressed the need for new perspectives within research and debate on children's health literacy. Such an imperative has no doubt been felt and expressed on multiple occasions where such researchers gather, but in this case ten of the presenters went on to write a shared paper that constitutes the present chapter. It is therefore an example of the 'embryonic' papers that are conceived through fruitful exchanges at conferences and the form that these might take if allowed to gestate more fully, as they were on the present occasion.

This process possibly illustrates what Steven Johnson (2010) describes in his book *Where Good Ideas Come From*. Johnson identifies 'the ground zero of innovation' as 'the conference table' (2010, p. 61) and emphasizes that 'the most productive tool for generating good ideas remains a circle of humans at a table,

A. Merchant
e-mail: almas.merchant@lbihpr.lbg.ac.at

D. Bruland
Institute for educational and health-care research in the health sector (InBVG),
FH Bielefeld University of Applied Sciences, Bielefeld, Germany
e-mail: dirk.bruland@fh-bielefeld.de

J. Bröder
Deutsche Gesellschaft für Ernährung e. V., Bonn, Germany
e-mail: broeder@dge.de

talking shop… an environment where new combinations can occur, where information can spill over from one project to another' (*ibid.*).

This chapter depicts how concepts like 'health literacy' can be critically explored by a group of researchers from different disciplines and contexts, who gather for a moment of intense interaction. The researchers generate vibrant ideas (the four topics discussed below, for example), relate these to the literature and offer a few significant cases with which they are familiar. After such an effervescent moment, the group typically disperses, individually or in clusters of researchers and—regrettably—the ideas that were collectively generated then dissipate. The present case provides an example of subsequent attempts to preserve some of the ideas through embodying them in a variant of an academic paper.

What might be some of the differences between such a product and a conventional journal article? The emphasis below is on capturing ideas with broad brush strokes, rather than compressing a broad debate into the format required of standard academic papers. Instead of an initial comprehensive overview of familiar definitions of health literacy, for example, this chapter takes one relevant definition (Pleasant 2014; see below) as its point of departure in order to use available space for wider exploration. In contrast to the required route of first summarizing available literature on adult health literacy, and given the dearth of studies on children's health literacy, the analysis below starts by directly addressing fallacies in debates on health literacy among children. Where conventional scholarship generally strives to give the impression of one sustained voice, this chapter attempts to capture a rich plurality of voices. Rather than cautiously presenting cases, the discussion below takes risks in juxtaposing children's realities as currently captured with the academic debate at its present stage.

The paper strives to synthesize coherently many ideas, allusions and connections, even if these could not be fully elaborated within the constraints of space. Its objective was to sensitize rather than to generalize (Wiener and Rosenwald 1993, p. 33). Such a piece might belong in the 'Perspectives' or 'Debate' or 'Opinion' section of a journal, but when the authors attempted to place it as such it appeared that the piece contained too many references for an 'Opinion' piece, yet not sufficient references for a standard article given that the wide span of discussion called for a tremendous sweep of citations. These challenges might have been addressed by extensively lengthening the paper, but it would then have been far too long for a conventional article—and the authors felt that brevity facilitated the cogency of argument made necessary by the prevalent neglect of children's health literacy, both within scholarly analyses and public policy, as well as by the insufficient attention paid to children's agency in what little debate took place on the subject.

The cross-disciplinary nature of the discussion further complicated the choice of journal for potential publication—because a paper that simultaneously addressed public health, the sociology of childhood and literacy studies attempted to bring together audiences that do not easily converse with one another. To cite Johnson again, the process involved 'far more open-ended and contentious meetings... and far more dialogue between people versed in different disciplines, with all the translation difficulties that creates' (Johnson 2010, p. 171) on top of all the related publication constraints.

The present chapter then takes its place amongst the others in this volume in evoking some 'voices along the way' within the HLCA project's first phase (notably through a dialogue with the WISHES network), voices that share insights about children's health literacy in a provocative manner. It evokes a moment of stimulating exchange early in the HLCA project, in the project's first year from 2015 to 2016, that has now—three years on—been grounded by rigorous 'PRISMA' type scrutiny of systematic reviews and meta-analyses within health literacy by some of the same authors (Bröder et al 2017; Okan et al 2018; see below). Many questions of course remain (Pinheiro et al 2018), and perhaps the time has come for another effervescent moment to engage with them again.

'Ideas rise in... liquid networks where connection is valued' Johnson tells us (2010, p. 245), where 'we open our minds to... many connected environments' (*op. cit.*, p. 21), where ideas 'connect, fuse, recombine... crossing conceptual borders' (*op.* cit., p. 22), through a 'spillover' whereby ideas flow from mind to mind, essentially liquid in a conducive setting (*op. cit.*, p. 53). Such an analogy resonates with allusions to 'fluid' and 'flow' in the preceding paragraphs, and indeed Johnson writes that '"flow"... suggests the essential fluidity that good ideas so often need' (*op. cit.*, p. 64). It is for this reason that the chapter is subtitled 'Debate from a "liquid network"', and our concluding paragraph will link this to Johnson's reference to the 'coffee house model of creativity' (op. cit., p. 169).

In the following six sections we'd like to share the debates and arguments that were generated within a liquid network when some members of HCLA and WISHES gathered at the pre-conference described above to discuss health literacy in childhood.

2   Presenting the main Arguments

Health literacy in childhood, this chapter argues, is as much about childhood and literacy as it is about health, and therefore the analytical pathways that underpin conventional health literacy research require reconsideration, as do the social policies that are based on such research. More recent insights from the sociology of childhood and from the new literacy studies can help to re-orient current approaches to health literacy in childhood (e.g. Fairbrother et al. 2016). Health literacy is presented here as much more than the processing of health information by individuals, and it is urged that health literacy assessments be broadened beyond simple vertical rankings of 'high' and 'low' health literacy. Social and cultural contexts need to be explored in greater depth and detail, with more attention paid to economic and political inequalities. Insights from the new literacy studies enable health literacy to be analysed in terms of literacy events and related social practices, giving language a central place and examining children's meaning-making processes with reference to well-being and quality of life. The chapter focuses on school-age children, provides examples and suggests that the arguments put forward about the analysis of health literacy apply more widely, including to adults. Health literacy—when viewed in the context of active citizenship and reflective practice—can be analysed as self-education through coaching and co-learning, including co-learning with children.

'Health literacy' refers to phenomena that are not directly observable and that are created through social practices and human choice in the face of social realities. Descriptions of health literacy as a 'complex social construct' (Pleasant 2014) highlight these characteristics. In this chapter, we extend this view to health literacy in childhood and argue that this composite term weaves together three complex social constructs—namely health, literacy and childhood. Secondly, we argue that the analytical pathways towards a robust construction of 'health literacy in childhood' have implications beyond scholarly analysis, and hold critical relevance for public debates around responsibilities for health literacy and related policies and programmes. Crucially, we emphasize that social constructions of health literacy in childhood should enable understanding of the ways in which children use language in its various forms to support health and well-being.

To elaborate these arguments, we start by outlining common trends within current constructions of health literacy in school-aged children. We do this on the basis of two reviews of literature embarked on in 2015 by some of the present authors (and now published as Bröder et al. 2017 and Okan et al. 2018). Systematic retrieval within scientific literature identified 32 references around theories and concepts, and another 15 references within the field of methodology. Preliminary findings highlight the following common features of current social constructions of health literacy within childhood:

1. Personal attributes such as knowledge and skills are the main focus, especially individual characteristics that are required in order to respond to societal and situational demands. Briefly summarized, these demands concern how health

information is gathered, understood, appraised and used, in terms of minimum standards for children's health. Conceptualization of health literacy in childhood within the literature surveyed is fairly similar to the majority of definitions and conceptualizations for adults, where (a) health literacy is seen as mainly located within the individual, (b) rational thinking and acting are emphasized and (c) the internal abilities of individuals are assessed in relation to external demands.

2. Social and cultural conditions or environments are widely acknowledged to be relevant but related discussions are far less refined than the elaborations on personal attributes.

3. Childhood is usually distinguished from adulthood through reference to developmental issues and tasks, drawing on concepts from developmental psychology rather than on sociological approaches. While past efforts have applied Piaget's age-oriented developmental phases to health literacy, there have been only a few attempts to explain how, when and through what circumstances children develop skills and acquire knowledge, including in the area of what we denote as health literacy.

4. Assessments of health literacy tend to rate personal attributes in terms of hierarchical ranking systems that distinguish between high and low—or adequate and inadequate—levels. It is hard to find assessments of health literacy for school-aged children that classify cases without ordering them within a hierarchy.

Undoubtedly there are some arguments to support the analytical pathways that have just been outlined, but we voice our scepticism about their sufficiency and we urge that these pathways be placed in a wider context. In pursuance of such an approach, this chapter contributes some critical reflections that challenge the prevalent understandings of health literacy in childhood and the paradigms that frame them. We regret that space constraints restrain us from providing more examples to illuminate complex discussions. For the same reason, this chapter concentrates on school-age children and does not focus on older adolescents and young adults. We argue that:

- ideas about 'health literacy in childhood' should be expanded beyond a prevalent focus on health and should take greater account of perspectives used in childhood studies as well as in literacy research,
- the analysis of health literacy must centre on meaning-making processes that relate to multiple forms of language, rather than merely on the use and processing of health information,

- the unit of observation has to shift from the individual to health literacy events and practices in order to explore related social practices, identify personal and contextual determinants and analyse social structures and backgrounds,
- vertical/hierarchical assessments of health literacy in childhood—based on rankings from 'low' to 'high'—need to be complemented with horizontal/non-hierarchical assessments,

The four sections of the chapter that follow develop our key themes: Sect. 1 argues that health literacy in childhood is as much about childhood and literacy as it is about health. Sect. 2 demonstrates how health literacy is more than only the individual processing of health information. Sect. 3 maintains that understanding health literacy is about capturing literacy events and related social practices. Sect. 4 notes that health literacy assessments need to be broadened beyond simple vertical rankings of 'high' and 'low' health literacy. The 'Discussion' section synthesizes the previous sections—advocating 'inclusiveness' but using 'inclusive' in a radically different sense from the more prevalent usages of the term within conventional health literacy research and within social policies that are based on such conventional research.

3 Health Literacy in Childhood is as much about Childhood and Literacy as it is about Health

Current conceptualizations of health literacy in childhood have mainly evolved in the fields of health research, notably within health care and public health. Not yet fully considered and discussed has been a wide range of relevant findings from childhood research and literacy research that provide important opportunities for rethinking current conceptualizations of childhood health literacy. Childhood studies extend across multiple strands, from psychological discussions (Grusec and Hastings 2006; Denzin 2009) to sociological analyses (Hurrelmann et al. 2015). Similarly, research into literacy spans a broad range of perspectives such as cognitive, psycholinguistic and sociocultural approaches (see e.g. Kennedy et al. 2012). Given the significant bias in current constructions of health literacy towards perspectives originating from health research, and the resultant neglect of other important points of reference, useful counterpoints are provided by work in the sociology of childhood (Brady et al. 2015) and the New Literacy Studies (Street 2003).

Many essential processes of cognitive, physical and social-emotional development take place during early, middle and late childhood. Children are therefore more engaged than adults with their own biological, cognitive, psychological, emotional and social development. They are busy understanding themselves and the worlds in which they live, and connecting internal with external demands. While children are generally dependent on their parents for economic resources and social support, they are already active agents in their own social worlds (Brady et al. 2015). Viewing children as social agents draws attention to children's perspectives on health and their health-related behaviour within different social contexts and cultures. Children continuously develop and change through socialization processes and interaction with their environment, including with parents, other adults and peers. How we view children depends largely on our own perception of childhood and the social role we attribute to children in everyday interactions, such as between teachers and students or between doctors and child patients.

This section highlights what is called the 'new sociology of childhood': changed perspectives within childhood research (Prout 2011) that present children as social 'beings' and not any longer as social 'becomings' that need to be filled with knowledge and skills as if they were empty vessels (Alanen 1998). Children are structurally significant within society (Qvortrup et al. 1994) even though they are relatively powerless in relation to political and social structures (Mayall 1998). Children constitute a social minority and a group of their own which merits the same attention that is paid to other social groups and minorities (Mayall 1994). They must therefore be recognized as social actors who are agents and citizens in their own right and co-constructors of their worlds (James and Prout 1990).

The key theme of children as social actors (Bühler-Niederberger 2010) is framed by the generational order that includes the intergenerational conflicts which occur when children interact with adult society, given the unequal distribution of power between children and adults (Huijsmans et al. 2014). Traditional and generally accepted postulates about childhood are thus questioned. Addressing children's agency within the dynamics of power relations between children and adults gains in importance when the social construction of health literacy defines children's active participation in decision-making as a major goal (Mayall 1998; Borzekowski 2009). Such new options within health literacy research enable the recognition of children as active agents and require that they always be seen in interaction with others, notably within intergenerational relationships. Let us consider an example, in this case of positive interaction with teachers.

Teachers play a major role in children's development. They get to see the children almost every day, so they can recognize behavioural changes and health problems—including mental health problems—and they are in a position to offer support to burdened children. An ongoing research project on teachers' mental health literacy explores the extent to which teachers' formal or informal health literacy extends to pupils in middle and late childhood whose parents are mentally ill (Bruland et al. 2016). It notes the vulnerability of children of mentally ill parents as a population at high risk of developing mental disorders. Teachers' knowledge about children's home situations becomes especially important here. Children often respond to such family stresses with symptomatic behaviour, and their school lives will reflect the burdens that set them apart from their classmates, as well as their attempts to cope. A systematic review of literature found only three studies that specifically focus on teachers mental health literacy and children with mentally ill parents (Bruland et al., submitted for publication). The scarce data highlights the difficulties that teachers encounter in identifying burdened pupils, but if they are able to do so they are usually troubled by the child's situation (Bibou-Nakou 2004; Reupert and Maybery 2007; Brockmann 2014). The findings from initial qualitative research confirm these insights, and show how poorly prepared teachers are without the required training or knowledge about where to turn for structured assistance to such children. Their professional role increasingly emphasizes knowledge transfer and encouragement of learning through management of large classes, rather than individual support to children in need. Questions remain: Do schools provide sufficient opportunities to promote children's health and for teachers to respond to pupils' life circumstances? Positive answers to these questions seem to be supported by research—so what policy implications and actions should follow?

## 4	Health Literacy is more than Individual Processing of 'Health Information'

Our critical review of current health literacy definitions and models finds, at their core, an emphasis on how individuals must function in order to meet prescribed standards that are set for particular situations. Such a focus highlights individual skills, abilities and competencies, while disregarding the social practices of health literacy that reflect the processes whereby meaning is created from the given information. Neither does this kind of approach address questions broader than individual needs for health literacy, nor the effects on health literacy of the sociocultural structures in which children and adults are embedded.

In contrast, literacy research is mainly concerned with language (whether spoken, written or body language), unlike research on health literacy where the term *language* has rarely been used as a key word. Health literacy research instead much more commonly uses the term *health information*. This merits further investigation, and we argue that a narrow focus on health information limits discussion to information processing and ignores the inherently interactive nature of health literacy. The term *health information* also proves inadequate when addressing the contribution of contextual factors to health literacy practices, practices that can be better captured when the notion of language is more centrally placed. We therefore suggest a shift in focus away from the use of health information, and towards direct attention to the processes at work when meaning is created within the use of multiple forms of language.

Meaning making in health literacy highlights how children understand and make sense of health-related messages, as do the adults who are significant in children's everyday lives. Health literacy definitions and conceptualizations—as in many other theoretical fields—have been developed by researchers or professionals who draw on available theoretical constructs and practical experiences. Such an 'expert concept' treats health information as largely objective. For most health-related subjects, however, especially those that are considered health promotion issues, a sufficiently rigorous evidence base to support content and information is difficult to establish. Instead, it seems that health information often conveys highly normative messages that imply what society expects of its members or parents of their children. We simply do not know enough about how and through whom children receive information, what sources they actively seek out, or the extent to which information is presented in a manner that children of various ages can engage with.

A major milestone in the sociology of childhood was the publication of anthropologist Myra Bluebond-Langner's book *The Private Worlds of Dying Children* in 1978. Based on her studies of terminally ill children aged three to nine, she revealed how these children perceived their illness and coped with it, and how they were capable of autonomously constructing the social reality of their inevitable deaths (Bluebond-Langner 1978). Her study highlights how the truth about children's deaths is not faced by professional medical staff and these children's families. She listened to these children during their most critical stage of life, and let them share their thoughts as she observed their actions in medical health care settings. Today, one can see that her study profoundly influenced and changed both the sociology of childhood and 'deterministic' theories about the socialisation of children (Ryan 2008) through its illumination of children's capacities to process and understand reality. On similar lines, health literacy for children with disabilities might primarily involve learning strategies to cope with the stereotypes that constitute an important part of their everyday experience, more than improving their health information seeking behaviour.

Models of health literacy as information processing are typically used to present a unidirectional logic from sender to receiver. This is in sharp contrast to the interaction between individuals and institutions—as in families or schools—where children negotiate their everyday realities and status (Bauer 2012; Alanen et al. 2015); the other actors in these negotiations are, of course, adults. Intergenerational relations include the unequal distribution of power in favour of adults, and through this interplay children are challenged every day to consolidate and assert their own status in society. These actions are influenced by social practices and power relations, and are significantly shaped by individual factors. Such consolidation processes and negotiations are an everyday reality for all children, within their daily practices that need to be understood. To support the analysis of these everyday negotiations, Bourdieu's theories of field, habitus and capital offer a valuable framework (see e.g. Bauer 2012) to understand health-related social practices involving children. Perspectives on literacy as event and as social practices (1984, 2003; Papen 2009) also highlight the relevance of Bourdieu's sociological approach to understanding social interactions and power relations. Approaches to health literacy in childhood should therefore recognise children as active participants in decision-making processes that are related to health. Health policies should apply democratic values and practices in daily life, by communicating on an equal footing, hearing children's perceptions and voices—and taking them seriously—as well as being careful not to act only upon adult perceptions of childhood.

The following case is relevant here:

Some fifteen years ago, a curriculum was developed for children as active citizens within health literacy—even though children were at that time not recognized as active citizens and the term 'health literacy' was not in wide use. A physiotherapist felt that physiotherapy could enable people of all ages to feel comfortable within their own bodies, to build on their strengths and to work on their limitations. It seemed wise to begin with children, in order to help them from early on to understand their bodies and to use them well, and to ground such understanding in the everyday classrooms activities of—also for children to learn all this through fun during class. For this purpose, a team was formed of children's physiotherapists as well as occupational, speech and drama specialists. The programme that was developed was called *The Class Moves!* and provided a curriculum of health literacy for children in primary school. Through play, mime and song, they built up sound physical habits that simultaneously stimulated cognitive development and social-emotional openness. By taking ten-minute breaks at various time throughout the school day, they learned in later life not to sit in front of a computer for hours but to move their body regularly and actively.

The eight months of the school year were each allocated a theme that recurred for each class at an appropriate developmental level as children grew older. At the beginning of the school year the theme was 'expressing emotions' followed by 'bodily awareness'. The exercises were available on a calendar, and later on an electronic page. For those who wished to understand the principles behind the exercises and the unfolding programme, a manual provided accessible text and illustrations. The programme encouraged children literally to *exercise* their rights, to be *active* citizens and to experience *moving* moments in all senses of the word 'moving' (Sijthoff 2014).

5   Understanding Health Literacy is about Capturing Literacy Events and Related Social Practices

Shifting the focus regarding health literacy towards processes of meaning making has implications for methodological approaches within health literacy research, including alterations in the unit of observation. Following sociocultural perspectives on literacy (e.g. Perry 2012), we suggest shifting the unit of observation from personal attributes of a child—which is the current mode in health literacy research—to health literacy events and practices that children are involved in. This connects to the new literacy studies where the research framework is organised around the notion of literacy events and practices.

A health literacy event can be defined as any occasion in which any form of language—whether spoken, written or body language—that is used to transmit a health-related message is integral to the nature of the participants' interactions and their interpretative processes (see Street 2003 for this adaptation of Heath's concept of literacy events). Analysing health literacy in terms of literacy events illuminates literacy practices, here defined as social practices that can be observed in a literacy event and that represent what people actually do when they are exposed to language. The investigation of social practices informs us about an individual's set of skills and knowledge and provides insights into beliefs and dispositions as well as values, attitudes, feelings and social relationships. Disposition, for example, is an individual attribute that in this context is defined as a state of readiness or a tendency to act in a specified way. Dispositions are influenced by the social context in which a child is embedded and reflect the impact of social structures on the processes of meaning making. Analyses of health literacy—as framed by literacy events and practices connected to meaning making—will consider willingness and readiness to act, as well as issues around a particular child's needs for health literacy.

Using health literacy events and practices as the main analytical framework allows us to outline at least three domains of research:

1. Personal attributes (skills, knowledge, understanding, beliefs, dispositions, values, attitudes, feelings, and social relationships) of the people who act in the health literacy event and who encode or decode health information by using multiple forms of language. Such research addresses the personal characteristics of the child, usually considered to be the receiver—and also those of the person who acts as the sender;
2. Attributes of the forms of language that are used in an event and attributes of the health-related content of language (e.g. multimodality, signs and symbols, content and evidence of health information, purpose);
3. Attributes of the context in which the interaction takes place or within which people are embedded (cultural and social attributes of the context, interrelationships and power relations between the people who act, their social agency).

Understanding health literacy in childhood involves grasping how children are placed and perceived within social structures and in relation to other social groups and generations (Huijsmans et al. 2014). This is inextricably linked to recognizing the social agency of children as fundamental to how children deal with health, well-being and the use of language in everyday life. A theoretical framework for health literacy that is adapted to age further requires the analysis of power relations and the ways in which children are listened to and taken account of in different social settings (e.g. family, health care, school), as well as analysis of the discourses and images of children in social and health policy and within related interventions.

One major goal of strategies to promote health literacy should be to identify and achieve the best balance between participation and protection for any child. In care—including health care—children depend more than adultson attachment figures such as caregivers or other adults. Thus, relevant adults must be incorporated into the analytical framework of health literacy as providers in a literacy event. Donald Schön developed the concept of reflective practice through self-education supported by coaching and co-learning (Schön 1987), and this has been adapted by George to examine relationships between children and the adults who are closest to them (George 2013). According to George's arguments, health literacy—notably in childhood but also in adulthood—can be presented as reflective practice and self-education facilitated by coaching and co-learning, giving rise to disciplined freedom within democratic spaces (*ibid.*).

A recent study of children at middle school level in Austria who were considered to be overweight used focus groups instead of questionnaires, in order to understand the perspectives and expectations of these children—and their caretakers in separate groups—rather than to 'assess' the health literacy of both groups (Kahlert and Merchant 2015). The research was oriented towards capturing the perceptions of children and their families who participated in a programme directed towards weight reduction through diet, physical activity and group therapy. Research questions focused on how children and families experienced the programme, what the personal goals of the children were, the extent to which they could achieve their goals, and the support provided by families, in addition to more conventional questions about barriers and stimuli towards behavioural change.

Focus group discussions both at the beginning and the end of the programme illuminated goals beyond those of weight reduction, a changed diet and increased physical activity. Children responded with their own goals, of participation around realistic targets and of improved social functioning related to positive developments of making more friends and having fun as well as proactively countering bullying. Parents however monitored improvement in the overall health of their child and were less aware of changes in their child's social functioning. Kahlert and Merchant (*ibid.*) discuss the pros and cons of focus groups for children of various ages, as well as other interactive exchanges through individual or telephone interviews, journal keeping and 'photo voices'.

6   Health Literacy assessment needs to be Broadened beyond Simple Rankings of 'High' and 'Low' Health Literacy

Vertical or hierarchical ranking systems of health literacy dominate most assessment tools in childhood, and reflect the normative nature of current conceptualizations of health literacy. Distinctions are made between high/low (or adequate/inadequate) levels of health literacy that guide the identification of children at risk for poor health outcomes. Such assessment procedures however disregard the multiple health literacy practices to which quantified ratings cannot be applied. We ask accordingly that conventional health literacy assessments be complemented by horizontal non-hierarchical assessment procedures.

Health can be related to literacy in different ways. It can specifically address the management or prevention of diseases. In such biomedical or pathogenic approaches, health is about treatment and risk management of diseases in order to restore health or to avoid disease, and health literacy processes instruct people on how to avoid life-threatening situations and therefore justify rating health literacy practices in terms of vertical or hierarchical rankings.

Vulnerability and susceptibility vary over the life course. Children differ significantly from the adult population and even amongst themselves in disease and disability patterns as well as in risk factor profiles. The notion of risk factors encompasses the range of social determinants of children's health and wellbeing. Social inequalities in health must be understood, as must be the impact on a child's development, health and care of being poorly equipped with socio-economic resources. For instance, a national study on children's health in Germany found a strong correlation between low parental social status and the prevalence of overweight and psychological problems in children (Robert Koch-Institut 2008). Highlighting the importance of personal as well as social and community resources implies that the promotion of health literacy must include both personal and social factors that impinge on children's lives. Health literacy practices have therefore to be related to empowerment strategies. We should bear in mind the risk of blaming children (or low-income parents) for apparently unfavourable health literacy practices and we must insist that 'dissemination' strategies squarely face the issues raised here.

A recent survey asked some 400 ninth and tenth graders—in a set of schools that spanned all the way from technical to vocational and special education in one German province—about their media health literacy, based on self-reporting and eight items from the German translation of the European Health Literacy Survey (Gerdes et al. 2016). An average of 75% of the students—although they were not at schools categorized at the most 'academic' level—reported that they found it easy or very easy to find and evaluate health information from media sources. Such self-reported health literacy was not significantly correlated with school type, gender, social and cultural background or school performance. However, around 25% of the students reported difficulties in locating and assessing health information through the media. Conventional health promotion approaches would try to 'empower' this latter group, for example through information campaigns or school-based curricula intended to strengthen their 'health literacy'.

At least three issues can be raised here:

- Conventional approaches concentrate on attitudes rather than on behaviour. A student may score extremely low on media health literacy items but can act in a very healthy way. Another student might have low health literacy scores but only because she or he is very well aware of difficulties in deciding what healthy behaviour is, given contradictory health research findings. This may—ironically—be assessed as low health literacy. Conversely, high scores could be related to lack of awareness of how complicated evaluating health information can be.
- Concentrating on the 25% of low scorers produces a 'target group'. Such a classification could negatively affect the self-description of school students as well as others' perceptions of them. Identifying target groups risks clubbing together individuals who have little in common except for one single attribute (if that).
- Conventional research focuses on certain assumed deficits, in this case among the 25% of students who reported difficulties with health information provided by the media.

Health can also be addressed in a way that is decoupled from any specific disease, through social models of health that address the social determinants of health and the impact of the social environment on individual health and well-being. Social models of health overlap with pathogenic health models but also connect to salutogenic approaches that are concerned with the origins of health and well-being. They address factors and processes that support individuals in responding to stimuli from internal and external environments in ways that promote their own quality of life. Salutogenesis is grounded in the comprehensibility, manageability and meaningfulness of internal and external demands (see e.g. Antonovsky 1987), and assumes that any balance between internal and external environments results from critical appraisal of internal or external stimuli. Social and salutogenic approaches to health, therefore, support the use of horizontal, non-hierarchical assessments of literacy practices. Such assessment practices are probably more appropriate to health promotion issues than the use of vertical rating systems.

The salutogenic approach can also be used as an analytical matrix for literacy events and practices that are not explicitly about health-related information, and it can thereby address literacy practices as such and their contribution to health and well-being. Broadening inquiry into health literacy practices beyond questionnaires also allows research to engage appropriately with persons who are able to read the world around them but may not (yet) be able to read and answer the words in a questionnaire. Children fall into this category, especially younger children. If we award respect and recognition to children, this may prove the start to an extension of our frontiers that will allow us to recognise and respect people whose circumstances do not easily allow the reading and writing of words, notably people with disabilities, whether those disabilities are physiological or reflect inequities within the society around. Here, the discussion of health literacy expands into debates on 'inclusion', a subject that we will return to at the end of the next section.

7 Disscussion

The complex social constructions of 'health', 'literacy' and 'childhood' have been scrutinised in this chapter, in terms of the different pathways that can be followed in analyzing them. Current discussions of health literacy in childhood—that are oriented primarily towards public health, that equate literacy with information processing and that rank health literacy along a vertical axis from low (inadequate) to high (adequate)—have been questioned in the present chapter. Instead we have argued for broad perspectives on children's health literacy that draw on the sociology of childhood as well as on the new literacy studies that position 'language' and 'meaning-making' more centrally within literacy than 'information', that emphasize literacy events and the related social practices, and that include case studies of children's health literacy to enable us to understand different contexts and that do not rank children's health literacy in a simple one-dimensional hierarchy.

The narrow approach measures health literacy by 'administering' questionnaires, and then ranking individuals on a hierarchical axis based on their answers and with the use of quantitative techniques. Quantitative research based on sound questionnaires can be very helpful, but there is a clear need for a complementary understanding of the existing competencies of children (and adults) that are independent of their existing shortcomings in some health-related competencies. Such respectful approaches recognize the resources of the disadvantaged and provide a basis for alternative policy approaches. People—including children—can only exercise health literacy when opportunities to engage in health-related activity are combined with participation in everyday decision-making.

We have therefore drawn attention to perspectives on health literacy practices in everyday life as a continuous interaction between personal and societal habits and norms, individual competences and skills, as well as the different opportunities individuals have in the light of unequal living conditions and resources. We argue that available health literacy concepts lack a sufficiently comprehensive approach to the unique characteristics of children, including their needs, social position and perceptions of health (and the same criticism can be applied to available health literacy concepts in relation to the unique characteristics of various groups of adults). Future research efforts should strive towards health literacy concepts for childhood that represent children's viewpoints and that are sensitive to their social worlds and life circumstances.

One promising approach—we have maintained—is to recognize children as active citizens in the context of health literacy, within a children's rights perspective that balances children's participation and their right to protection. This approach is very compatible with the new sociological paradigm that presents children as social agents and co-constructors of their worlds (e.g. Bühler-Niederberger 2011). Current understandings in the sociology of childhood could help health literacy researchers understand everyday actions by children that maintain or impede their physical, mental, social and emotional health and well-being. Our arguments for attention to and recognition of children as social actors within health literacy urge that rethinking health literacy in childhood should be the start to rethinking health literacy more generally, including for adults and especially for adults who experience relative powerlessness within their socio-political contexts.

Children tend to be excluded from the analysis of their health literacy, although they are major actors who can really tell us about their world, which in turn we need to learn about and to conceptualise, to operationalise, to measure and to assess within our studies. Health literacy should enable children to develop the competencies to decide and act for themselves which help them to identify a personal idea of a good life as well as to cope with challenges that are part of their socialization. This way, we will recognize children as persons and citizens, and we will further recognize that people in general need support to develop personal ideas of a good life and to exercise their right to participate in decisions that affect their lives.

Here, the understanding of 'citizenship' will have to go much deeper than as a synonym for 'becoming a good and responsible person' that puts pressure on individuals. Instead, acknowledging that children are citizens is an important part of striving to create spaces for children to pursue their own understanding of the world, whereby they are inspired to approach their own health and that of others in an informed, empowered and ethically responsible way (Paakkari and Paakkari 2012). Children should be encouraged to reflect upon the validity and reliability of health information, both in terms of sources and content, and to relate information to their individual situations, needs and beliefs, exploring the possibilities for acting upon information in a health promoting manner.

Debates around health literacy therefore need to move on from questions that ask: "When do we consider an adult to be health literate?", and relatedly: "When do we consider a child to be health literate?" Wider questions should also be addressed, such as 'When do we consider multidisciplinary research to be health literate, i.e. literate in the realities of people's—including children's—everyday lives?' and 'When do we consider policy makers to be health literate in terms of grasping the daily realities of different groups of citizens, including children?' Health literacy on these lines would mean that policy makers and multidisciplinary researchers engage in self-education and co-learning with different categories of citizens, including co-learning with children (to return to the adaptation of Schön's work by George 2013, cited earlier). The answer to both questions will raise issues of inclusion—*not* 'inclusion' in the sense of programmes that ensure that everyone adheres to certain dominant norms about 'healthy behaviour,' but inclusion through research that explores different children's and adults' conceptions and experiences of what is healthy for them, and through social policies that are based on such research.

8   Conclusion

When Johnson writes about 'the collisions that happen when different fields of expertise converge in some shared physical or intellectual space' (2010, p. 163), he does not refer only to formal spaces but highlights environments where ideas can be 'tossed around... in a more playful setting' (*op. cit.*, p. 169). As an example of 'new hubs for intellectual collaboration,' (*op. cit.*, p. 228), he draws attention to the role that coffee houses played during the Enlightenment. This chapter can be said to apply Johnson's 'coffee house model of creativity' (*op. cit.*, p. 169) to a pre-conference that provided 'a cross-disciplinary coffeehouse environment' (*op. cit.*, p. 171) to generate the ideas and arguments, presented above. In closing then, it seems appropriate to cite Johnson's advice: 'frequent coffee houses and other liquid networks; follow the links; let others build on your ideas...' (*op. cit.*, p. 246).

References

Alanen, L. (1988). Rethinking childhood. *Acta Sociologica, 31*(1), 53–67.
Alanen, L., Brooker, L., & Mayall, B. (2015). *Childhood with Bourdieu*. London: Palgrave Macmillan.
Antonovsky, A. (1987). *Unraveling The Mystery of Health*. San Francisco: Jossey Bass.
Bauer, U. (2012). *Sozialisation und Ungleichheit. Eine Hinführung*. Wiesbaden: VS Verlag.

Bibou-Nakou, I. (2004). Helping teachers to help children living with a mentally ill parent. Teachers' Perceptions on Identification and Policy Issues. *School Psychology International, 24*(1), 42–58.

Bluebond-Langner, M. (1978). *The private worlds of dying children.* Princeton: Princeton University Press.

Borzekowski, D. L. (2009). Considering children and health literacy: a theoretical approach. *Pediatrics, 124*(3), 282–288.

Brady, G., Lowe, P., & Olin Lauritzen, S. (2015). Connecting a sociology of childhood perspective with the study of child health, illness and wellbeing: Introduction. *Sociology of Health & Illness, 37*(2), 173–183.

Brockmann, E. (2014). *Kinder psychisch erkrankter Eltern in der Schule.* Katalog der Deutschen Nationalbibliothek. http://d-nb.info/1069092843/34. (last accessed 12 Aug. 2015).

Bröder, J., Okan, O., Bauer, U., Schlupp, S., Bollweg, T., Saboga-Nunes, L., et al. (2017). Health literacy in childhood and youth: A systematic review of definitions and models. *BMC Public Health, 17*(1), 1–25.

Bruland, D., Pinheiro, P., Bittligmayer, U. H., & Bauer, U. (2016). "Teacher's Mental Health Literacy": Forschungsprojekt zur schulischen Gesundheitsförderung von Kindern psychisch erkrankter Eltern. *Prävention und Gesundheitsförderung, 11*(2), 73–79.

Bühler-Niederberger, D. (2010). Introduction: Childhood Sociology – Defining the State of the Art and Ensuring Reflection. *Current Sociology, 58*(2), 155–164.

Bühler-Niederberger, D. (2011). *Lebensphase Kindheit: Theoretische Ansätze, Akteure und Handlungsräume.* Weinheim: Beltz Juventa.

Denzin, N. K. (2009). *Childhood socialization.* New Brunswick and London: Aldine Transaction.

Fairbrother, H., Curtis, P., & Goyden, E. (2016). Making health information meaningful: Children's health literacy practices. *SSM-Population Health, 2,* 476–484.

George, S. (2013). *Children As Self-Educators, Parents As Coaches: Disciplined Freedom And Democratic Spaces.* Working Paper Series 2012–2013/ III. University of Delhi. http://www.du.ac.in/du/uploads/Academics/centres_institutes/13032013_DSkothari_Working_paper_3.pdf (last accessed 22 June 2016).

Gerdes, J., Bittlingmayer, U. H., Osipov, I., Sahrai, F., Faßhauer, U., Riegel, C., & Immerfall, S. (2016). *Die Entwicklung individueller Life Skills im Schuljahresverlauf.* Freiburg: University of Education, Freiburg, https://www.ph-freiburg.de/fileadmin/dateien/fakultaet3/sozialwissenschaft/Soziologie/LiST_2._Zwischenbericht_Life_Skills-Entwicklung_im_Schuljahresverlauf.pdf (last accessed 23 June 2016).

Grusec, J. E., & Hastings, P. D. (Eds.). (2006). *Handbook of Socialization. Theory and Research.* New York: The Guilford Press.

Huijsmans, R., George, S., Gigengack, R., & Evers, S. (2014). Theorizing Age and Generation in Development: A relational approach. *European Journal of Development Research, 26*(7), 163–174.

Hurrelmann, K., Bauer, U., Grundmann, M., & Walper, S. (Eds.). (2015). *Handbuch Sozialisationsforschung.* Weinheim: Beltz-Juventa.

James, A., & Prout, A. (1990). *Constructing and reconstructing childhood: Contemporary issues in the sociological study of childhood.* London: Falmer Press.

Johnson, S. (2010). *Where good ideas come from: The natural history of innovation*. New York: Riverhead Books.

Kahlert, R., & Merchant, A. (2015). *Methods in health literacy as applied to children and young people: Focus group research report*. Vienna: Ludwig Boltzmann Health Promotion Institute.

Kennedy, E., Dunphy, E., Dwyer, B., Hayes, G., McPhillips, T., Marsh, J., O'Connor, M., & Shiel. G. (2012). *Literacy in early childhood and primary education (3–8 years). NCCA Research Report No. 15.* Dublin: National Council for Curriculum and Assessment.

Mayall, B. (Ed.). (1994). *Children's childhoods: Observed and experienced.* London: Falmer Press.

Mayall, B. (1998). Towards a sociology of child health. *Sociology of Health & Illness, 20*(3), 269–288.

Okan, O., Lopes, E., Bollweg, T.M., Bröder, J., Messer, M., Bruland, D., Bond, E., Carvalho, G.,S., Sorensen, K., Saboga-Nunes, L., Levin-Zamir, D., Sahrai, D., Bittlingmayer, U.H., Pelikan, J,. Thomas, M., Kessl, F., Bauer, U., & Pinheiro, P. (2018). Generic health literacy measurement instruments for children and adolescents: a systematic review of the literature, *BMC Public Health, 18*(1), 1–19.

Paakkari, L., & Paakkari, O. (2012). Health literacy as a learning outcome in schools. *Health Education, 112*(2), 133–152.

Papen, U. (2009). Literacy, Learning and Health – A social practices view of health literacy. *Literacy and Numeracy Studies, 16*(2) and *17*(1), 19–34.

Perry, K. H. (2012). What is literacy? – A critical overview of sociocultural perspectives. *Journal of Language and Literacy Education, 8*(1), 50–71.

Pinheiro, P., Bittlingmayer, U.H., Bröder, J., Okan, O., & Bauer, U. (2018). *A review of health literacy of children and young people: definitions, interpretations, and implications for future research and practice initiatives.* Aberystwyth, A Child's World International Conference.

Pleasant, A. (2014). Advancing Health Literacy Measurement: A Pathway to Better Health and Health System Performance. *Journal of Health Communication, 19*(12), 1481–1496.

Prout, A. (2011). Taking a step away from modernity: Reconsidering the new sociology of childhood. *Global Studies of Childhood, 1*(1), 4–14.

Qvortrup, J., Bardy, M., Sgritta, G., & Wintersberger, H. (Eds.). (1994). *Childhood matters: Social theory, practice and politics.* Avebury: Aldershot.

Reupert, A., & Mayberry, D. (2007). Strategies and issues in supporting children whose parents have a mental illness within the school system. *School Psychology International, 28*(2), 195–205.

Koch-Institut, Robert (Ed.). (2008). *Lebensphasenspezifische Gesundheit von Kindern und Jugendlichen in Deutschland.* Berlin: Robert Koch-Institut.

Ryan, P. J. (2008). How new is the "new" social study of childhood? The myth of a paradigm shift. *Journal of Interdisciplinary History, 38*(4), 553–576.

Schön, D. A. (1987). *Educating the Reflective Practitioner.* San Francisco: Jossey-Bass.

Sijthoff, S. (2014). Exercising rights and active citizenship: Children, physical activity and learning – in the classroom and beyond. In M. Thomas (Ed.), *A Child's world: Contemporary issues in education* (pp. 39–58). Aberystwyth: Aberystwyth University.

Street, B. (1984). *Literacy in theory and practice.* New York: Cambridge University Press.

Street, B. (2003). What's "new" in New Literacy Studies? Critical approaches to literacy in theory and practice. *Current Issues in Comparative Education, 5*(2), 77–91.

Weiner, W. J. (1993). A moment's monument: The psychology of keeping a diary. In R. Josselson & A. Lieblich (Eds.), *The narrative study of lives* (Vol. One). Newbury Park: Sage Publications.

Mental Health Literacy—Do We Need Another Health Literacy Concept?

Dirk Bruland and Patricia Graf

1   Introduction

Worldwide, mental illnesses account for about 14% of the burden of disease (Prince et al. 2007). The relevance of this topic is going to increase in the next years if one considers the forecast by the WHO predicting that e.g. depression will become the most common illness in the Western world by the year 2030 (WHO 2011). Due to this, mental disease prevention is very important and, regarding the WHO's definition of health, mental health promotion is necessary as well to reach a 'state of complete physical, mental and social well-being' (WHO 1948). Therefore, it is important to include mental health explicitly when discussing Health including Health Literacy. There are different definitions of Health Literacy, the most common are:

> *"Health Literacy has been defined as the cognitive and social skills which determine the motivation and ability of individuals to gain access to understand and use information in ways which promote and maintain good health. ... Health Literacy means more than being able to read pamphlets and successfully make appointments. By improving people's access to health information and their capacity to use it effectively, health literacy is critical to empowerment"* (WHO 1998).

D. Bruland (✉)
FH Bielefeld University of Applied Sciences, Bielefeld, Germany
e-mail: dirk.bruland@fh-bielefeld.de

P. Graf
Faculty of Educational Sciences, Bielefeld University, Freiburg, Germany
e-mail: patricia.wahl@uni-bielefeld.de

> *"Health literacy is linked to literacy and it entails people's knowledge, motivation and competences to access, understand, appraise and apply information to take decisions in everyday life in terms of healthcare, disease prevention and health promotion to maintain and improve quality of life during the life course"* (Sørensen et al. 2012, p. 3).

Despite the vagueness of the Health Literacy concept and the great variety of definitions, the underlying understanding of illness and health often remains unclear (Sørensen et al. 2012; Malloy-Weir et al. 2016), especially the relevance of mental health. Sometimes authors refer explicitly to mental health as a state of well-being, but this component often remains underrepresented. Jorm (2015) clearly points out: "First, the health literacy field ignored mental disorders. ... The second reason was that the mental health field ignored health literacy" (p. 1166). A relevant factor for the promotion of mental health and the prevention of mental disorders could be the concept of mental health literacy (MHL), which was first defined by Jorm et al. in 1997. In this article, Anthony Jorm's concept of mental health literacy is introduced and discussed with regard to its meaning for and relation to general health literacy. For this, we first introduce in the definition of Mental Health Literacy the way it is measured, staying close to the original work by Jorm et al. (1997). As a next step we show the understanding of prevention to discuss open questions concerning Mental Health Literacy and the relationship between Health Literacy and Mental Health Literacy.

2 Mental Health Literacy

In reference to Health Literacy, Jorm et al. (1997) defined the term Mental Health Literacy as

> *"knowledge and beliefs about mental disorders which aid their recognition, management or prevention"* and includes *"the ability to recognize specific disorders; knowing how to seek mental health information; knowledge of risk factors and causes, of self-treatments, and of professional help available; and attitudes that promote recognition and appropriate help-seeking"* (p. 182).

Jorm later described mental health literacy as "knowledge that benefits the mental health of a person or others including: knowledge of how to prevent a mental disorder; recognition of disorders when developing; knowledge of effective self-help strategies for mild-to-moderate problems; and first aid skills to help others" (Kutcher and Wei 2016, p. 155).

The basic idea of Mental Health Literacy was to increase the general public's knowledge and skills in particular with regard to identification and management in dealing with mental disorders (Jorm 2015). Up to then the focus in dealing with mental disorders had usually been on professionals in the primary health care system (especially GPs). The high prevalence of mental disorders is cited as the reason for targeting the general population. Jorm et al. (1997) assumed that everyone experiences some mental illness in the course of his or her life, either by being affected themselves, or through contact with others who are affected. Therefore, Mental Health Literacy is not limited to one's own person, it is linked to the possibility of action to benefit one's own mental health as well as that of others. In addition, there is a lack of disease awareness on the part of the individual that he/she has a mental disorder and the majority does not take up therapy offers or rather take a long time for seeking professional help (Gulliver et al. 2010). So Jorm (2011) reports "evidence that people with a mental disorder are more likely to seek professional help if someone else suggests it" (p. 5). The concept of Mental Health Literacy implied raising the skills for management and help seeking in the society/social environment with the aim for early recognition of mental disorders as well as a previous access to health care systems and interventions.

Mental health literacy usually has its theoretical place assigned as part functional Health Literacy. In addition to reading and calculating skills knowledge about psychiatric diseases and their treatment was added (Mårtensson and Hensing 2012). Like Health Literacy, it also refers to health-related knowledge and seeking health-related information, without evidence whether knowledge actually leads to better action. However, it is assumed that, as with Health Literacy, raising Mental Health Literacy enables a person to use resources and to make healthy choices in everyday life for oneself, and especially for others. See Table 1 for a comparison of both concepts. It is considered an argument in favour of a specific mental health concept within Health Literacy, that a very different understanding of health is needed regarding the special symptoms and consequences of mental illnesses compared to those of purely physical illnesses (Jorm 2015). There are different help systems and existing legal bases that, for example, enable the use of services like psychotherapy. Another aspect is that interventions have to be evaluated using domain-specific assessments that are relevant for the field of mental health.

Table 1 Comparison Health Literacy and Mental Health Literacy; own compilation

	Health Literacy	**Mental Health Literacy**
Definition	Functional Health Literacy: the degree to which individuals have the capacity to obtain, process and understand basic health information and services needed to make appropriate health decisions (means mostly to read and understand health information).(National Action Plan to Improve Health Literacy, U.S. Department of Health and Human Services 2010) Expanded Health Literacy Health literacy is linked to literacy and it entails people's knowledge, motivation and competences to access, understand, appraise and apply information to take decisions in everyday life in terms of health-care, disease prevention and health promotion to maintain and improve quality of life during the life course. (Sørensen et al. 2012)	1) knowledge and beliefs about mental disorders which aid their recognition, management or prevention. Mental health literacy includes the ability to recognize specific disorders; knowing how to seek mental health information; knowledge of risk factors and causes, of self-treatments, and of professional help available; and attitudes that promote recognition and appropriate help-seeking (Jorm et al. 1997)
Level	(mostly) Individual Level	(mostly) Population / interpersonal Level
Aim	(in reference to functional level) Understand mathematical concepts (for example sugar levels in food) such as probability and risk Navigate the healthcare system, including filling out complex forms and locating providers and services Share personal information, such as health history, with providers Engage in self-care and chronic-disease management (U.S. Department of Health and Human Service, Fact Sheet) and in an expanding understanding: increase the personal abilities to navigate the health care setting	Improving knowledge and beliefs towards mental illness & facilitate access to treatment

(continued)

Table 1 (continued)

	Health Literacy	Mental Health Literacy
Background	Health literacy is a core competence and a high level of health literacy is considered of substantial benefit for maintaining one's health (Berkman et al. 2011). Health literacy describes a person's knowledge and competence to meet the complex demands of health in modern society. (Sørensen et al. 2012)	Because of the high prevalence of mental disorders over the lifetime, it has been argued that everyone will either develop one of these disorders themselves or have close contact with someone else who does. Consequently, members of the public need to have some knowledge to allow them to recognize, prevent and seek early help for mental disorders. They also need to have the skills to support other people in their social network who develop a mental disorder.
Application	General (some special Health Literacy like Digital Health Literacy), mostly not disease-specific	Focus on mental health problems [but it seems that the focus is only on mental **diseases not** on mental **health**- (mostly no specific mental diseases)]
Assessment	Functional: REALM, TOFLA; Complex: HLS-EU-Q, HLQ	MHL-Q: Structured interviews using case vignettes (cases developed based on medical DSM-Symptoms)

3 Measuring MHL and Results of the First Assessment

Measurement

There are different questionnaires to measure MHL, such as the Mental Health Knowledge Schedule (MAKS), the World Psychiatric Association (WPA) "Open the Doors" (WPA-OD) questionnaire, the Depression Literacy Scale (DLS), the Knowledge about Schizophrenia Questionnaire (KASQ), the Schizophrenia Knowledge Questionnaire (SKQ), and the 'In Our Voices' (IOV) knowledge measure. Still the most used questionnaire is the Mental Health Literacy Questionnaire (MHLQ) by Jorm and colleagues (1997) (Wei et al. 2015). Because of this, we focus on the original MHLQ (Jorm et al. 1997). The MHL-Q starts with one of six different versions of case vignettes. Every version focusses on a different mental disease; depression, depression with suicidal thoughts, early schizophrenia, chronic schizophrenia, social phobia and PTSD. All vignettes were written to satisfy the diagnostic criteria according to the classification system DSM. Respondents were also randomly assigned to receive either male ("John") or female ("Mary") versions of the vignette. The names John and Mary are used because they are the most common names in Australia and are meant not to evoke cultural associations.

Example

> *"John is 30 years old. He has been feeling unusually sad and miserable for the last few weeks. Even though he is tired all the time, he has trouble sleeping nearly every night. John doesn't feel like eating and has lost weight. He can't keep his mind on his work and puts off making decisions. Even day-to-day tasks seem too much for him. This has come to the attention of his boss, who is concerned about John's lowered productivity"* (Jorm et al. 1997).

After being shown the vignette, respondents were asked two open-ended questions:

'What would you say, if anything, is wrong with John/Mary?' and 'How do you think John/Mary could best be helped?'.

The rest of the interview consisted of questions to determine the respondents' knowledge of and views about:

- Various people who could help (whether each category of person was likely to be helpful, harmful, or neither, for the person described);
- A range of possible treatments and non-pharmacological treatments (whether each treatment was likely to be helpful, harmful, or neither, for the person described);
- Knowledge of likely prognoses;
- Knowledge of risk factors; and
- Beliefs associated with stigma and discrimination.

Results of the first assessment

The aim of the first study on MHL was to measure the public's recognition of mental disorders and their beliefs about the effectiveness of various treatments. First results are that for many members of the public it is hard to recognize specific mental disorders. Laymen differ from mental health experts mostly in their beliefs about causes and effective treatments (Jorm 2011), which will be shown by two examples: a) For depression, more than half of laymen find vitamins, minerals, tonics or herbal medicines are helpful (about 57% of respondents). b) For the schizophrenia vignette, antidepressants were regarded as helpful by 38% of respondents, followed by vitamins and minerals (34%) and antipsychotics (23%). Regarding the results of the questionnaire Jorm (2000) comes to the conclusion:

> *"The public's belief about medication is in sharp contrast to both the evidence from randomised controlled trials and the views of mental health professionals that antidepressant and antipsychotic medications are effective. The public's negative views about psychotropic medication also contrast with their own positive views about medication for common physical disorders"* (p. 397).

This result has still been confirmed over time (Jorm 2011): "Surveys of public beliefs about professionals and treatments have been carried out in a range of countries and show that there are sometimes major discrepancies between public and professional views" (p. 3). The conclusion concerning Mental Health Literacy is that it should be increased among the public.

Measurement critics

The measurement has not remained without discussion. There are two main aspects a) using case vignettes and b) scientific standards. a) Case vignettes have advantages and disadvantages, which can be seen in Table 2.

b) In their survey study on measuring instruments for Mental Health Literacy O'Connor, Casey and Clough (2014) come to the conclusion that most of the studies and measurement instruments included

> *"failed to reported detailed information about the sample, measure development and testing to demonstrate the psychometric properties of their tool. There are substantial limitations in current ability to measure Mental Health Literacy and there is significant scope for the development and evaluation of psychometrically robust measures that assess the relevant attributes of MHL"* (p. 197).

O'Connor and Casey (2015) developed a new scale-based measure of mental health literacy, the MHLS. This instrument demonstrated good internal and test-retest reliability, but this tool must still prove its worth in (research) practice.

As with Health Literacy questionnaires, there are similar critiques, mainly concerning the HLS-EU. The most frequent criticism is that the questionnaire is not valid (e.g. Steckelberg and Meyer 2017). The kind of self-evaluation in this questionnaire must highly correlate with self-confidence (which is not assessed) and could be a major problem (bias). It is not clear how levels of Health Literacy (good or bad) are constructed—which is similar to the MHL-Q. Although there is much criticism regarding the MHL-Q by Jorm et al. (1997) discussion about case vignettes, it must be taken into account that this questionnaire has been tested in practice, is widely used and therefore has a high comparability of results.

Table 2   (Dis-)advantages of case-vignettes; own compilation based on Leighton (2010)

Pro	Contra
• makes abstract concepts such as mental health real	• using hypothetical situations designed to elicit assessment of possible responses raises questions as to how far one can generalize about normative beliefs or draw conclusions about respondents' own behaviour from this type of data
• A method of introducing sensitive topics which respondents might otherwise find difficult to broach	• their relative inability to capture the complex factors that influence attitudes
• They do not require participants to have indepth knowledge of topics and provides a focus for those without experience	• responses may not indicate with complete accuracy how respondents will act in real-life situations, therefore their practical relevance may be both unclear and limited
• They offer a way both of asking questions concretely and of distancing them from personal experience	• However, it is argued that social researchers cannot claim to access individuals' internal psychological beliefs. Instead, what they can justifiably lay claim to is verbal or written accounts of what is believed. Thus, the focus needs to be on respondents' accounts, rather than on their beliefs.
• They are a useful tool to highlight adolescents' own subjective definitions, meanings and ideas	• Finally, it is recommended that a three-pronged approach to establishing internal validity of vignettes: They are developed from the literature or based on clinical cases, submitted to a panel of experts for comment, and pretested to remove ambiguous questions.
• Participants generate their own responses	
• Some studies have concluded that people respond to vignettes in much the same way as they would if faced with a real life situation and that respondents are less likely to give socially acceptable responses than if asked directly	

The conducted studies show that the MHL-Q questionnaire can visualize knowledge and attitudes which hinder the recognition and management of mental health problems and confirm that mental health literacy can be improved (Jorm 2011).

Qualitative measurement of Mental Health Literacy
Little is known about measuring Mental Health Literacy using qualitative methods. By means of a contemporary secondary analysis Coe (2009) evaluated data from focus groups to review the answers regarding the MHL-dimensions.

"The results reveal that qualitative data added depth to what was known previously and provided a range of new insights into Mental Health Literacy. There are challenges about recognizing symptoms as they emerge, compared with 'with hindsight'; there is a subtle balance between stigma and barriers to help seeking; accumulated adversity is perceived to be a key risk factor; coping strategies and stigma are crosscutting themes; the general practitioner has significant influence in facilitating access to appropriate support" (Coe 2009, p. 34).

This approach seems to be very useful but using qualitative methods for measuring Mental Health Literacy is still an underestimated approach in measuring Mental Health Literacy (but this, it seems, is also the case with Health Literacy).

4   Prevention and Intervention

Jorm (2011) stated very clearly:

"Undoubtedly, the least developed area of mental health literacy is the area of prevention. A possible contributing factor is that we know less about what are the major modifiable risk factors for mental disorders than we know for cancer, heart disease, and diabetes. The one major risk factor that is known is traumatic life events, but reducing these is a social goal in its own right and often difficult to achieve. Nevertheless, there are modifiable risk factors for mental disorders that the public needs to know about. An important example is the association between cannabis use and risk of psychosis. ... Other examples concern the role of parenting in mental disorders. Parents need to know that a range of parenting behaviors affect the risk of their adolescent children misusing alcohol and other substances. There was agreement between young people and professionals about a range of prevention strategies: physical activity, keeping contact with family and friends, avoiding use of substances, and making time for relaxing activities. ... These findings show that there is fertile ground for preventive action by the public. However, in contrast to the situation with major physical diseases, nothing is known about what members of the public do in practice for prevention of mental disorders" (p 7).

Regarding this understanding of prevention there are different continuations leading to a) practical implementation regarding professionals and families (Schulze et al. 2019) b) deviant understandings and c) new MHL concepts.

a) Challenges with the Mental Health Literacy concept depend on different social contexts and professional conditions where this concept was used. There are different considerations on how the concept should be adapted for certain fields (families with a mentally ill parent, social workers, teachers), mainly how much and what needs to be known as well as the influence of organizations (Schulze et al. 2019).

b) Mental Health Literacy is not seen as an independent concept but rather as a relevant resource for processes like empowerment. In this way there are many possibilities to promote individual resources as well as resources in the social system (or public) and to shift Mental Health Literacy closer to prevention research (Wahl and Lenz 2016).

c) A new MHL concept was developed by the Canadian researcher Kutcher. The concept is close to Jorm et al. (1997) including understanding mental disorders and their treatments as well as enhancing help-seeking efficacy. In addition, the concept includes understanding how to obtain and maintain good mental health and decreasing stigma related to mental disorders (Kutcher et al. 2016). This definition has more relation to prevention and includes the discussion about how to prevent mental disorders in a way that is good for oneself, which is mostly used for school interventions. For Health Literacy health promotion and prevention are mostly taken into account. The WHO stated at the 7th Global Conference on Health Promotion that health education leads to Health Literacy, "which aims to influence not only individual lifestyle decisions, but also raises awareness of the determinants of health, and encourages individual and collective actions which may lead to a modification of these determinants."

5   Interventions

Interventions are hard to explain for Mental Health Literacy as well as for Health Literacy. The question is, what are Health Literacy or Mental Health Literacy interventions? Mainly all health related interventions focus on dealing with information and increase the knowledge and/or the skills for dealing with health related issues. Health Literacy interventions, which use the term health literacy, are very often related to thematic domains like diabetes, physical activity or nutrition. Mental Health Literacy is more targeted than Health Literacy interventions. The most far reaching are Mind-Matters and Beyond Blue.

Beyond Blue is a well-known institution in Australia. It aims to raise knowledge and change attitudes in the public concerning mental diseases like depression and suicide. The intervention consists in raising awareness with public activity like posters, advertising on television and in print media, offering educational videos, and having a website with a lot of information. There are a lot of partnerships with health services, schools, workplaces, universities, media and community organisations and service users participating in Beyond Blue.[1]

Mental Health Literacy in young people and their supporters (mostly teachers) is an important area of intervention. Hence, MindMatters aims to raise knowledge about mental health and managing mental health problems in secondary schools. MindMatters provides materials to schools in Australia, but the use of these is not standardised. Schools are encouraged to make the materials fit in with their own curriculum. In this way mental health literacy should be increased by the teachers and students themselves.[2] In a similar way Kutcher developed a school-based mental health literacy intervention for students and teachers in Canada with the aim to provide a good "pathway to care".[3]

---

6   Discussion

So far, we introduced the Mental Health Literacy concept and referred to Health Literacy. In the following final chapter, we will discuss questions that remain unanswered regarding the Mental Health Literacy concept on which we will focus first. In a second step we will discuss Mental Health Literacy with regard to its meaning for and relation to general health literacy.

Open questions

First, Mental Health Literacy is assigned to be a part of functional Health Literacy. Medical and disease-oriented knowledge is a key aspect in this understanding of Mental Health Literacy. For example, the MHL-Q is based on a medical perspective and compares results concerning the public's belief with evidence from randomised controlled trials and the views of mental health professionals. There are two questions arising from that point: a) There is no known discussion about how much mental health literacy is sufficient for laymen. For example, teachers often have contact to people with mental health problems (children,

---

[1]For more information: https://www.beyondblue.org.au/home for adults and for children https://www.youthbeyondblue.com/.

[2]For more information: https://www.mindmatters.edu.au/.

[3]For more information: http://teenmentalhealth.org.

parents as well as colleagues), but they are usually not trained to work with persons suffering from mental health issues. In practice, other things become more crucial than to know about diagnoses, causes, risk factors or management/self-treatments, that is to say they have to recognize something is wrong and to be a gatekeeper to mental health professionals. The work of Schulze et al. (2018) shows impressively how Mental Health Literacy depends on the scope of professional roles and framework conditions. b) Following up on this, the aim that the general population be better informed about mental health issues will indisputably lead to better management of mental health issues. However, can this also lead to a 'psychologisation' of society as a side effect in a way that the behaviour of people would be directly linked to a mental health issue? If teachers e.g. are more sensitized to mental health issues, this is good at first glance because if the teacher recognizes that something is wrong, he/she will react to this. But what if they know more about diagnoses, will they more often reduce behaviours to medical causes instead of viewing them in the light of normal reactions to living conditions, e. g in case of the sadness of a student over a little time or the "strange behaviour" of parents? A worker in a child and adolescent psychiatry expressed the view that if the system is overloaded, children often get transferred to his institution sooner because "… with the diagnosis you can work with pills. If the young people are discharged, they can be described as mental ill…" (Bruland 2017, p. 136). This is a very functional perspective, and it has to be discussed, how much knowledge is appropriate for which area and to look at the specific area. Basically, it must be discussed whether knowledge leads to action and/or seeking help? And if it does, how can this concept be protected from being misused as purely an activation method? In a study of our own, a lot of people with mental health issues stated they knew about professional help but did not use it in order to maintain the family situation and avoid stigma (Bruland et al. 2019). It is an ethical question, who and at which point may interfere with the rights of another person and act as a guardian for them (of course if there is no sign of harm or aggression towards themselves or others).

Apart from that, a typical question arises, how we can uncover blind spots? Frameworks of specific areas have already been mentioned, but there is also a connection between health and social conditions. For example, social inequality is not explicitly evident in the mental health literacy concept. Those aspects are important to make political changes without the medicalization of society. To uncover blind spots, it would also be necessary to enhance the discussion of a critical mental health literacy. Graham, Killoran and Parekh (2016) stated that critical mental health literacy could encourage communities "to new ways to (re) conceptualize, (re)discuss, and, ultimately, (re)think" (p. 9) mental health and wellbeing. Following the description of the Canadian Alliance on Mental Illness and Mental Health (CAMIMH 2007), critical mental health literacy could be developed through education to critically appraise information of relevance to health and to develop skills to critically analyse and use information to mobilize people for social and political action, as well as individual action. Professionals in different areas (and people concerned) could question, examine, and transform their practice rather than be only compliant with mental health information. Community empowerment can be seen as an important factor in health promotion as well as in health literacy. It could be in Mental Health Literacy as well, including the development of strategies adequate to the practice field, "the development of a broad range of strategies to enhance personal skills and capacities for informed choice, and critical analysis and collective empowerment for action on the social and environmental determinants of mental health. It would support social as well as individual benefits, building social capital, and promoting social and economic development" (CAMIMH 2007, p. 36). So, the open question is, how can users of the systems participate by understanding the mental health literacy concept and how can the systems learn from their users e.g. what is helpful to increase mental health, wellbeing and quality of life in communities?

Do we need another (mental) health literacy concept?

Looking at the definition and state of the art in mental health literacy research it is an independent domain, with only little relation to Health Literacy (Jorm 2015). HL focuses explicitly on physical health, does not deny the psychological aspect, but has gaps in its theoretical design and empirical findings in connection with mental illness, which makes a special understanding of Health Literacy for mental diseases necessary. Following Jorm (2015), we can therefore, answer the question: "Do we need another health literacy concept?" with a resounding yes. In our contribution it can be seen how mental health literacy has a special view on psychiatric diseases and their treatment, which cannot be taken into account in such a way by research on general health literacy.

However, looking at the open questions above Mental Health Literacy can benefit a lot from Health Literacy knowledge and research results. Maybe Mental Health Literacy is more similar to complex Health Literacy than would appear at first glance, and the open question can be answered regarding health literacy research. Mackert et al. (2015) called for a "general" Health Literacy perspective rather than a fragmentation of literacies (e.g. specific illnesses/conditions, specific populations, different information channels).

"As a result, numerous definitions and measures of health literacy exist. This fragmentation and inconsistency create a barrier to conceptualizing, measuring, and

understanding health literacy across health domains and fields. Improving the understanding of health literacy in one context is less helpful if the research cannot more broadly inform knowledge in contexts" (Mackert et al. 2015, p. 1161).

We come to the conclusion that we need a Mental Health Literacy concept for the specific conditions of the mental health domains, but on the other hand we also need a broader understanding of mental health literacy to answer open question with good evidence. Based on the knowledge and experience with Mental Health Literacy, we bring up a definition of Mental Health Literacy to hopefully open a discussion in Mental Health Literacy. It is closer to Health Literacy, uses intersections of both domains and respects the special field of mental health:

Mental Health Literacy includes an individual's or a group's knowledge, attitudes, beliefs and competencies relevant to maintain, promote (or restore) mental health. Mental Health Literacy interacts with contextual factors like organizational, social and political conditions. Knowledge is understood as an awareness of oneself (self-reflexion) and others (empathy) and includes not merely knowledge about symptoms and diagnoses. Competencies that help promote mental health and deal with mental health issues are self-help strategies and first-aid interventions for others, formal and informal help-seeking as well as competencies to access, understand, appraise and apply mental health-related information.

References

Berkman, N. D., Sheridan, S. L., Donahue, K. E., Halpern, D. J., & Crotty, K. (2011). Low health literacy and health outcomes: An updated systematic review. *Annals of Internal Medicine, 155,* 97–107.

Bruland, D. (2017). Patientenorientierter Bedarf im Alltag der Kinder- und Jugendpsychiatrie. Eine empirisch explorierende Untersuchung zu pädagogischen Handlungsgrundlagen Sozialer Arbeit in der Kinder- und Jugendpsychiatrie. Bielefeld: Universität Bielefeld. https://pub.uni-bielefeld.de/record/2911896.

Bruland, D., Gross, E., Langer, S., & Wahl, P. (2019). Hilfe(auf)suchprozesse in von psychischen Gesundheitsproblemen eines Elternteiles betroffenen Familien. *Eine qualitative Studie zur Familienperspektive. Verhaltenstherapie mit Kindern und Jugendlichen - Zeitschrift für die psychosoziale Praxis, 15*(1):7–19.

CAMIMH – Canadian Alliance on Mental Illness and Mental Health (2007). MENTAL HEALTH LITERACY in Canada: Phase One Draft Report Mental Health Literacy Project. http://camimh.ca/wp-content/uploads/2012/04/Mental-Health-Literacy_-_Full-Final-Report_EN.pdf.

Coe, N. (2009). Critical evaluation of the mental health literacy framework using qualitative data. *The international journal of mental health promotion, 11*(4), 34–44.

Graham, D., Killoran I., & Parekh, G. (2016). Supporting students' mental health and emotional well-being in inclusive classrooms. In: Gordon, M. (Eds.), *Challenges surrounding the education of children with chronic diseases. A volume in the book series: Advances in early childhood and k-12 education.* IGI Global, Hershey PA, p. 86–116.

Gulliver, A., Griffiths, K.M., & Christensen H. (2010). Perceived barriers and facilitators to mental health help-seeking in young people: a systematic review BMC Psychiatry 10:113 https://bmcpsychiatry.biomedcentral.com/track/pdf/10.1186/1471-244X-10-113.

Jorm, A. F., Korten, A. E., Jacomb, P. A., Christensen, H., Rodgers, B., & Pollitt, P. (1997). "Mental health literacy": A survey of the public's ability to recognise mental disorders and their beliefs about the effectiveness of treatment. *Medical Journal of Australia, 166,* 182–186.

Jorm, A. F. (2000). Mental health literacy: Public knowledge and beliefs about mental disorders. *British Journal of Psychiatry, 177,* 396–401.

Jorm A. F. (2011). Mental health literacy: Empowering the community to take action for better mental health. American Psychologist. Advance online publication. https://doi.org/10.1037/a0025957.

Jorm, A. F. (2015). Why we need the concept of "Mental Health Literacy". *Health Communication, 30*(12), 1166–1168. https://doi.org/10.1080/10410236.2015.1037423.

Kutcher, S., Wei, Y., & Coniglio, C. (2016). Mental health literacy: Past, present, and future. *The Canadian Journal of Psychiatry, 61*(3), 154–158.

Leighton, S. (2010). Using a vignette-based questionnaire to explore adolescents' understanding of mental health issues. *Clinical Child Psychology and Psychiatry., 15*(2), 231–250.

Mackert, M., Champlin, S., Su, Z., & Guadagno, M. (2015). The many health literacies: Advancing research or fragmentation? *Health Communication, 30*(12), 1161–1165.

Malloy-Weir, L.J., Charles C., Gafni, A., & Entwistle, V. (2016). A review of health literacy: Definitions, interpretations, and implications for policy initiatives. *Journal of Public Health Policy, 37*(3), 334–352.

Mårtensson, L., & Hensing, G. (2012). Health literacy – a heterogeneous phenomenon: A literature review. *Scandinavian Journal of Caring Sciences, 26*(1), 151–160.

O'Connor, M., Casey, L., & Clough, B. (2014). Measuring mental health literacy – a review of scale-based measures. *Journal of Mental Health, 23*(4), 197–204.

O'Connor, M., & Casey, L. (2015). The Mental Health Literacy Scale (MHLS): A new scale-based measure of mental health literacy. *Psychiatry Research, 30,* 229(1–2), 511–516.

Prince, M., Patel, V., Saxena, S., Maj, M., Maselko, J., Phillips, M. R., et al. (2007). No health without mental health. *Lancet, 370*(9590), 859–877.

Schulze, K., Wahl, P., Bruland, D., Harsch, S., & Rehder, M. (2019). An empirical perspective on the concept of 'Mental Health Literacy' in the field of families with parental mental illness. In O. Okan, U. Bauer, D. Levin-Zamir, P. Pinheiro, & K. Sørensen (Eds.), *International handbook of health literacy research, practice and policy across the life-span.* Bristol: Policy Press Bristol University Press.

Sørensen, K., Van den Broucke, S., Fullam, J., Doyle, G., Pelikan, J., Slonska, Z., & Brand, H. (2012). Health literacy and public health: A systematic review and integration of definitions and models. *BMC Public Health, 72,* 80. https://bmcpublichealth.biomedcentral.com/track/pdf/10.1186/1471-2458-12-80.

Steckelberg, A., Meyer, G., & Mühlhauser, I. (2017). Questionnaire Should not Be Used any Longer Dtsch. *Ärzteblatt International, 114*(18), 330.

U.S. Department of Health and Human Services. (o. J.). Quick Guide to Health Literacy. https://health.gov/communication/literacy/quickguide/factsbasic.htm#one.

U.S. Department of Health and Human Services. (2010). National Action Plan to Improve Health Literacy. https://health.gov/communication/HLActionPlan/pdf/Health_Literacy_Action_Plan.pdf.

Wahl, P., & Lenz, A. (2016). Mental Health Literacy – Ein hilfreiches Konzept für die psychosoziale Praxis Verhaltenstherapie und psychosoziale Praxis, 48(4).

Wei, Y., McGrath, P. J., Hayden, J., & Kutcher, S. (2015). Mental health literacy measures evaluating knowledge, attitudes and help-seeking: A scoping review. *MC Psychiatry, 15*, 291–310. Advance online publication. https://doi.org/10.1186/s12888-015-0681-9.

World Health Organization – WHO. (1948). 'Constitution of WHO: principles'. http://www.who.int/about/mission/en/.

World Health Organization – WHO (1998). Health Promotion Glossary. http://www.who.int/healthpromotion/about/HPR%20Glossary%201998.pdf.

World Health Organization – WHO (2011). 'Global burden of mental disorders and the need for a comprehensive, coordinated response from health and social sectors at the country level'. http://apps.who.int/gb/ebwha/pdf_files/EB130/B130_9-en.pdf.

World Health Organization – WHO. (2009). 7th Global Conference on Health Promotion. Health Literacy Track. http://www.who.int/healthpromotion/conferences/7gchp/track2/en/.

Health Literacy and its Determinants in 11 and 12-year-old School Children in Germany

Agnes Santha, Uwe H. Bittlingmayer, Torsten M. Bollweg, Jürgen Gerdes, Orkan Okan, Gözde Ökcu, Paulo Pinheiro, Igor Osipov and Diana Sahrai

A. Santha (✉)
Faculty of Technical and Human Sciences, Sapientia Hungarian University of Transylvania, Tirgu Mures, Romania
e-mail: santhaagnes@ms.sapientia.ro

U. H. Bittlingmayer · J. Gerdes · G. Ökcu
Institute of Sociology, University of Education Freiburg (Germany), Freiburg, Germany
e-mail: uwe.bittlingmayer@ph-freiburg.de

J. Gerdes
e-mail: juergen.gerdes@ph-freiburg.de

G. Ökcu
e-mail: goezde.okcu@ph-freiburg.de

T. M. Bollweg · O. Okan · P. Pinheiro
Faculty of Educational Sciences, Bielefeld University, Bielefeld, Germany
e-mail: t.bollweg@uni-bielefeld.de

O. Okan
e-mail: orkan.okan@uni-bielefeld.de

P. Pinheiro
e-mail: paulo.pinheiro@uni-bielefeld.de

I. Osipov
Institute of Educational Research, Wuppertal University, Wuppertal, Germany
e-mail: osipov@uni-wuppertal.de

D. Sahrai
School of Education, University of Applied Sciences and Arts Northern Switzerland, Institute of Special Education and Psychology, Muttenz, Switzerland
e-mail: diana.sahrai@fhnw.ch

© The Editor(s) (if applicable) and The Author(s), under exclusive license to Springer Fachmedien Wiesbaden GmbH, part of Springer Nature 2021
L. A. Saboga-Nunes et al. (eds.), *New Approaches to Health Literacy*, Gesundheit und Gesellschaft, https://doi.org/10.1007/978-3-658-30909-1_10

183

1   Introduction

In the adult population, Germany ranks at about the middle of the European health literacy table, with almost 20% of its population having excellent and only 11% inadequate health literacy (HLS-EU Consortium 2012, p. 6). A more recent nationwide study found only 7.3% excellent health literate Germans, 9.7% with inadequate health literacy, and more than 50% with limited knowledge (Schaeffer et al. 2017). The consequences of low health literacy are harsh: poorer health status, less use of preventive services, increased hospitalization, longer recovery periods and increased mortality rates (Betz 2007; Wolf et al 2010). Furthermore, people with low health literacy have less knowledge about health outcomes, behaviours and health practices. In this way, health literacy is a contributing factor to health inequalities (Bravemen and Barclay 2009).

Based on a systematic review of the existing literature, DeWalt and Hink (2009) point out that children with low health literacy generally display worse health behaviours. Low health literacy in parents leads to detrimental health behaviour and poor health outcomes in their children. Both parent and child literacy are associated with important health outcomes, and health literacy is a mediating variable between parental and child health. Most importantly, lower-than-average health literacy among adolescents seems to be related to more risky health behaviours.

Health-related knowledge, attitudes and behaviours developed during childhood are increasingly being recognised as deeply rooted and responsible for resistance to change in later adulthood. Although there is some indication that health literacy might increase to some extent with age (Tiller et al. 2015), enhancing it is key to improving health-promoting behaviour from a young age (Schmidt et al. 2010). Studies measured child health literacy in different age groups and found that while child obesity, for instance, is mostly associated with parental factors, mostly with parental obesity and health literacy, adolescent obesity is strongly associated with the adolescents' own health literacy (Chari et al. 2013). So, starting from secondary school age, children increasingly take the responsibility for their own health. This fact justifies the necessity of dealing with child health literacy and its determinants. At ages 11 to 15 children and adolescents make the transition to self-management, and care responsibilities are also transferred from parents to the self-care of children, so child health literacy gains importance. What is more, children aged 11 to 12, precisely the age group in the focus of the present study, are already highly involved in their medical self-care (Alderson et al. 2006).

The focus of this paper is the health literacy of German children aged 11-12, pupils in the 6th grade. The central research question is to what extent do personal-structural (demographic, socio-economic) and situational (school-system-related) agents impact upon health literacy in children. The aim is not to predict, but to explain differences in health literacy across important inequality variables. A clear limitation of this study is that it does not allow inferences regarding health behaviours to be made from health literacy.

2 Data and Methods

In the year 2017, during the third wave of the Lions Quest Erwachsen werden[1] project, the health literacy of 6th grade children was assessed in a sample size of 1671 (3rd wave of a longitudinal survey; we refer here to cross-sectional data). Drawing on the HLS-EU conceptual model of health literacy (Sørensen et al. 2012) and based on the original 47-item Health Literacy Model HLS-EU-47 (Sørensen et. al. 2013), a scale measure of health literacy suitable for school-aged children was created of 16 Likert-scale type questions (see Appendix for the items). The questionnaire adapted to this age group includes questions related to competences (access, understand, appraise and apply) as well as to the domains healthcare, disease prevention and health promotion. More details on the child questionnaire are provided by Bollweg et. al. (2019a, b).

Raw data percentage is used for presenting descriptive statistics and reliability test, whereas for the explanatory analysis, a summed health literacy scale of factor scores is used. Higher factor scores indicate better health literacy. A reliability test was performed on the questionnaire items. Cronbach alpha indicate that the scale is a good measurement tool in terms of internal consistency. Cronbach's alpha, the measure of internal consistency for Likert-type scales showed that

---

[1]The Lions Quest school programme is extremely wide-spread internationally. It comes originally from the United States, where it is named Skills for Action, and the original background was the prevention of addictions. The German version of the programme developed the original one further and has been revised four times. It is nowadays one of the most used school-based prevention programmes in Germany, mostly used in grades 5 to 7. Between 2016 and 2019 Uwe H. Bittlingmayer, Jürgen Gerdes and Gözde Ökcu conducted an evaluation study in a quasi-experimental pre-/post-follow-up-design, aiming at measuring the impact of the Lions Quest programme on the development of life skills among the students; cf. for details Gerdes et al. 2017; Gerdes et al. 2018. The incorporation of a health literacy-scale was used only in the follow up-survey.

the scale reached good reliability ($\alpha = 0.87$). All items included in the analysis appeared to be worthy of retention, as the deletion of none of them would have resulted in an increase of the measure's internal consistency.

Exploratory factor analysis was performed to find the latent structure behind health literacy variables with polichoric correlation that takes into account an assumed categorical data structure. Our factor solution consists of 16 items. Factor scores obtained this way were being saved and missing values were estimated with a maximum likelihood algorithm for persons who had "I don't know" answers for less than 20% of the questions (3 questions). The other respondents with "I don't know" answers to more than 3 questions were excluded from calculation following the standard procedure (HLS-EU-Consortium 2012). The health literacy factor scores are considered standardized variables with normal distribution.

Scale validity was checked with confirmatory factor analysis, and the one factor model fit is acceptable. The comparative fit index in R higher than 0.95 indicates a good fit. The CFI model fit test was significant but research shows that in large samples this test is oversensitive. Comparative fit index would then be higher than 0.95, RMCA lower than 0.05, SRMR lower than 0.08.

Descriptive characteristics reveal the main first-glance differences in health literacy across the selected groups. Variables along which basic descriptive statistics are performed are later included in the regression analysis, which assesses the explanatory power of variables one by one, adjusted for the effect of all other covariates. These are gender, socioeconomic status, mother's education, language spoken at home, family structure, school performance, school type and finally, federal state.

Gender is a priori important in health research, and therefore remains in the regression model throughout the whole model building algorithm.

In recent years, studies have adopted the family affluence scale (FAS) as an adequate measure of parental socieconomic status. The measure was developed and validated in the HBSC study (Boyce et al. 2006), and widely used in geographically diverse samples of child populations (Kehoe and O'Hare 2010; Hartley et al. 2016). The scale, rather than parental educational level, profession or income has proven to be a valid construct for measuring socioeconomic status of school-aged children. The Family Affluence Scale items are also much easier to answer at this age, and they result in fewer missing answers than do classic measures of socioeconomic status. Several studies point to the direct causal relationship between socioeconomic status measured with the FAS scale and some aspects of child and adolescent health, in particular, eating habits (Fismen et al. 2012; Voráčová et al. 2014).

The mother's education level was used as a proxy for cultural capital, whereas home language was relied upon to indicate the acculturation of the child - his/her proficiency in German culture, which is considered a prerequisite for processing information regarding health. Several researchers on migrant health point out that linguistic obstacles in understanding health issues and accessing health services result in less recourse to these services (Iglesias et alii 2012, p. 14) and implicitly, worse health outcomes.

Based on the findings of previous studies, family structure is supposed to impact upon health literacy (Locker 2007; Kumar et al. 2014). Family structure— allegedly significant for health literacy—was approached in the simplest way possible, namely whether a child is being raised by two parents or in a single-parent family. The Federal Statistical Office also uses this differentiation on family forms, however, given the purpose of this study, the legal foundation of a parental relationship was disregarded, and two-parent families encompass both married and cohabiting couples raising children of their own, of one of them, or adopted children. We proceed from the assumption that single parent-families are more at risk where general health literacy, health behaviour and health outcomes of children are concerned.

The German secondary school system is highly structured along school types, ranging from the most prestigious grammar schools to the stigmatized special needs schools, mostly overlapping but also crossing social inequalities and the share of students with migration background in the different school types. Our data include school type as a possible predictor of inequalities in health literacy.

School performance is measured using the grades obtained in the latest semester. To assess global school performance, a scale was constructed using the grades of the most important subjects, with a range of 12 units (minimum 4, maximum 16).

The program and the questionnaire were used in seven German federal states, as follows: Brandenburg and Saxony Anhalt from the former German Democratic Republic, North Rhine-Westphalia, Lower Saxony, Hessen, Bavaria und Baden-Württemberg from the former Federal Republic of Germany. Baden-Württemberg is not part of this analysis due to the low case number. In regression analysis, these were used as dummy variables, using North Rhine-Westfalia, the most populated federal state, as a baseline (reference) category.

During the regression analysis we aimed to find the best fitting and most parsimonious causal model, using the variable selection procedure. Following Kleinbaum et al. (2007), the model was first simplified leaving out the non-significant interaction effects one by one. Thereafter an automatized variable selection algorithm was used. Apart from gender, the remaining variables were allowed to be sorted out by the algorithm. Enter selection method was used, setting the threshold at 5% for inclusion and at 10% for exclusion. The final model was subjected to multicollinearity diagnostics, monitoring the VIF and Tolerance indicators.

Ordinal variables with less than 10 categories—in our case, family affluence, school performance and school type—were examined for whether to use them as continuous or categorical variables in the form of dummies. The first one assumes linear effect, which might be too rigorous a restriction, while the latter does not use the hierarchy of categories. Technically this was done as follows: in the final model the ordinal variables were tested. Two models were fitted, in the first case variables were used as continuous, in the second one as categorical variables using dummies. The more parsimonious model was chosen using the AIC information criteria indicator, so that in the final model, school type was used as a dummy, whereas family affluence and school performance were used in their original continuous forms.

3   Results

As first indicators of health literacy in the target population, the Figs. 1, 2 and 3 sum up the basic distributions of the responses to each Likert-type item measuring the components of health literacy.

Among the components of health literacy, children claim to be most familiar with the consequences of smoking, with the importance of vaccination and with the need to relax.

A health literacy scale was computed from the above 16 components, and factor scores were used in the further analysis, higher factor scores indicating better health literacy. Table 1 displays the mean factor scores and standard deviations of health literacy along selected groups of school children.

Results on the means and dispersion along socio-demographic categories in Table 1 seem to reconfirm some of our assumptions as well as the findings of previous research. More prestigious school types are associated with better scores in health literacy. The worse scores as well as the broadest ranges are to be observed in special schools. Very good school performance is directly reflected in better health literacy scores. At this descriptive level, mother's higher education and outstanding family affluence are also associated with better child health literacy. It also seems that children with German home language have an advantage in health literacy: on average, the scores of children with migration background are worse than those of native Germans.

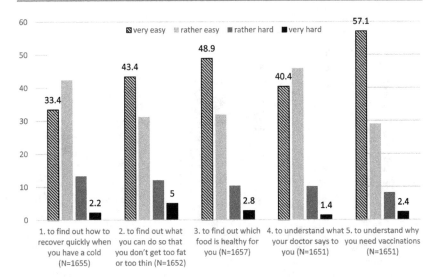

Fig. 1 Distribution of answers given to health literacy items, 1–5 (%). (Source: own depiction)

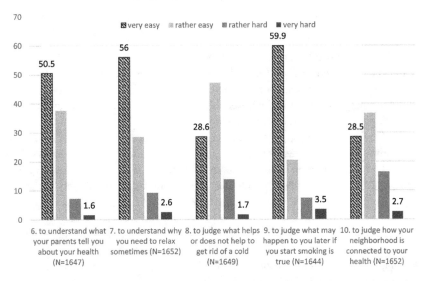

Fig. 2 Distribution of answers given to health literacy items, 6–10 (%). (Source: own depiction)

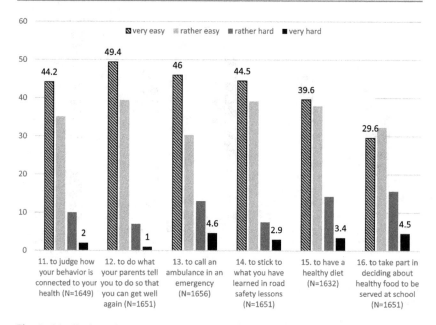

Fig. 3 Distribution of answers given to health literacy items, 11–16 (%). (Source: own depiction)

Some of the results, however, also contradict our expectations. Girls seem to have somewhat worse health literacy scores than boys and two-parent families have no advantage in child health literacy compared to single parents. Among federal states, the former Federal Republic of Germany states Hessen and Lower Saxony have slightly better scores than the rest.

However, these descriptive results do not allow far reaching conclusions to be drawn. In order to identify the personal-structural and situational agents that impact health literacy in school children adjusted to co-variates, a linear regression model was called upon, which measures the impact of explanatory variables one by one, controlling for other effects.

Socio-demographic and school-related variables introduced in the regression model explain a total of 9.2% of the total variance in health literacy, the F statistic is significant, and neither VIF nor tolerance values indicate multicollinearity among variables. Table 2 displays the model with the largest explanatory power and the variables with significant effects.

Table 1 Mean factor scores of health literacy along socio-demographic and situational categories. N = 1624. (Source: own depiction)

Category	HL factor score mean	STD	Category	HL factor score mean	STD
Total	*0.35*	*0.99*	School: grammar	0.262	0.92
Girls	–0.059	0.90	School: elementary + comprehensive	–0.112	0.86
Boys	0.055	0.94	School: middle	0.114	0.92
Single-parent family	0.018	0.99	School: lower secondary	0.026	0.92
Two-parents family	–0.056	0.90	School: special	–0.236	1.16
Home language: German	0.019	0.92	School performance: very good	0.171	0.86
Home language: other	–0.217	0.91	School performance: good	0.078	1.00
Mother's education: none	–0.180	0.99	School performance: moderate	–0.018	0.87
Mother's education: lower secondary	–0.30	0.89	School performance: poor	0.075	0.89
Mother's education: secondary	0.026	0.86	State: North Rhine-Westphalia	0.044	0.94
Mother's education: A-levels	0.171	0.95	State: Saxony-Anhalt	–0.272	0.91
FAS: lowest quartile	–0.187	0.91	State: Brandenburg	–0.120	1.01
FAS: second quartile	–0.060	0.84	State: Lower Saxony	0.111	0.83
FAS: third quartile	0.070	0.96	State: Hessen	0.120	0.93
FAS: highest quartile	0.122	0.94	State: Bavaria	0.10	0.95

Observing the absolute Beta (β) values it can be stated that there are five variables that have a significant effect upon health literacy. It is the regional differences that are the most striking (Beta $= -0.278$), so that the largest difference

Table 2 The determinants of health literacy. Linear regression, N = 1546. (Source: own depiction)

Explanatory variables	Non-standardized B	p	Standardized β (Beta)
School type/ Grammar vs. elementary + comprehensive	−0.394	0.028	−.136
Family affluence	0.059	0.004	.173
Federal state/ NR-W vs. Brandenburg	−1.154	0.000	−.278
School performance	0.056	0.030	.171
Gender (0: girl, 1: boy)	−0.174	0.042	−.094
Constant	*0.112*	*0.000*	*8.716*

Adjusted R^2 = 0.92, F = 3.756, p = 0.000
The decrease in the case number is due to the fact that in the linear regression model only entails those cases with valid answers on each item included

in health literacy between two children at the age of 11-12 is explained solely by their place of residence. The scores of Brandenburg pupils are far behind those of North Rhine-Westphalia, used as reference category in the analysis. In the descriptive statistics above there were other states that scored even lower, however, only the disadvantage of Brandenburg remains significant after controlling for the other co-variates (B = −1.154). No greater differences are revealed between federal states. Although the study was carried out in a restricted number of federal states in Germany, data reveals the advantage of regions from the former Federal Republic of Germany (West) over those from the former German Democratic Republic (East).

The impact of region on child health literacy is (surprisingly) far ahead of family affluence (Beta = −0.173) and school performance (Beta = 0.171). The wealth of the family of origin causes remarkable differences: an increase of only one unit on the 17-point Family Affluence Scale leads to an increase of 0.059 points (B = −0.059) on the health literacy scale. Health literacy is to a large extent positively associated with school performance. One unit difference in school performance represents half a unit difference in health literacy (B = 0.056).[2]

---

[2]The value of non-standardized B is positive, because school performance is measured by grades, where smaller values represent better grades in the German school system, and for health literacy, smaller numbers also represent better scores.

Ranking fourth, school type also impacts health literacy, causing significant and large differences (Beta = −0.136). Compared to grammar school pupils (Gymnasium), children attending elementary and comprehensive schools (Gesamt-/Grundschule) score as much as 0.4 points lower on the health literacy scale (B = −0.394). The advantage of grammer school pupils is significant.

Finally, the a priori important predictor, gender, has an impact in itself on health literacy (Beta = −0.094). Compared to sixth-grade boys in the same federal state, same type of school, with similar family affluence, home language, cultural capital and school performance, girls score higher on the health literacy scale. A boy is significantly less health literate than a girl (B = −0.174), given similar social and situational conditions.

4   Discussion

The instrument we adapted from Torsten Bollweg et al. (2019a, b) was originally designed for 4th-graders, the children of our survey were older. Furthermore, because the Health Literacy-instruments in Bielefeld and Freiburg were not developed a in a parallel, or aligned fashion, we could not directly compare our results with the Bielefeld working group. However, we assume independently from the Bielefeld study that our results are valid since the coherence of our scale is satisfying and the results are generally convincing. We conclude that the Health Literacy-instrument that we used and that was originally developed in Bielefeld is suitable not only for 4th-graders but also for 5th- and 6th-graders.

Between children with similar socio-economic background, same schooltype, similar school performance, and even of the same gender, an immense difference of 1154 points is measured on the health literacy scale (factor score), due only to the region they come from, i.e. the fact that they live in Brandenburg and not elsewhere in Germany. To date, these results are the first findings to show regional differences in health literacy in Germany, no previous studies have considered this aspect, neither in the general population nor in children.

The Lions Quest evaluation research project assessed regional differences with regard to the life skills of children, both participating states from the former German Democratic Republic (Brandenburg and Saxony Anhalt) scoring lower on some of the life skills as well (Gerdes et al. 2017). Hence further analysis appears to be called for. However, in a first approach, the lower health literacy scores in some states might be due to school curriculum differences.

The socioeconomic status of the family of origin has a significant effect, so that the health literacy scores of children coming from better-off families are higher than those of their counterparts from a less advantegeous background. Considering two pupils on the extreme poles of family wealth (6 and 23 points on the Family Affluence Scale), their difference in health literacy is a considerable $(23-6)*(-0.059) = 1.003$ points.

A similar study carried out in Germany's eastern part with a different methodology found that children from higher social status families showed a better knowledge of health topics (Schmidt et al. 2010). In the adult German population, health literacy was positively associated with educational level, net household income and self-perceived social position (Tiller et. 2015), and international studies attest that parent health literacy also correlates with these factors (Alderson et al. 2006).

Differences among German school types with regard to learning progress have been detected by Baumert et al. (2006) and with regard to general literacy and reading skills by Szczesny and Watermann (2011). PISA studies indicate that there is a two-way association between reading skills/literacy and school type, better literacy skills largely increasing the chance of choosing the most prestigious secondary school type, the grammar school, especially in Germany (Maaz et al. 2007). Our data on health literacy echo the findings on general literacy. School differences contribute to the inequalities in health literacy, grammar school pupils having a considerable advantage over other school types, among which the disadvantage of elementary and comprehensive school pupils remain significant even when controlling for co-variates. To sum up, school type differences work independently of social factors such as family affluence.

The observed relationship between health literacy and school performance echoes the findings of previous research among the German adult population (Schaeffer et al. 2017). This is no surprise, particularly considering that most measures of health literacy are associated with generic reading tests and largely focus on reading skills (DeWalt and Hink 2009). A novelty of the Lions Quest survey was that the questionnaire items on health literacy measured not only functional skills, but interactive and critical engagement with health issues as well. Also, school performance was measured with the complex indicator of school grades in four different subjects, which reach far beyond functional literacy skills in the German language. The strong impact of school performance on health literacy is a fact: the better the school performance, the better the health literacy.

Gender has its well-established place in health research, and this is also true of health literacy. Although descriptive statistics have already revealed higher means for boys compared to girls, linear regression has confirmed the impact of gender on health literacy in favor of girls. Due to its a priori significance, the regression model building algorithm was generated in a way that retained gender in all models until the very end and not did allow of its exclusion. The impact of gender is significant: girls have better health literacy skills than boys, all other conditions being the same. In the general German population encompassing all age groups, research has found the reverse result, a lower health literacy score among women compared with men (Tiller et al. 2015), but in an East German study on child health literacy, gender predicted health knowledge in line with our findings (Schmidt et al. 2010). However, and this is important to point out, the better knowledge of girls is not reflected in their health behaviours. For instance, a nationwide survey assessed similar smoking and alcohol consumption trends in children and adolescents (Lampert and Thamm 2007; Schmidt et al. 2010).

In international research, limited parent health literacy has been associated with ethnic minority status, low educational level, low income, lack of child insurance or public insurance and single parenthood (Bennett et. al 2003; Janisse et al. 2010). Poorer oral health was found in children living in single-adult households than in children from multi-adult households (Locker 2007). A systematic review of scientific articles also identified family structure as important for child oral health (Kumar et al. 2014), children raised by single parents having worse outcomes. Despite the well-founded assumption, family structure does not explain health literacy differences.

Mother's education was introduced in the analysis, on the assumption that cultural capital and competences of the family are reflected in the health literacy scores of the child. Although multicollinearity diagnostics did not reveal any methodological query in this respect, in the model building algorithm cultural capital was left out from the very first regression model. The reason might be that the family affluence scale as used in this study already entailed some information on cultural capital (the number of books at home), or that cultural capital largely correlates with family affluence itself, which remained significant even in the last explanatory model. Cultural capital in its turn predicts the school performance of children (Szczesny and Watermann 2011), and this latter has also proven to be a determining factor in health literacy.

For Germany, Maaz et al. (2007) identified family language as the second best predictor for entering the prestigious grammar school. Based on this finding, we assumed that the language spoken at home is a differentiating agent in other aspects, too, and it should also impact on health literacy, in the sense that if coinciding with school language, it increases the likelihood of better health literacy, whereas a different family language represents a risk to adequate health literacy. The data do not provide evidence for this assumption. Moreover, descriptive results indicate somewhat better health literacy scores for immigrant children, and in regression analysis family language does not impact upon health literacy scores in any sense. Although the lack of acculturation is proven to impact negatively upon health (Jaber et al. 2003; Wändell et al. 2003), no such effect was supported by our data with regard to the health literacy of school-aged children. Assessing differences in the health literacy of Germans, starting from adolescence, Berens et al. (2016) did indeed find an association of migrant background with limited perceived health literacy, but only among adults, and such an effect was not registered among adolescents. Our data provides fresh evidence for a very young, pre-adolescent age group, indicating that second generation immigrants, even if their home language is not German, are not disadvantaged in health literacy compared to their native German counterparts. In the United States, results are contradictory, and besides evidence for the impact of language spoken at home on health literacy, there have been studies that have found no association between the two (Martin et al. 2009).

5   Summary and Conclusions

This study provides new insights into the mechanisms by which both personal-structural and situational variables influence the health literacy of German school children in the 6th grade. Some allegedly important predictors such as migration background, family structure and cultural capital do not directly impact upon health literacy, others lead to considerable differences between children. Most importantly, there are immense differences between federal states, pupils in the state of Brandenburg scoring much lower on the scale than those in other states, despite similar social and school-related conditions. Assessing this regional difference is the key finding of our study. The analysis reconfirmed the role of family affluence and gender, widely recognised as impacting health literacy, whereas school-related agents such as school type and performance also prove relevant.

With respect to the measurement of health literacy, it is important to note that children actively construct meaning from health information through their own embodied experiences. In relation to food and health, for instance, Fairbrother et al (2016) found that children aged only 11-12 do not passively absorb information but rather work with it to create meaning, through their engagement in critical and interactive health literacy. Our study is one of the few that also consider these critical and interactive aspects when measuring child health literacy. Nevertheless, future research should increasingly consider the fact that health literacy is a dynamic rather than a static construct.

Appendix

The questionnaire measured child health literacy with answers on a 5-point Likert-type scale to the following questions:
How easy or difficult it is for you to:

1. find out how to recover quickly when you have a cold?
2. find out what you can do so that you don't get too fat or too thin?
3. find out which food is healthy for you?
4. understand what your doctor says to you?
5. understand why you need vaccinations?
6. understand what your parents tell you about your health?
7. understand why you need to relax sometimes?
8. judge what helps or does not help to get rid of a cold?
9. judge whether what adults say may happen to you later if you start smoking is true?
10. judge how where you live (neighborhood, district, street) is connected to your health?
11. judge how your behavior (exercise and diet) is connected to your health
12. do what your parents tell you to do so that you can get well again?
13. call an ambulance in an emergency?
14. stick to what you have learned in road safety lessons?
15. have a healthy diet?
16. take part in deciding whether healthy food is served at school?

References

Alderson, P., Sutcliffe, K., & Curtis, K. (2006). Children as partners with adults in their medical care. *Archives of Disease in Childhood, 9,* 300–303.
Baumert, J., Stanat, P., & Watermann, R. (2006). Schulstruktur und die Entstehung differenzieller Lern- und Entwicklungsmilieus. In: Ids. (eds.): Herkunftsbedingte Disparitäten im Bildungswesen: Differenzielle Bildungsprozesse und Probleme der Verteilungsgerechtigkeit. Vertiefende Analysen im Rahmen von PISA 2000.
Berens, E.-M., Vogt, D., Messer, M., Hurrelmann, K., & Schaeffer, D. (2016). Health literacy among different age groups in Germany: Results of a cross-sectional survey. *BMC Public Health, 16,* 1151.
Betz, C. (2007). Health literacy: The missing link in the provision of health care for children and their families. *Journal of Pediatric Nursing, 22*(4), 257–259.

Bollweg, T. M., Orkan, O., Fretian, A. M., Bröder, J., Domanska, O., & Jordan, S. et al. (2019a, in press). Adapting the European Health Literacy Survey Questionnaire for 4th-grade Students in Germany. Validation and Psychometric Analysis. In: *Health Literacy Research & Practice* 3.

Bollweg, T. M., Orkan, O., Pinheiro, P., Bröder, J., Bruland, D., & Fretian, A. M. et al. (2019b, in press). Adapting the European Health literacy survey questionnaire for 4th-grade students in Germany. Questionnaire Development and Qualitative Pretest. In: *Health Literacy Research & Practice* 3.

Boyce, W., Torsheim, T., Currie, C., & Zambon, A. (2006). The Family Affluence Scale as a measure of national wealth: Validity of an adolescent self-report measure. *Social Indicators Research, 78*, 473–487.

Bravemen, P., & Barclay, C. (2009). Health disparities beginning in childhood: A life-course perspective. *Pediatrics, 124*, 1.

Chari, R., Warsh, J., Ketterer, T., Hossain, J., & Sharif, I. (2013). Association between health literacy and child and adolescent obesity. *Patient Education and Counseling*, 61–66.

Fairbrother, H., Curtis, P., & Goyder, E. (2016). Making health information meaningful: Children's health literacy practices. *SSM Population Health, 2*, 476–484.

Fismen, A.-S., Samdal, O., & Torsheim, T. (2012). Family affluence and cultural capital as indicators of social inequalities in adolescent's eating behaviours: A population-based survey. *BMC Public Health, 12*, 1036.

Gerdes J., Bittlingmayer, U. H., Osipov, I., & Okcu, G. (2017). Die Verteilung von Life Skills nach sozialstrukturellen Merkmalen und Aspekten der Schulperformanz. Eine Auswertung der 1. Erhebung im Projekt „Zur Evidenzbasierung in der schulischen Gesundheitsförderung, Primärprävention und inklusiven Beschulung" (EGePriB) 1. Zwischenbericht im Rahmen der Wirksamkeits- und Akzeptanz-Evaluation des schulischen Unterrichtsprogramms „Erwachsen werden" von Lions Quest (4. Ausgabe) in 5. Klassen verschiedener Schulformen in sechs Bundesländern. Pädagogische Hochschule Freiburg.

Hartley, J. E. K., Levin, K., & Currie, C. (2016). A new version of the HBSC Family Affluence Scale – FAS III: Scottish Qualitative Findings from the International FAS Development Study. *Child Indicators Research, 9*, 233–245.

HLS-EU CONSORTIUM (2012). Comparative report of health literacy in eight EU member states. The European Health Literacy Survey HLS-EU. Online publication: http://www.health-literacy.eu.

Kehoe, S., & O'Hare, L. (2010). The reliability and validity of the Family Affluence Scale. *Centre for Effective Education, Queen's Univer. Effective Education,2*(2), 155–164.

Kleinbaum, D., Kupper, L., Nizam, A., & Muller, K. E. (2007). *Applied regression analysis and other multivariable method.* Duxburry Press.

Kumar, S., Kroon, J., & Lalloo, R. (2014). A systematic review of the impact of parental socio-economic status and home environment characteristics on children's oral health related quality of life. *Health quality life outcomes*, 12–41.

Lampert, T., & Thamm, M. (2007). Tabak-, Alkohol- und Drogen konsum von Jugendlichen in Deutschland. Ergebnisse des Kinder- und Jugendgesundheitssurveys (KiGGS). *Bundesgesundheitsblatt Gesundheitsforschung Gesundheitsschutz, 50*, 600–608.

Locker, D. (2007). Disparities in oral health-related quality of life in a population of Canadian children. *Community Dentistry Oral Epidemiology, 35*, 348–356.

Maaz, K., Watermann, R., & Baumert, J. Familiärer Hintergrund, Kompetenzentwicklung und Selektionsentscheidungen in gegliederten Schulsystemen im internationalen Vergleich. *Eine vertiefende Analyse von PISA Daten. Zeitschrift für Pädagogik 53*(4), 444–462.

Martin, L. T., Ruder, T., Escarce, J. J., Ghosh-Dastidar, B., Sherman, D., Elliott, M., et al. (2009). Developing predictive models of health literacy. *Journal of General Internal Medicine, 24,* 1211.

Nutbeam, D. (2000). Health literacy as a public health goal: A challenge for contemporary health education and communication strategies into the 21st century. *Health Promotion International, 15,* 259–267.

Schaeffer, D., Berens, E.-M., & Vogt, D. (2017). Health Literacy in the German Population. Results of a Representative Survey. *Deutsches Ärzteblatt 114*(4), 53–60.

Schmidt, C. O., Fahland, R. A., Franze, M., Splieth, C., Thyrian, J. R., Plachta-Danielzik, S., et al. (2010). Health-related behaviour, knowledge, attitudes, communication and social status in school children in Eastern Germany. *Health Education Research, 25*(4), 542–551.

Sørensen, K., Van den Broucke, S., Fullam, J., Doyle, G., Pelikan, J., Slonska, Z., & Brand, H. for (HLS-EU) Consortium Health Literacy Project European. (2012). Health literacy and public health: A systematic review and integration of definitions and models. *BMC Public Health, 12,* 80.

Sørensen, K., Van den Broucke, S., Pelikan, J.M., Fullam, J., Doyle, G., Slonska, Z., Kondilis, B., Stoffels, V., Osborne, R.H., & Brand, H. on behalf of the HLS-EU Consortium. (2013). Measuring health literacy in populations: Illuminating the design and development process of the European Health Literacy Survey Questionnaire (HLS-EU-Q). *BMC Public Health, 2013*(13), 948.

Szczesny, M., & Watermann, R. (2011). Differenzielle Einflüsse von Familie und Schulform auf Leseleistung und soziale Kompetenzen. *Journal for educational research online, 3*(1), 168–193.

Tiller, D., Herzog, B., Kluttig, A., & Haertin, J. (2015). Health literacy in an urban elderly East-German population – results from the population-based CARLA study. *BMC Public Health, 15,* 883.

Voráčová, J., Sigmund, E., Sigmundová, D., & Kalman, M. (2014). Family Affluence and the Eating Habits of 11- to 15-Year-Old Czech Adolescents: HBSC 2002 and 2014. *International Journal of Environmental Research & Public Health., 13*(10), 1034.

DeWalt, D., & Hink, A. (2009). Health literacy and child health outcomes: A systematic review of literature. *Pediatrics, 124*(3), 265–274.

Wardle, J., Robb, K., & Johnson, F. (2002). Assessing socioeconomic status in adolescents: The validity of a home affluence scale. *Journal of Epidemiol. Community Health, 56,* 595–599.

Wolf, M. S., Feinglass, J., Thompson, J., & Baker, D. W. (2010). In search of low health literacy: Threshold vs. gradient effect of literacy on health status and mortality. *Social Science and Medicine, 70,* 1335–1341.

Some Cultural Dimensions of Health Literacy

The Importance of New Media and eHealth Information in the Everyday Life of Female Adolescents with Turkish Migration Background in Germany

Zeynep Islertas

1 Introduction

With a population of 13 million, children and adolescents make up 16% of the population in Germany (Statistisches Bundesamt 2018). Childhood and adolescence are important stages of life regarding health, because health behavior in this developmental stage affects highly the health in later adulthood (Bundeszentrale für gesundheitliche Aufklärung 2018; Quenzel 2015; Robert Koch Institut 2018).

Health is closely connected to different socio-demographic dimensions (Birkner et al. 2013; Bittlingmayer 2016; Niederbacher and Zimmermann 2011). According to the current literature, a high socioeconomic status is positively associated with health-promoting behavior. The differences between persons of "high" and "low" socioeconomic status with regard to their health status and health behavior are referred to as "health inequality" in the literature (Hurrelmann and Richter 2009; Robert Koch Institut 2017). Hence, members of socially disadvantaged groups are more often affected by chronic illnesses and discomfort, estimate their own health and health-related quality of life worse than do members of more privileged groups. Also, they die more often prematurely.

Persons with a migration background are described as vulnerable, they are more likely to have a lower socioeconomic status than the indigenous population

Z. Islertas (✉)
Institute of Sociology, University of Education Freiburg (Germany), Freiburg, Germany
e-mail: zeynep.islertas@ph-freiburg.de

© The Editor(s) (if applicable) and The Author(s), under exclusive license to Springer Fachmedien Wiesbaden GmbH, part of Springer Nature 2021
L. A. Saboga-Nunes et al. (eds.), *New Approaches to Health Literacy*,
Gesundheit und Gesellschaft, https://doi.org/10.1007/978-3-658-30909-1_11

(Hurrelmann and Richter 2009; T. Lampert et al. 2013; Robert Koch Institut 2017). The socioeconomic status of children and adolescents is derived primarily from their parents (Danielzik and Müller 2006). Children and adolescents with a two-side migration background live significantly more often in a socially disadvantaged situation compared to children and adolescents without or with only a one-sided immigrant background (Sachverständigenrat deutscher Stiftungen für Integration und Migration 2016; Stanat and Edele 2011). It should be noted that persons with a migration background are not a homogeneous group. Therefore, within the migrant population, the social milieu affiliation should be differentiated. Children and adolescents with a Turkish migration background are by far more likely to belong to the lowest social stratum than children and adolescents with an Italian, Spanish or Portuguese immigrant background in Germany (Bundeszentrale für politische Bildung 2016).

The vulnerability of this target group is additionally underlined by the state of their health. That is why children and adolescents with a Turkish migration background are more likely to be in poor health compared to autochthonous children and adolescents. They are more often overweight and obese (Robert Koch Institut 2008; Schenk et al. 2007; Ünal 2011), they are less vaccinated as recommended (Robert Koch Institut 2008) and they more often commit suicide (Bundeszentrale für politische Bildung 2010; Robert Koch Institut 2008) compared to children and adolescents without a migration background.

Numerous studies have shown that people with a migrant background seldom participate in prevention and health promotion programs (such as early detection and screening). Some of the explanations provided by the existing research are the following: complicated access to health promotion programs caused by information deficits on the part of both the organizer and the potential participant, culturally specific peculiarities in disease and health behavior, different communication behavior and language difficulties. In order for this to be improved in the long term, practitioners should carry out a differentiated target group analysis when planning and implementing measures to determine their (the migrant's) interests and needs (Borde and Blümel 2015; Bundeszentrale für gesundheitliche Aufklärung 2011).

In a recent article Lampert describes the possibility to reach children and adolescents via the internet (C. Lampert 2018). Nevertheless female adolescents with Turkish migration background are not targeted and the question if this target group can also be reached by electronic health offers needs clarification.

Numerous studies describe the use of the television as the main media used by the female and male adolescents with Turkish migration background and the importance that the adolescents attach to it (Radyo ve Televizyon Üst Kurulu

2007; Trebbe et al. 2010). Insights into the use of New Media by the target group are hardly discoverable. Furthermore the importance that adolescents ascribe to the New Media and whether and how they use it to get health information is currently a research desideratum.

This chapter focuses an ethnographic youth health study that aims to answer the following questions: 1) What New Media are accessible to female adolescents with Turkish migration background? 2) Do female adolescents with a Turkish migration background use New Media and, if so, what do they use them for? 3) What significance is attributed to the New Media by this target group? 4) Do female adolescents with Turkish migration background use New Media to get health information and if so, in what way?

In the first step—within this chapter—the digital devices owned by the adolescents with and without migration background in Germany are presented. This pursues the question whether digital inequality is to be found among the target group. The following section discusses the importance that adolescents attach to different hardware and software, before we move on to demonstrate the relevance of New Media and Internet access to the acquisition of information on health by adolescents. Furthermore, the terms eHealth and eHealth Literacy will be discussed before describing the relationship between eHealth Literacy and health through various studies. Results from an ethnographic youth health study on "New Media and the health of female adolescents with a Turkish migration background" can be found in the penultimate section. Finally, based on the theoretical and empirical findings, recommendations for media aiming at health promotion will be presented in order to create target group specific electronic health information and to better reach the "vulnerable group".

2   Media Equipment of Adolescents

Adolescents grow up with a wide range of media devices. Smartphone, computer/laptop and WiFi are available in nearly all families. Furthermore, 96% of the households have got a television, two in three families own a stationary game console, and 63% of the households a tablet-PC (Medienpädagogischer Forschungsverbund Südwest 2019). Adolescents are often tied to the equipment of the family household. They also state a high satisfaction concerning their available media devices and can hardly mention devices which they would still need – apart from general updates and new device versions (Calmbach et al. 2016).

Comparing "groups of adolescents" and their media equipment, there is a difference between the "younger" and the "older" ones. According to the latest

"Youth, Internet, (Multi-) Media" -Study (JIM-Study) (2019), 84% of the 12 to 13-year-old adolescents and 96% of the 16 to 17- year-olds already own a smartphone.

A clear increase with age also appears with regard to the possession of private laptops, stationary game consoles and computers. While 29% of 12 to 13-year-olds possess a laptop, this increases to 49% at the ages of 16 to 17 (Medienpädagogischer Forschungsverbund Südwest 2019).

In contrast to age, differences in economic resources do not seem to imply "digital inequality" in the context of media equipment (Kutscher 2010; Marr and Zillien 2010; Zillien 2009). Thus, the JIM-study reports that access inequities to digital media are largely overcome (Medienpädagogischer Forschungsverbund Südwest 2017). Therefore, media devices are not exclusive to wealthy adolescents but adolescents of all social layers have access to them. In addition, there are no significant differences between the educational backgrounds of the adolescents and their media equipment (Medienpädagogischer Forschungsverbund Südwest 2019)

The target group of this chapter, adolescents with Turkish migration background, who have repeatedly been described as vulnerable (Blasius et al. 2008; Bundesamt für Migration und Flüchtlinge 2008; Butterwegge 2010; Weiss 2007) seem to be equipped with a smartphone at an average age of 15 (Trebbe et al. 2010). In addition, the television is in first place concerning available mass media among adolescents with a Turkish migration background, where a television is to be found in almost every household. In this target group, about 60 percent of 12 to 19-year-olds have their own TV device. At the individual level, the computer equipment rate of the adolescents with a Turkish migration background also reaches the values of television (Trebbe et al. 2010).

3 Importance of Hardware and Software in the Everyday Life of Adolescents

To the adolescents, devices which allow online applications seem to be more relevant than devices that do not allow access to the internet. The mobile phone (almost everybody owns some variation of a smartphone) represents undisputedly one of the most important things in the life of adolescents. In the study of German Federal Association for Information Technology, Telecommunications and the Research Association Southwest the adolescents highlighted especially the "all-in-one" feature when describing the importance of this device. The smartphone is described as an info center, a navigation device, an opportunity for entertainment and above all a communication medium within the peer group (Bundesverband Informationswissenschaft 2017; Medienpädagogischer Forschungsverbund Südwest 2017). The 14 to17-year-old adolescents who participated in the study "What makes teens tick" by Calmbach and colleagues, rarely mention the television as a central and important device. However, from descriptions of the media devices used in everyday life, it can be derived that the television is still used. The television is apparently a medium that has already become so self-evident that it is no longer worth mentioning. It is a device that does not receive undivided attention. It is considered an option to "relax" or to "chill out". Furthermore, compared with the television the adolescents show a much stronger emotional attachment to the game console. They prefer the game console to play online games and watch videos on the internet. Therefore, the television and the game console are important in the everyday life of the adolescents, but nowhere near so much as the smartphone (Calmbach et al. 2016).

Study results on adolescents with Turkish migration background also describe the importance of the smartphone in the everyday life of the adolescents: For the 12 to 15-year-olds the smartphone first and foremost serves as a communication medium and secondarily as a form of entertainment—a significant role in their daily lives. In this age group the possibility to stay in contact with their parents seems to be important. Among the 16 to 19-year-olds, the communication among friends is considered to be the most important function. In addition to communication the possibilities to listen to music, take photos and to be able to play games are considered important by the target group (Trebbe et al. 2010).

With regard to television use these adolescents use German and Turkish speaking television programs. In the group of 12 to 19-year-old adolescents there are more German speaking television program users than there are among the older population. The reasons for the use of Turkish television include the search for information about Turkey and films, soap operas and other programs that appeal to them better than those by German broadcasters. In addition, the Turkish television can be used to not forget the Turkish language and the "Turkish culture". On this occasion, male and older people over the age of 65 watch newscasts programs more often than do females. The third generation—especially the women—follow Turkish soap operas more often than do the males (Halm and Sauer 2006; Radyo ve Televizyon Üst Kurulu 2007). Even when using other media such as the internet, daily newspapers and the radio, German-speaking sources are preferred by the 12 to 19-year-old adolescents with a Turkish migration background (Trebbe et al. 2010).

In addition to age, there is also a connection between the use of German-language media services and the educational level of the target group, as the use of German-language media increases with the degree of education. Reversely, the educational level does not have a consistent impact on frequency of Turkish-language media use (Halm and Sauer 2006; Radyo ve Televizyon Üst Kurulu 2007). While the television is usually regarded as a "gap filler" or "parallel medium", the adolescents with Turkish migration background are more active in using the computer, especially to browse the Internet (Trebbe et al. 2010).

Most devices allow adolescents to access various programs that are subsumed as "software". In the software area, video sharing platform YouTube, communication platform WhatsApp and communication and entertainment platform Instagram are among the most important among adolescents. The fourth popular software among the adolescents is SnapChat. SnapChat's basic idea of making photos and other media visible to the recipient for a few seconds before they "destroy" themselves is the reason why it is considered one of the best platforms on the Internet (Medienpädagogischer Forschungsverbund Südwest 2017, 2019). Another favorite offer in the adolescents' opinion is the music platform Spotify (Medienpädagogischer Forschungsverbund Südwest 2019). If a distinction between female and male adolescents is also made regarding software, it can be stated that Whatsapp and Instagram are the most popular applications for both sexes. Snapchat is the second preference for girls and Youtube for boys. Furthermore, Instagram, SnapChat and Spotify use increases with age. The YouTube use decreases with age. WhatsApp has a comparable proportion of "fans" in the age group of 12 to 19-year-olds (Medienpädagogischer Forschungsverbund Südwest 2019). Study results describing the use of software by adolescents with a Turkish migration background are hard to find and represent therefore a research desideratum.

4   Timeframes and Reasons for using online offers

According to the latest JIM study, 89% of the adolescents go online daily (Medienpädagogischer Forschungsverbund Südwest 2019). Self- assessment of the time for daily internet surfing is 205 min on average. Male adolescents were—with 214 min daily—dedicating more time to online time than females with 194 min daily (Medienpädagogischer Forschungsverbund Südwest 2019). Self-estimated online time is highest among the 18 to 19-year olds (257 min); the average among 12 to 13-year-olds is 127 min. Regarding educational level, grammar school students spend less time online (198 min) than do adolescents attending secondary school (216 min) (Medienpädagogischer Forschungsverbund Südwest 2019). Adolescents with a Turkish migration background are considered as "root users" of the Internet regardless of their age, since they are online for more than four days a week (Trebbe et al. 2010).

Duration of online use can be considered in four dimensions: communication, information, entertainment, and games. Even if some blurring and overlapping can be seen—the largest share of adolescents' online time is spent on communication. The entertainment-oriented use accounts for 30% of the total usage (Medienpädagogischer Forschungsverbund Südwest 2019). One-fourth of the time, adolescents spent on online games, while the use of informative content accounts for ten percent. Total time share differs between female and male adolescents. Female adolescents attach the greatest importance to the possibility of communication via online portals. This accounts for almost 41% of the time spent online. 34% of the whole time of the female adolescents is to be assigned to entertainment possibilities, 14% for games, and 10% on the search for information. Male adolescents use 29% of the whole time for communication activities, 28% for entertainment, 34% for playing online games and ten percent on the search for information. Furthermore, with regard to school education, there are no significant differences. The communication activities are more important for all adolescents—no matter what level of education they have—than playing online games or searching for online information (Medienpädagogischer Forschungsverbund Südwest 2019). Insights into what software is used to what extent by female adolescents with a Turkish migration background in Germany are hard to find.

5   Internet and (Health) Information Acquisition

Adolescents only use spent ten percent of their online time searching for information. Using the query tool of search engines, YouTube and Wikipedia remain the main activity of adolescents when it comes to searching for information on the internet (Bundesverband Informationswissenschaft 2017; Bundesverband Informationswissenschaft, Telekommunikation und neue Medien e. V. 2011; Medienpädagogischer Forschungsverbund Südwest 2019). High-interest topics, on which adolescents search for information on the internet, are for instance "solution of personal problems" as well as information on current affairs. According to the JIM study, it is important for three out of four adolescents to learn something from "the world of music" and the field of "education and work" (Medienpädagogischer Forschungsverbund Südwest 2015). Besides, the Internet is one of the most important tools to receive health information (Kummervold et al. 2008). Research highlights that adolescents use the Internet to receive information on subjects such as wellness, lifestyle, pregnancy, fitness, nutrition, piercings/tattoos and on the subject skin (Wartella et al. 2016; Zschorlich et al. 2015). In addition to health apps, various search platforms and websites are used. Besides written online information, the Internet is seen as a direct channel of communication with health professionals and other stakeholders (Zschorlich et al. 2015). In the procedure of searching for information, age-specific differences can be found: For example, active research via the "Google" search platform or information retrieval via the "Wikipedia" website increases significantly with the age, especially among the 12 to 15-year-olds, while YouTube videos have similar relevance for adolescents in the age between 12 and 19. Otherwise no significant gender-specific differences are to be found within the online searching process of adolescents (Medienpädagogischer Forschungsverbund Südwest 2017). Information on female adolescents with a Turkish migration background is hard to find.

In summary, it can be concluded, that electronic health information can hold great potential to reach socially disadvantaged adolescents, as 1) the technical access is not a problematic issue to adolescents and 2) adolescents' use of New Media has a significant role in their everyday lives. The question that nevertheless needs to be investigated is if technical access suffices to deal adequately with electronic health information. Chesser and colleagues argue that digital health information is not accessible to all sections of the population. Hence, the authors summed up not only the technical possibilities favoring accessibility, but also competences that are necessary to be able to use the electronic health information adequately (Chesser et al. 2016).

6   EHealth & Health Outcome

The first web pages with medical contents occurred as early as 1993. Since then a growth of information on health-related online contents, as well as the number of those that use the Internet to procure information on health subjects or to be in touch with other users about health subjects has increased steadily (Rossmann 2010).

eHealth is a concept used to describe various Internet-based health services. However, a uniform understanding and use of the concept introduced in the 1990s does not exist. Often eHealth seems to serve as a buzzword for almost everything related to electronics and medicine. Depending on the author and target group, eHealth mixes with other terminology such as telemedicine, online health, cyber medicine or consumer health informatics (Eysenbach 2001). One reason for this might be the origin of the term, because eHealth was initially used mainly by industry in the style of e-commerce, e-business or e-solutions, to address and clarify the many potentialities of digital health media offers (Eysenbach 2001). Numerous definitions can be found in the literature trying to describe eHealth. One of the most cited is Eysenbach's definition (Eysenbach 2001). Eysenbach describes eHealth as: *"an emerging field in the intersection of medical informatics, public health and business, referring to health services and information delivered or enhanced through the Internet and related technologies. In a broader sense, the term characterizes not only a technical development, but also a state-of-mind, a way of thinking, an attitude, and a commitment for networked, global thinking, to improve health care locally, regionally, and worldwide by using information and communication technology."*(Eysenbach 2001 p. 1). Thus, it seems that, according to Eysenbach, eHealth subsumes all offers that facilitate communication within the healthcare system and the provision of health information and seems to support health care.

To be able to use this electronic health information adequately, different skills and kinds of knowledge are needed, which are summarized under eHealth Literacy. eHealth Literacy is a cognitive-based concept of skills and abilities that a person needs to deal with electronic health information adequately. Norman and Skinner (2006) summarize six competencies, subdivided into analytical and context specific skills. Among the analytical competencies, the authors subsume the traditional reading and writing skills, media literacy and information literacy. Health literacy, computer literacy and science literacy are summarized under the heading context-specific skills (Norman and Skinner 2006).

Numerous studies on eHealth Literacy describe that adolescents, those with a high level of education and who spend a lot of time on the internet, have a high eHealth Literacy level and are able to deal adequately with electronic health information (Richtering et al. 2017; Xesfingi and Vozikis 2016). Existing studies also indicate that the use of electronic health information may be related to multiple health behaviors (Dutta-Bergman 2004; Lee et al. 2015). In the study by Yang and colleagues, students with high eHealth Literacy demonstrated an increased likelihood of healthy eating habits, a high level of physical activity, and healthy sleep patterns compared to those with low eHealth Literacy levels (Yang et al. 2017).The study by Mitsutake and colleagues also describe the link between eHealth Literacy and positive health behavior. Nevertheless, they specified that this connection does not exist with harmful behavior patterns like smoking or excessive consumption of alcohol (Mitsutake et al. 2016). In addition to these positive correlations between the socioeconomic factors, eHealth Literacy level and the health behavior of individuals, Blackstock and colleagues call for caution when looking at this relationship. They found a positive connection between eHealth Literacy levels and health risk behavior, when different socioeconomic variables are controlled (Blackstock et al. 2016). However, in addition to quantitative studies, it is important to carry out qualitative work that explores the importance of electronic health information in the everyday life of adolescents, the link with socioeconomic factors and the health of the target group.

7 Qualitative Study on the use of New Media and Electronic Health Information by Female Adolescents with a Turkish Migration Background in Germany

The ethnographic research project "eHealth Literacy and Minority Health (ELMi)" aims to explore the understanding of health and the health behavior of female adolescents with a Turkish migration background. A main focus is the exploration of the connection of health with the usage of New Media in the everyday life of these adolescents. The study aims to understand and describe 1) New Media relevance and use by female adolescents with Turkish migration background in their everyday life and 2) in which way and why New Media is used by these adolescents to get health information. To answer these questions adequately, qualitative data was collected. The results, which are reported below, were based on a focus group interview and four guided individual interviews. For our data collection methodology we drew on the approach of Schulz and Colleagues (Schulz et al. 2012) and Helfferich (Helfferich 2014). Qualitative content analysis according to Mayring (Mayring 2010) helped us analyze the data adequately. The individual interviews with 16-year-old adolescents with two-side migration background, all of whom were aiming for O-level type school leaving certificates ("Mittlere Reife") at the time of the survey, were conducted in private households. For the focus group discussion, a space in the university was preferred as a neutral location. In order to comply with data protection regulations and to protect the privacy rights of participants, personal research data was processed through pseudonymization techniques (Liebig et al. 2014). The collected data—one part in German and one in Turkish, because the participating adolescents sometimes changed languages within the conversation—was translated into English by the author.

New Media and the Internet access in the everyday lives of female adolescents with Turkish migration background

In all households of the interviewed adolescents, there was at least one laptop, computer or tablet pc. A smartphone is owned by all adolescents participating in the study: *"Well I do have a smartphone. The laptop belongs to all of my family members. We do not have a computer" (Eda* 2016*); „Well I have a computer and a smartphone. Well we used to have a tablet- pc, but not anymore" (Kübra* 2016*); "Of course my smartphone first of all. Which I use the most, so to say. We also own two tablet-pc's, but only one of them is used and never by me, so it's more the domain of my father (Esra* 2016*).*

It is noteworthy that the adolescents only mention the smartphone as their own device. The laptop, computer or tablet pc seems to be available to all family members in all households. There are several reasons for the use of New Media by the participating female adolescents with a Turkish migration background. The computer, the laptop and the tablet pc are used by all respondents primarily for schoolwork and secondarily for watching videos via online platforms. The meaning of the Internet for the adolescents can be derived from the description of the use of these devices: *"(...) I use a laptop for school if I hand in a seminar paper or so, or have to write a documentation, then I use the laptop or also simply for Youtube, videos, or if I watch soap operas, I also like to use the laptop. And computer, our computer doesn't have internet access, so I use it, actually, only for printing"* (Leyla 2016). Esra describes her use of the computer in the same way as Leyla. The only addition is that she differentiates between the computer and the tablet pc in their household: *"I use our computer only for school stuff, when I have to write a documentation and the tablet I basically never use, because it that does not appeal to me. The computer does appeal to me, because I think it's better to do my school stuff on the computer, for example, than on the tablet. You can do it on the tablet also, but on the computer it's better (..) because you have a real keyboard and can type better" (Esra* 2016*).*

The smartphone is unanimously awarded the entertainment and communication function, which takes place primarily online. So the smartphone is used to be able to stay in contact with members of the peer group. In addition, the adolescents use the software-supported device to watch videos: *"Most of the time, I also use my smartphone to keep in touch with my friends. And also to watch my soap operas there" (Kübra* 2016*); "With the smartphone, I surf the internet, I chat with friends.. I actually use the smartphone for entertainment when I have free time. Of course, also to phone" (Leyla* 2016*).* The adolescents judge the smartphone as more important than the computer, laptop and tablet pc in their everyday life. All interviewed adolescents think they could not do without their smartphone. With their computer, laptop, and tablet pc the relationship is much more detached, since they can access software programs which are needed for doing the school duties on the smartphones as well. The importance of the smartphone is underlined additionally by the adolescents, as it enables them to stay in touch with their peer group: *"(..) because you just need a laptop for school but a* *smartphone is also an everyday thing, which you always use. I think I could not do without the phone. Without a computer yes, but not without the smartphone. Because there, with the smartphone, I'm not the kind of person who plays on the smartphone or has a lot of games on it or something, its more for me that I'm really in touch with my friends (Leyla* et al. 2016); *"The homework you can also do on the smartphone" (Kübra* 2016). The difference between the importance that the adolescents ascribe to the computer, laptop and tablet pc and the smartphone is also recognized by the self-estimated time of daily use of these devices. Thus, a longer time period is spent daily on the smartphone than on any of the other devices: *"Ehm, 8-9 h. Maybe, seven hours of the day I use my smartphone. I think the computer less than the smartphone, maybe six or seven hours" (Leyla* 2016); *"I do not spend any time on the computer. I use the computer only when I'm doing a presentation or something else for school, but not for any additional time. On the smartphone I spend 24 h. No, I don't know, just always when I have leisure time or I don't have anything else to do, then I am actually always on the smartphone" (Kübra* 2016).

The communication with friends is done primarily via the software "WhatsApp". This application is used by all interviewees: *"So most of the time I'm in contact with friends on WhatsApp. You have your own groups and everything"* (Leyla et al. 2016); *"Yes, exactly. I use apps only to keep in touch with friends. Actually I do not have any other apps to stay in touch"* (Leyla et al. 2016). In addition to the communication platform "WhatsApp" the software Instagram, SnapChat, Twitter and Facebook are used by the adolescents. Only one of the interviewed adolescents has an account on Facebook and Twitter and uses these platforms rarely: *"Actually, I only communicate on WhatsApp (…) and I do Facebook, but I use it very rarely." (Leyla* et al. 2016); *"(..) I still use Twitter. But I use it rarely. To follow some stars" (Leyla* et al. 2016).

Compared with websites, the opportunities that different apps provide are attributed a higher priority by the adolescents. Web pages are used by the adolescents exclusively to do school duties, to download songs or make online purchases: *"(…) I actually spend no time on any website. Well, only for school"* (Leyla et al. 2016); *„Or when you download songs"*(Leyla et al. 2016); *"For shopping, for clothes, for example, if I want to order something, then I prefer websites but only sometimes"* (Leyla et al. 2016).

German-speaking or Turkish-speaking pages are used by the adolescents depending on the topic, with German-speaking pages being preferred because they are considered more comprehensible: *"While preparing for the FÜK exam [interdisciplinary competence evaluation], when searching for Turkish Halay [Turkish folk dance], I searched Turkish websites"* (Kübra 2016); *"That totally depends. Well, I don't pay much attention to that, I do of course make sure that it´s in German, so I understand everything, but sometimes it´s also Turkish (…) so it´s different every time"* (Esra 2016); *"I cannot read Turkish, well I can read but not every single word and then I don't understand it"* (Kübra 2016). It seems that the adolescents, who seem to have no difficulties orally communicating in Turkish can classify themselves less competent in written Turkish. Thus German-speaking homepages are preferred for written information. On the other hand soap operas are viewed in Turkish: *"Yes, I only watch Turkish soap operas"* (Esra 2016); *"Then mostly [I watch the soap operas] on YouTube, or just on their pages. For example, on Kanal D [Turkish television broadcaster] or ShowTV [Turkish television broadcaster]"*; *"Well, the Turkish soap operas, because we don't receive Turkish-speaking TV channels, I watch on YouTube (…) (Leyla et al. 2016)"*

Online research by female adolescents with Turkish migration background

In addition to the entertainment and communication opportunities, the interviewed female adolescents with a Turkish migration background use the opportunity to get online information on everyday questions and questions that arise when completing their homework. The search platform "Google" is primarily used and additionally the "Wikipedia" and "Gutefrage.com" ("goodquestion. com") homepages are known and used to get information. It is especially important for the interviewed adolescents that the homepage is understandable and to promptly receive an answer: *"On Google I write what I'm looking for and then there are different pages mostly always at first Wikipedia and there—you check mostly there first. And then, if I do not really understand it, I just look at pages where it´s explained maybe in a way that is a little bit easier to understand and is written in a simpler way".* (Esra 2016); *"Recently I asked a question, for our school, because of the FÜK [interdisciplinary competence evaluation]. A question wasn't answered, I put that then simply on [goodquestion.com] and I got an answer immediately"* (Leyla et al. 2016); *"or if I have a question, for example whether I can return something to the shop, that I have already worn, that´s just an example, then I´ll just ask that [gutefrage.com] if I cannot ask at home at the moment or I need to get an answer quickly"* (Leyla et al. 2016). In addition to the comprehensibility of pages, the wording used by the author seems to be crucial in the evaluation of the content: *"I think that it depends on how the person wrote it. If the content is written objectively, then I just think it helps me more than if somebody wrote it in 'youth words'"* (Leyla 2016).

On health issues, two adolescents also use the internet to obtain information. In this context the searching platform "Google" is used, just as with other information. The participant Leyla also points to the importance of her "mother" in health issues and explains why and when she uses which "source of information": *"So my first idea is actually Google, because I enter my question and usually I get answers. But if it´s about stuff I do not know, which I'm not so often confronted with and where I just know where my mother has experience with it and then I actually ask her. But rather Google than my mother because I believe that on this homepage even doctors answer or someone else who knows something about that. I don't know, I don't mean to say, I trust Google more than my mother, but she didn't suffer all those illnesses, or all the symptoms and so that she could have an answer to everything"* (Leyla 2016). The mother and other members of their social network are also named by the other participants as people to be contacted on health issues. They play the role of the first point of contact for health issues. Thus the internet takes a second-rate role for them: *"At first my mother and if she doesn't know, then my relatives, my aunts or others and if they don't know either, then internet"* (Kübra 2016); *"Mum is important in health issues. Well, for example, if I have a headache, for three hours and, then I first go to my mother and ask her what it might be. And then she tells me, for example, drink a lot of water or take a medication if it´s really not bearable. If it is already one, two or three days, then I would search on the internet for information"* (Eda 2016). The adolescents don't only distinguish between the internet and the social contact persons, but also within the social contact persons and the questions they ask them. For example, in the case of youth-specific health questions, friends are preferred instead of the mother: *"Especially at puberty or something, some questions may be more embarrassing, and you´re more likely to ask friends who may have experience with it"* (Leyla 2016). The medical doctor is mentioned only by one participant as a contact person for health issues: *"Of course, [I ask] the medical doctor, that is normal. Sometimes on the internet (…) sometimes I ask my friends, if they have experienced something like that, and then of course my mother"* (Esra 2016).

It should be noted that the experience that people from the social network have on various health-related issues, in addition to the topic-specific specification of the contact persons, are a selection criteria for the adolescents. Thus, they trust the people from their social environment and their dealing with health-related events and their acquired experience, but they trust information on the internet as well.

8   Conclusion

At least one television, computer, laptop or tablet pc is present in the household of the adolescents taking part in the study. In addition, all interviewees own a smartphone. Only the smartphone they call their own device. To all other devices all members of the family have access. Most devices allow internet access in all households. The smartphone, which is primarily used to maintain communication between peer group members and for entertainment purposes, is also given greater importance than the other devices. In addition, the importance of the smartphone can be derived from the amount of time which the adolescents spend with their device in their everyday life. These findings support existing results of studies that describe the importance of New Media in the daily life of adolescents. Also the results regarding the most popular and widely used software underline the existing findings and at the same time these represent a new research result, since there are hardly any studies explicitly focusing on adolescents with Turkish migration background. Thus, there seems to be no significant difference in the selection and use of software between the autochthonous and the adolescents with Turkish migration background in Germany. The female adolescents also use the online communication and entertainment platforms—referred to as "popular" in the existing studies.

The internet is also viewed as a source of information by adolescents with Turkish migration background. They use the internet to answer acute questions they are dealing with in their everyday lives. In contrast to what the available studies describe, the target group doesn't use mainly videos to get information. They prefer online sources which provide written information. It is important for the interviewed adolescents to find quickly understandable information. It should be noted that the participating adolescents with Turkish migration background prefer German-speaking websites to receive information. As a reason for this preference they mention better intelligibility. The adolescents, who seem to be able to communicate fluently in Turkish, seem to be able to switch languages in conversations (from German to Turkish and back again) and watch Turkish-speaking soap operas in their everyday lives, seem to feel more competent in the German written language than in written Turkish. Thus, Turkish language skills are preferred for entertainment purpose and German skills in correspondence.

In this context, it should be added that when searching for health information it is not just the internet that the adolescents draw on. The social network, and especially the mother and the peer group, seem to play a significant role in the search for health information, so that the opportunities to seek health information on the internet are not the "only option" but a possibility alongside the "social network".

9   Recommendations for eHealth Promotion Programs

The participating adolescents attached value to various hardware and software. Thus, the internet offers opportunities to present a platform for providing target group specific health information. In order to extend access not only to the technical area but also to the content level as described by Cheeser and colleagues (Chesser et al. 2016) the comprehensible processing and presentation of electronic health information is imperative. In addition, quick findability and the scientific processing of content seem to be important. Consequently, the possibility to create an "electronic" way to reach the "population" which is described by the existing health promotion programs as "difficult to reach" with target group specific access (content adapted to needs and easy to understand), can be one way to reduce the health inequality in Germany.

References

Birkner, B., Hurrelmann, K., Buchner, F., Gerber, U., Brand, A., Schnabel, P. E., Wasem, J. (2013). *Gesundheitswissenschaften*. Berlin: Springer.

Bittlingmayer, U. H. (2016). Strukturorientierte Perspektive auf Gesundheit und Krankheit. In M. Richter & K. Hurrelmann (Eds.), *Soziologie von Gesundheit und Krankheit* (pp. 23–40). Wiesbaden: Springer VS.

Blackstock, O. J., Cunningham, C. O., Haughton, L. J., Garner, R. Y., Norwood, C., & Horvath, K. J. (2016). Higher eHealth literacy is associated with HIV risk behaviors among HIV-Infected women who use the internet. *The Journal of the Association of Nurses in AIDS Care: JANAC, 27*(1), 102–108.

Blasius, J., Friedrichs, J., & Klöckner, J. (2008). *Doppelt benachteiligt?*. Wiesbaden: VS Verlag.

Borde, T., & Blümel, S. (2015). Gesundheitsförderung und Migrationshintergrund. https://www.leitbegriffe.bzga.de/bot_angebote_idx-156.htm.

Bundesamt für Migration und Flüchtlinge. (2008). Schulische Bildung von Migranten in Deutschland. https://www.Publikationen/WorkingPapers/wp13-schulische-bildung.pdf; jsessionid = 0420850640CDA878A3CD96C23534766.1_cid359?__blob = publicationFile.

Bundesverband Informationswissenschaft. (2017). Kinder und Jugend in der digitalen Welt. https://www.bitkom.org/Presse/Anhaenge-an-PIs/2017/05-Mai/170512-Bitkom-PK-Kinder-und-Jugend-2017.pdf.

Bundesverband Informationswissenschaft, Telekommunikation und neue Medien e.V. (2011). Jugend 2.0: Eine repräsentative Untersuchung zum Internetverhalten von 10-bis 18-Jährigen. https://www.bitkom.org/Bitkom/Publikationen/Studie-Jugend-20.html.

Bundeszentrale für gesundheitliche Aufklärung. (2011). Migration, Prävention, Gesundheitsförderung: Empfehlungen für fachkräfte. https://www.medbox.org/migration-pravention-gesundheitsforderung/download.pdf.

Bundeszentrale für gesundheitliche Aufklärung. (2018). Kinder- und Jugendgesundheit: Gesund aufwachsen. https://www.bzga.de/bot_jugendgesundheit.html.

Bundeszentrale für politische Bildung. (2010). Deutschland: Studie über hohe Suizidrate bei Frauen türkischer Herkunft. http://www.bpb.de/gesellschaft/migration/newsletter/57051/deutschland-studie-ueber-hohe-suizidrate-bei-frauen-tuerkischer-herkunft.

Bundeszentrale für politische Bildung. (2016). *Datenreport 2016: Ein Sozialbericht für die Bundesrepublik Deutschland. Schriftenreihe der Bundeszentrale für Politische Bildung.* Bonn: BpB.

Butterwegge, C. (2010). *Armut von Kindern mit Migrationshintergrund.* Wiesbaden: VS Verlag.

Calmbach, M., Borgstedt, S., Borchard, I., Thomas, P. M., & Flaig, B. B. (2016). *Wie ticken Jugendliche 2016?: Lebenswelten von Jugendlichen im Alter von 14 bis 17 Jahren in Deutschland.* s.l.: Springer. http://www.doabooks.org/doab?func=fulltext&rid=19074.

Chesser, A., Burke, A., Reyes, J., & Rohrberg, T. (2016). Navigating the digital divide: A systematic review of eHealth literacy in underserved populations in the United States. *Informatics for Health & Social Care, 41*(1), 1–19.

Danielzik, S., & Müller, M. J. (2006). Sozioökonomische Einflüsse auf Lebensstil und Gesundheit von Kindern. *Deutsche Zeitschrift Für Sportmedizin, 57*(9). https://www.researchgate.net/profile/Manfred_Mueller3/publication/242732709_Soziookonomische_Einflusse_auf_Lebensstil_und_Gesundheit_von_Kindern/links/54a13fbc0cf257a636027771/Soziooekonomische-Einfluesse-auf-Lebensstil-und-Gesundheit-von-Kindern.pdf.

Dutta-Bergman, M. J. (2004). Health attitudes, health cognitions, and health behaviors among Internet health information seekers: Population-based survey. *Journal of Medical Internet Research, 6*(2), e15.

Eda (2016, June 15). Interview by Z. Islertas.

Esra (2016, August 28). Interview by Z. Islertas.

Eysenbach, G. (2001). What is e-health? *Journal of Medical Internet Research, 3*(2), E20.

Halm, D., & Sauer, M. (2006). Almanya´daki Türk Medyası. http://www.konrad.org.tr/Medya%20Mercek/04halm.pdf.

Helfferich, C. (2014). Leitfaden- und Experteninterviews. In N. Baur & J. Blasius (Eds.), *Handbuch Methoden der empirischen Sozialforschung* (pp. 559–574). Wiesbaden: Springer VS.

Hurrelmann, K., & Richter, M. (2009). *Gesundheitliche Ungleichheit: Grundlagen, Probleme, Perspektiven (2* (aktualisierte ed.). Wiesbaden: VS Verlag / GWV Fachverlage GmbH Wiesbaden.

Kübra (2016, June 27). Interview by Z. Islertas.

Kummervold, P. E., Chronaki, C. E., Lausen, B., Prokosch, H.-U., Rasmussen, J., Santana, S., ··· Wangberg, S. C. (2008). Ehealth trends in Europe 2005–2007: A population-based survey. *Journal of Medical Internet Research, 10*(4), e42.

Kutscher, N. (2010). Digitale Ungleichheit: Soziale Unterschiede in der Mediennutzung. In G. Cleppien & U. Lerche (Eds.), *Soziale Arbeit und Medien* (1st ed., pp. 153–164). Wiesbaden: VS Verlag.

Lampert, C. (2018). Gesundheitsangebote für Kinder und Jugendliche im App-Format ("Health offers for children and adolescents in the App-Format"). *Prävention Und Gesundheitsförderung, 34,* 74.

Lampert, T., Kroll, L. E., von der Lippe, E., Müters, S., & Stolzenberg, H. (2013). Sozioökonomischer Status und Gesundheit: Ergebnisse der Studie zur Gesundheit Erwachsener in Deutschland (DEGS1) [Socioeconomic status and health: results of the German Health Interview and Examination Survey for Adults (DEGS1)]. *Bundesgesundheitsblatt, Gesundheitsforschung, Gesundheitsschutz, 56*(5–6), 814–821.

Lampert, T., Hoebel, J., Kuntz, B., Müters, S., & Kroll, L. E. (2018). Messung des sozioökonomischen Status und des subjektiven sozialen Stauts in KiGGS Welle 2. *Journal of Health Monitoring, 3*(1).

Lampert, T., & Mielck, A. (2008). Gesundheit und soziale Ungleichheit: Eine Herausforderung für Forschung und Politik. *Gesundheit Und Soziale Ungleichheit, 6*(2), 7–16.

Lampert, T., Müters, S., Stolzenberg, H., & Kroll, L. E. (2014). Messung des sozioökonomischen Status in der KiGGS-Studie: Erste Folgebefragung (KiGGS Welle 1) [Measurement of socioeconomic status in the KiGGS study: first follow-up (KiGGS Wave 1)]. *Bundesgesundheitsblatt, Gesundheitsforschung, Gesundheitsschutz, 57*(7), 762–770.

Lee, Y. J., Boden-Albala, B., Jia, H., Wilcox, A., & Bakken, S. (2015). The association between online health information-seeking behaviors and health behaviors among Hispanics in New York City: A community-based cross-sectional study. *Journal of Medical Internet Research, 17*(11), e261. https://doi.org/10.2196/jmir.4368.

Leyla (2016, June 28). Interview by Z. Islertas.

Leyla, Esra, & Kübra (2016, June 17). Interview by Z. Islertas.

Liebig, S., Gebel, T., Grenzer, M., Kreusch, J., Schuster, H., Tscherwinka, r., ··· Witzel, A. (2014). Datenschutzrechtliche Anforderungen bei der Generierung und Archivierung qualitativer Interviewdaten. https://www.ratswd.de/dl/RatSWD_WP_238.pdf.

Marr, M., & Zillien, N. (2010). Digitale Spaltung. In W. Schweiger & K. Beck (Eds.), *Handbuch Online-Kommunikation* (pp. 257–282). Wiesbaden: VS Verlag.

Mayring, P. (2010). Qualitative Inhaltsanalyse. In G. Mey & K. Mruck (Eds.), *Handbuch Qualitative Forschung in der Psychologie* (1st ed., pp. 601–613). s.l.: VS Verlag (GWV).

Medienpädagogischer Forschungsverbund Südwest.. (2015). JIM-Studie 2015: Jugend, Information, (Multi-)Media. https://www.mpfs.de/fileadmin/files/Studien/JIM/2015/JIM_Studie_2015.pdf.

Medienpädagogischer Forschungsverbund Südwest. (2017). JIM-Studie 2017: Jugend, Information, (Multi-)Media Basisstudie zum Medienumgang 12-bis 19-Jähriger in Deutschland. https://www.mpfs.de/fileadmin/files/Studien/JIM/2017/JIM_2017.pdf.

Medienpädagogischer Forschungsverbund Südwest. (2019). JIM-Studie 2019: Jugend, Information, Medien. https://www.mpfs.de/fileadmin/files/Studien/JIM/2019/JIM_2019.pdf.

Mitsutake, S., Shibata, A., Ishii, K., & Oka, K. (2016). Associations of eHealth literacy with health behavior among adult internet users. *Journal of Medical Internet Research, 18*(7), e192.

Niederbacher, A., & Zimmermann, P. (2011). *Grundwissen Sozialisation: Einführung zur Sozialisation im Kindes- und Jugendalter* (4., überarbeitete und aktualisierte Auflage). Wiesbaden: VS Verlag / Springer Fachmedien Wiesbaden GmbH Wiesbaden.

Norman, C. D., & Skinner, H. A. (2006). Ehealth literacy: Essential skills for consumer health in a networked world. *Journal of Medical Internet Research, 8*(2), e9.

Quenzel, G. (2015). *Entwicklungsaufgaben und Gesundheit im Jugendalter.* Zugl.: Bielefeld, Univ., Habil.-Schr., 2014. Weinheim: Beltz Juventa.

Radyo ve Televizyon Üst Kurulu. (2007). Almanya´da yaşayan Türklerin Televizyon izleme eğilimleri Kamuoyu Araştırması. https://www.rtuk.gov.tr/assets/Icerik/Alt-Siteler/almanyada-yasayan-turklerin-televizyon-izleme-egilimleri-kamuoyu-arastir-masi-14-kasim-20070056.pdf.

Richtering, S. S., Hyun, K., Neubeck, L., Coorey, G., Chalmers, J., Usherwood, T., … Redfern, J. (2017). Ehealth Literacy: Predictors in a Population With Moderate-to-High Cardiovascular Risk. *JMIR Human Factors, 4*(1), e4.

Robert Koch Institut. (2008). Schwerpunktbericht der Gesundheitsberichterstattung des Bundes: Migration und Gesundheit. https://www.rki.de/DE/Content/Gesund-heitsmonitoring/Gesundheitsberichterstattung/GBEDownloadsT/migration.pdf?__blob=publicationFile.

Robert Koch Institut. (2017). Gesundeheitliche Ungleicheit in verschiedenen Lebensphasen. https://www.rki.de/DE/Content/Gesundheitsmonitoring/Gesundheitsberichter-stattung/GBEDownloadsB/gesundheitliche_ungleichheit_lebensphasen.pdf?__blob=publicationFile.

Robert Koch Institut. (2018). Kinder- und Jugendgesundheit. https://www.rki.de/DE/Con-tent/Gesundheitsmonitoring/Themen/Kinder_und_Jugendgesundheit/KiJuGesundheit_node.html.

Rossmann, C. (2010). Gesundheitskommunikation im Internet. Erscheinungsformen, Potenziale, Grenzen. In W. Schweiger & K. Beck (Eds.), *Handbuch Online-Kommuni-kation* (pp. 338–363). Wiesbaden: VS Verlag.

Sachverständigenrat deutscher Stiftungen für Integration und Migration. (2016). Doppelt benachteiligt? Kinder und Jugendliche mit Migrationshintergrund im deutschen Bil-dungssytem: Eine Expertise im Auftrag der Stiftung Mercator. https://www.stiftung-mercator.de/media/downloads/3_Publikationen/Expertise_Doppelt_benachteiligt.pdf.

Schenk, L., Ellert, U., & Neuhauser, H. (2007). Kinder und Jugendliche mit Migra-tionshintergrund in Deutschland. Methodische Aspekte in Kinder- und Jugendge-sundheitssurvey (KiGGS) [Children and adolescents in Germany with a migration background. Methodical aspects in the German Health Interview and Examination Survey for Children and Adolescents (KiGGS)]. *Bundesgesundheitsblatt, Gesundheits-forschung, Gesundheitsschutz, 50*(5–6), 590–599.

Schulz, M., Mack, B., & Renn, O. (Eds.). (2012). *Fokusgruppen in der empirischen Sozial-wissenschaft: Von der Konzeption bis zur Auswertung.* Wiesbaden: Springer VS.

Stanat, P., & Edele, A. (2011). Migration und soziale Ungleichheit. In H. Reinders (Ed.), *Empirische Bildungsforschung: Gegenstandsbereiche* (1st ed., pp. 181–192). Wies-baden: VS Verlag / Springer Fachmedien Wiesbaden GmbH Wiesbaden.

Statistisches Bundesamt. (2018). Bevölkerung - Zahl der Einwohner in Deutschland nach Altersgruppen am 31. Dezember 2016 (in Millionen). https://de.statista.com/statistik/daten/studie/1365/umfrage/bevoelkerung-deutschlands-nach-altersgruppen/.

Trebbe, J., Heft, A., & Weiß, H.-J. (2010). *Mediennutzung junger Menschen mit Migrationshintergrund: Umfragen und Gruppendiskussionen mit Personen türkischer Herkunft und russischen Aussiedlern im Alter zwischen 12 und 29 Jahren in Nordrhein-Westfalen. Schriftenreihe Medienforschung der Landesanstalt für Medien Nordrhein-Westfalen: Bd. 63.* Düsseldorf, Berlin: LfM, Landesanstalt für Medien Nordrhein-Westfalen (LfM); Vistas.

Ünal, A. (2011). Ernährung bei Familien mit Migrationshintergrund: Warum sind türkische Kinder oft so dick? *MMW-Fortschritte Der Medizin, 153*(43), 50–53.

Wartella, E., Rideout, V., Montague, H., Beaudoin-Ryan, L., & Lauricella, A. (2016). Teens, health and technology: A national survey. *Media and Communication, 4*(3), 13.

Weiss, H. (2007). *Leben in zwei Welten: Zur sozialen Integration ausländischer Jugendlicher der zweiten Generation.* Wiesbaden: VS Verlag / GWV Fachverlage GmbH.

Xesfingi, S., & Vozikis, A. (2016). Ehealth literacy: In the quest of the contributing factors. *Interactive Journal of Medical Research, 5*(2), e16.

Yang, S.-C., Luo, Y.-F., & Chiang, C.-H. (2017). The associations among individual factors, eHealth literacy, and health-promoting lifestyles among college students. *Journal of Medical Internet Research, 19*(1), e15.

Zillien, N. (2009). *Digitale Ungleichheit.* Wiesbaden: VS Verlag. https://doi.org/10.1007/978-3-531-91493-0.

Zschorlich, B., Gechter, D., Janßen, I. M., Swinehart, T., Wiegard, B., & Koch, K. (2015). Gesundheitsinformationen im Internet: Wer sucht was, wann und wie? [Health information on the Internet: Who is searching for what, when, and how?]. *Zeitschrift fur Evidenz, Fortbildung und Qualitat im Gesundheitswesen, 109*(2), 144–152.

Health without formal Education?

Health Literacy, Quality of Life and Health Behavior Among Male Heads of the Household in Four Districts of the Ghazni Province, Afghanistan

Stefanie Harsch, Asadullah Jawid, M. Ebrahim Jawid,
Luis A. Saboga-Nunes, Uwe H. Bittlingmayer,
Diana Sahrai and Kristine Sørensen

The authors gratefully acknowledge the support of the participants in Ghazni province, the interviewers and particularly Mrs. Sharifa Jawid; furthermore we would like to thank the Afghan Ministry of Public Health for welcoming this study.

S. Harsch (✉) · U. H. Bittlingmayer
Institute of Sociology, University of Education Freiburg (Germany), Freiburg, Germany
e-mail: stefanie.harsch@ph-freiburg.de

U. H. Bittlingmayer
e-mail: uwe.bittlingmayer@ph-freiburg.de

A. Jawid
Institute of Mathematics and Statistics, American University of Afghanistan, Kabul, Afghanistan

M. E. Jawid
Director Shuda Hospital, Ghazny (Afghanistan), Shuhada Organization, Ghazny, Afghanistan
e-mail: ebrahim.jawid@shuhada.org

L. A. Saboga-Nunes
Institute of Sociology, Public Health Research Centre, University of Education Freiburg (Germany), Freiburg, Germany
e-mail: luis.saboga-nunes@ph-freiburg.de

1   Introduction

In our global and complex world, various factors have a negative impact on our health, and attaining the highest status of health is essential to leading a fulfilling, prosperous and productive life. So, to cope with negative impacts and promote health, its determinants, health literacy and quality of life are essential. Although many studies demonstrate the relationship between health literacy, education and health behavior, little is known about its relationship with the quality of health or the situation in crises-affected low-income countries. People living Ghazni share a multitude of burdens such as poor prerequisites for health, low formal education, an inadequate health system, and several pathological but preventable health issues (e.g. leishmaniasis (Stahl et al. 2014)). This study aims to contribute to the growing number of health literacy assessment worldwide and is also innovative by focusing on the relationship between health literacy and people's literacy and quality of life.

By reducing complexity at the individual level, linear and simple theoretical models explain the relationship between various health concepts, for example, health education leads to health literacy, which results in a good health decision, demonstrated in health behavior and leads to good health (e.g. Nutbeam 2000). Moreover, the concept of health literacy needs to be defined as more than the ability to read and understand health information but as the ability to find, understand, appraise and apply information to make health decisions and thus empower to manage health (Nutbeam 1998). To describe the level of health literacy, inform governments, identify vulnerable groups, and tailor health interventions, studies on health literacy have increasingly been conducted worldwide such as in the US, Scandinavian countries and other European countries (Bröder et al. 2017; European Commission 2014; Jordan and Hoebel 2015; Okan et al. 2017; Pelikan 2012) but also recently increasingly in countries of the global South like Iran and Pakistan (Duong et al. 2017; Ghaddar et al. 2012; Haerian et al. 2015; Haghdoost et al. 2015). Most studies reveal that a remarkably large group of people with a

D. Sahrai
School of Education, Institute of Special Education and Psychology, University of Applied Sciences and Arts Northern Switzerland, Muttenz, Switzerland
e-mail: diana.sahrai@fhnw.ch

K. Sørensen
Director of the Global Health Literacy Academy, Risskov, Denmark
e-mail: contact@globalhealthliteracyacademy.org

poor level of health literacy live in European as well as in Asian countries, partly over 50% of the population. Each study replicated a (greater or minor) association between the level of health literacy and educational attainment or health behavior, and sometimes age effects or gender effects could also be found (Duong et al. 2017; Pelikan et al. 2012). The cross-country comparison revealed that people in low-income countries are likely to have a lower level of health literacy (on average) compared to high-income countries (Duong et al. 2017)). Two plausible explanations are, on the one hand, the higher level of education, making it more likely for people to perceive the interaction with health information to be easy or, on the other hand, the instrument in use (HLS measuring tool) is better tailored to people in high-income countries where it was first used. Despite the increase in empirical evidence from around the world, conflict- and crisis-affected countries and states with a high illiteracy rate, such as Afghanistan, are rarely studied. A thorough search of the relevant literature yielded only one article on the health literacy of Afghan people emigrated to Sweden but not in Afghanistan itself (Wångdahl 2017).

In general, Afghanistan is afflicted by many difficult circumstances such as geographical conditions, conflict, corruption, poverty, migration and climate change, and many other poor prerequisites of health (WHO 2015) which affect the reported 'quality of life'. In the Human Development Index, this country is one of the poorest in the world (ranking 169th out of a total 188). Living conditions are challenging (gross national income per capita is $ 1 871), health is poor (life expectancy at birth is 64.0 years) and education is at a low level (mean years of schooling is at 3.8 years) (UNDP 2019). Thus, a very high percentage of people never attended school and is illiterate (on average only 38.2% Afghans are literate [52% men, 24.2% women] (CIA 2019). Afghanistan is among the leading countries in providing insufficient health services in rural and remote areas, and public health indicators such as under-five mortality are three to five times higher than in neighboring countries. Various barriers to health care exist: Availability, transportation and costs, but also cultural considerations (for example) determine that the choice of health behavior is not merely made by the individual him/herself, but also within the family, who decide on the appropriacy/feasibility of health management strategies. Besides the important role of the oldest women in the family, one key-decision maker in the family is the male head of the household, which is why his health literacy level is relevant to all his family members (see the study in Pakistan (Sabzwari 2017)). Furthermore, traditional treatment and the consultation of the mullah is also very widespread in rural areas. Empirical data on Afghanistan should be studied cautiously, as most studies – including those in the health care sector – are conducted in major cities and safe places and rarely anything is known about health issues of the 3 out of 4 people (73%) living in rural and remote areas. To gain a better understanding of the health situation of those mostly neglected but highly at risk people, we wanted to explore the level of health literacy and of quality of life of (il)literate people in remote areas and their health behavior.

Based on a literature review, we assumed the level of health literacy in Afghanistan might be low, but still illiterate people might be able to report good health behavior and high quality of life. To the best of our knowledge, empirical data on health literacy and quality of life comes from patient studies and mostly from studies with functional measures such as TOFHLA (Parker et al. 1995) but not from comprehensive measures of, e.g., HL such as the HLS-EU-Q, with the exception of one where HL is associated with the entire QoL-scale and the physical and mental subscale (Jovanić et al. 2018). It is controversial whether the relationship between health literacy and health behavior in Afghanistan is consistent, strong, or even at all existent. Furthermore, we assumed that contextual and socio-demographic indicators could have an impact on health literacy but also on health behavior and quality of life.

2   Aim and Research Questions

The purpose of this study was to assess the level of health literacy and quality of life of Afghan men, to explore associated factors – in particular education attainment – and to discuss the complex relationship between illiteracy, health literacy, health behavior, determinants of health and quality of life. The guiding research questions were:

1. Constructs
   1.1.   What is the level of education in Afghanistan?
   1.2.   What is the level of health literacy in Afghanistan?
   1.3.   What is the level of quality of life in Afghanistan?
   1.4.   Are educational attainment, health literacy and quality of life associated?
2. What sociodemographic and contextual factors are associated with health literacy and quality of life in Afghanistan?
3. What health behavior is associated with health literacy and quality of life?

It is plausible to assume that the level of health literacy among heads of the household may be low, based on other studies demonstrating health literacy to be associated with educational attainment, socio-economic status, age, health system capacity, proximity to health centers and health behavior. The various difficulties in Afghanistan suggest that the quality of life might be low. Furthermore, we presumed education may not be the one dominating determinant and many people may demonstrate reasonably good health behavior. Besides, we assessed the religious beliefs and patient empowerment (see forthcoming articles) and explored a salutogenic perspective on the health literacy and health behavior of people with no or low levels of education.

3   Data and Methods

For this multi-site study, we developed a questionnaire consisting of 102 items from the following instruments: 45 general health-related items, 15 health literacy items from the *HLS-EU-Q16*, 18 items from *Quality of Life* (WHOQOL-BREF) (WHO 1996), 8 items from the *Spirituality, Religion, Personal Beliefs Questionnaire* (WHOQOL-SRPB-BREF) (Skevington, Gunson, and O'Connell 2013) and 16 items from the *Questionnaire for patient empowerment measurement* (Ünver and Atzori 2013*)*. The items and supplementary questions were selected based on their content, cultural appropriateness and relevance.

We measured health literacy using the HLS-EU-Q developed by Pelikan, Soerensen et al. (Pelikan et al. 2012) shortened to the HLS-EU-Q16 by Röthlin et al. (2013) and slightly modified and translated into Dari using the pioniering work by Wångdahl et al. (2014; Wångdahl 2017). We also translated it into Pashtu. In both translations we excluded one item because of its practical irrelevance in this area of Afghanistan. Concerning the validation of internal consistency, the Cronbach alpha in our sample is $\alpha = .860$ (Items: 15, Cases: 391). This value is fairly high and can be regarded as evidence of appropriate internal consistency of the indices (Sørensen et al. 2015). We calculated health literacy levels based on the average of the answers given and excluded all respondents under 15 years of age and with more than 20% missing answers. Detailed information on the scale and the calculation strategies (Harsch et al. 2020).

We measured the quality of life using the *Quality of Life Scale* (WHOQOL-BREF) (WHO 1996) and chose 18 items from it. The total mean and subscale means were calculated for all participants completing the entire scale as suggested in the standard procedure (Röthlin et al. 2013).

Participants reported on educational attainment in a three-item gradation: Illiteracy, basic education, formal and higher education. Regarding health behavior, we focused on the predominant issues in Afghanistan, such as help-seeking, family health, and nutrition, and developed appropriate questions based on the daily experience in the hospital in Afghanistan.

3.1   Research Area

We conducted research in the Ghazni province in four of the most densely populated districts Jaghori, Malistan, Nahoor, and Qarabagh (see Fig. 1). Only one hospital, the Shuhada hospital, and 25 health centers serve these districts to answer population needs. These districts are representative of the geography of most of Afghanistan with a study area of about 7355 square kilometers in width and an altitude difference of more than 2000 meters.

3.2   Sample and Data Collection

We employed a two-stage stratified sampling strategy. In the first stage, we selected a number of community development councils (CDC) from the list of all CDCs in each district using a simple random sampling. In the second stage, we randomly selected a specific number of households from each selected CDC.

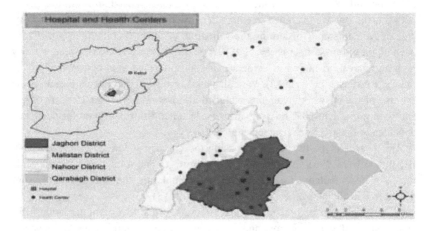

Fig. 1 Research Area - Hospital and Health Centers *(source: own depiction)*

Table 1 Population distribution in the study district and number of interviewees *(source: own depiction)*

No.	District	No. of Households	Population	No of CDC	No of Interviewees (male)
1	Jaghori	33837	167082	27	227
2	Malistan	35556	169379	8	109
3	Nahoor	29225	100845	27	147
4	Qarabagh	2881	23048	2	19
5	Total	101499	460354	64	502

We calculated the number of CDCs and participants from each district based on the share each district had in the total population sample of all four districts (cf. Table 1 below). Two trained male interviewers travelled to the villages and conducted the interviews orally with the head of the household in Dari or Pashtu. We adhered to the inclusion criteria defined by the HLS-EU consortium and limited the sample to participants aged 15 years and above. Table 1 illustrates the distribution of the population in the study districts[1] as well as the number of CDCs and the number of male respondents from each district.

3.3 Statistical Analysis

Prior to data analysis, we excluded 16 of the 502 respondents because they replied "I don't know" to more than 20% of the 15 health literacy-items (equivalent to more than three items). We calculated the level of health literacy based on the mean of all the answers given by a person, the calculated means, and the standard deviations for groups and population. For international comparison, we converted all scores to a standardized metric from 0 to 50 points. 0 represents the 'lowest possible' and 50 represents the 'best possible' health literacy score. Additionally, we defined the three levels 'inadequate' (0–25), 'problematic' (>25–37.5), 'sufficient' (>37.6–50) health literacy according to the common established classification. To identify vulnerable groups, the 'inadequate' and 'problematic' levels were combined into a single level called 'limited health literacy' (0–37.5). (Duong et al. 2017; Pelikan et al. 2012; Sørensen et al. 2015). Many indicators

---

[1]The data was provided by the "National Solidarity Program" of the Ministry of Rural Rehabilitation and Development.

in Afghanistan are very low, therefore the use of international cut-off values can lead to large differences in group size and limit comparison. Since we wanted to explore the explanations for the differences within our sample, we converted the indicators into dichotomous variables. Hence, we aggregated basic and formal education into one education category (= none and some education) and split the sample into two halves by dividing the HLS-EU-Scale by the median (here 22.22 on a scale from 0 to 50) and the Quality of life by the median of 51 (on a scale from 38 to 70). This allowed us to perform a detailed analysis of behavior in relation to the indicators discussed. We computed univariate and multivariate analyses (multivariate linear regression models) and controlled for possible covariates (age, education). Furthermore, we calculated odds ratio, confidence intervals etc. for the comparison of groups of illiterates and literate men.

Sample:
502 male heads of the household in the villages from the following districts participated in the survey: Jaghori (N = 227), Malistan (N = 109), Nahoor (N = 147), and Qarabagh (N = 19). The male respondents are on average 48.18 years old (range between 16 and 90 years) with most participants between 50-59 years (N = 127 participants) followed by 60-69 years old (N = 85). As many as 43 participants are aged 70 and above. The majority of respondents are married (95.8%), live in a household of about 8.5 people (ranging from 2 to 27) with an average of 2.2 literate people. The most common occupation is farming (65.14%) and working at home (8.8%) or being a shopkeeper (7.4%). The main sources of income are farming (46.2%), business (40.8%) and also remittances (money sent by relatives living abroad) (11.0%). Their daily living and health behavior take place in a certain location with particular contextual characteristics. Only 14% of men have access to a river (14%), a road (85%) and a car (18%). Access to electronic communication is also limited, partly because only about half the population has electricity (45%), and partly because devices such as phones (57%), TV sets (25%) and the Internet (5%) are only accessible to a few.

4   Results

4.1   Educational Attainment

Educational attainment is generally low with 51.6% of illiterates (N = 251), 18.5% with basic education (N = 90) and about three tenths with formal education (29.8%) (N = 145). Education is negatively correlated with the age

$r = -.252$, p<.001. For example, in the group aged over 60, 78 people are illiterate, but with even distribution there should be only 66.1 people. In contrast, only 24 people in this age group have formal or higher education, although 38.2 people could have been expected. In the age group up to 30, the pattern is inversely the same, significantly more people have formal and higher education and fewer are less educated than expected. (χ^2 (12) = 62 891, p<.001). Thus, calculated in decades, older men are more likely to be illiterate than younger men.

4.2 Health Literacy Level

In the four districts in Ghazni province, male heads of the household have low (self-reported) health literacy (see Fig. 2). Of the 486 respondents, only 1.0% have sufficient health literacy as measured by the HLS-EU-Q15. The majority (72.4%) have an inadequate health literacy-level and around one quarter (26.5%) have a problematic level of health literacy. Health literacy is not correlated with age ($r = -.059$, p = .196). Not all activities related to health literacy are described as difficult. In general, the activity perceived as easy by the majority of respondents is "to understand the advice on health given by family member" (Item 14) (44.12% perceived it as fairly or very easy). By contrast, only about a quarter of the male heads of the household living in the villages consider it easy "to find information on treatments that concern them" (Item 1) (27.54%) followed by "to find out where to go to get professional help" (Item 2) (30.99%). Of those without education, 74.5% consider it difficult "to find information on treatment that concerns you", but 42.7% say it is easiest "to understand advice on health given by family members or friends" (2.4). So in general, understanding health information received from people nearby is much easier compared to any other general health-related task.

HL Level of Afghan Male Heads of the Household
(N=486; in %)

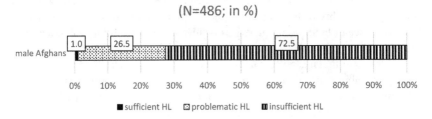

Fig. 2 Percentage of HL level of Male Afghans *(source: own depiction)*

5   Quality of Life

The mean quality of life level – measured using the relevant indicators – is M = 2.89, SD: .339, with a minimum of 1.69 and maximum of 4.25. The entire scale is not correlated with age (r = −.043, p = .345). Variance exists between the four subscales of the quality of life scale: physical, psychological, social and environment. "Social relationship" has the strongest support M = 3.545 SD = .856, followed by physical health M = 3.128, SD = 309; environment M = 2.578, SD = .56 and psychological M = 2.505, SD = .472. The majority of respondents agreed with items expressing satisfaction with sexual life and personal relationships. Whereas the lowest number of people stated that they were "satisfied (…) with their access to health services" (M = 2.1955, SD = .89), 60.9% were not satisfied (at all), only 5.1% reported to be satisfied and 34.0% did not specify how they felt.

5.1   Association between Education, Health Literacy and Quality of Life

The education level has a weak association with health literacy (r = .133, p = .003). Three out of four illiterate men have inadequate level of health literacy and one of four illiterate men have a problematic level of health literacy. Overall, the education level is also associated with the quality of life (r = .180, p < .001). *Yet the quality of life (total score) is not associated with the level of health literacy.*

5.2   Determinants of and Factors Associated with Literacy, Health Literacy or Quality of Life

To explore the relationship between the determinants of health, literacy, health literacy and quality of life, we calculated (partial) correlations. The groups with more/less health literacy and more/less quality of life vary from each other. (see Table 2)

Overall, our findings reveal that the sociodemographic data and context factors are comparably poor and the distance to the nearest health centers is immense. The men in our sample live far away from the nearest health center (on average 14.86 h by car, answers range from one to 65 h).

Table 2 Relationship between Sociodemographic Data and Health Literacy and Quality of Life *(source: own depiction)*

Male heads of the Household (in villages)	Health Literacy				Quality of Life		
	General (N=486)	High HL (N=245)	Low HL (N=241)	Sig.	High QoL (N=240)	Low QoL (N=223)	Sig.
Socio-demographic data							
Age (in years)	47.92 (±15.6) (R: 16–90)	47.07 (±14.6)	48.78 (±16.4)	n.s.	48.77 (±15.1)	49.29 (±14.3)	n.s.
Marital status (married)	95.7	96	95	n.s.	100	100	n.s.
Education (%) _illiterate (I) _basic education (BE) _formal education (FE)	I: 51.6 BE: 18.5 FE: 29.8	I: 46.9 BE: 20.8 FE: 32.2	I: 56.4 BE: 16.2 FE: 27.4	n.s.	I: 45.7 BE: 20.2 FE: 34.1	I: 60.4 BE: 18.8 FE: 20.8	$\chi^2(2)=12.243$, p=.002
Main occupation (%) _farmers (F) _others (O) _work at home (H) _shopkeeper (S) _teacher (T) _gvt/NGO employee (E)	F: 65.14 O: 14.1 W: 8.8. S: 7.4	F: 64.1 O: 15.9 W: 9.4 S: 7.3 T: 2.4 E: 0.8	F: 66.4 O: 12.9 W: 7.5 S: 7.1 T: 4.1 E: 2.1	n.s.	F: 58.7 O: 17.5 W: 10.8 S: 8.5 T: 3.6 E: 0.9	F: 75.0 O: 10.4 W: 6.7 S: 5.0 T: 0.8 E: 2.1	$\chi^2(5)=18.25$, p=.003
Main source of income (%) _farming (F) _business (B) _remittances (R) _employed (E)	F: 45,9 B: 41,6 R: 10,5	F: 35.5 B: 49.4 R: 13.5	F: 56.4 B: 33.6 R: 7.5	$\chi^2(3)=$ 23,47, p<.001	F: 48.0 B: 39.0 R: 9.9 E: 3.1	F: 44.2 B: 43.8 R: 11.8 E: 0.8	n.s.
Household size (Mean, SD, range)	8.5 (±7.2) (R: 2–27)	8.81 (±9.6)	8.22 (±3.8)	n.s.	8.80 (±10.24)	8.37 (±3.1)	n.s.

(continued)

Table 2 (continued)

Male heads of the Household (in villages)	Health Literacy				Quality of Life		
	General (N=486)	High HL (N=245)	Low HL (N=241)	Sig.	High QoL (N=240)	Low QoL (N=223)	Sig.
Literates in household (mean)	2.18 (±1.80; R: 0–9)	2.24 (±1.8)	2.2 (±1.8)	n.s.	2.39 (±1.98)	1.97 (±1.6)	r=.132, p=.011
Access to infrastructure							
Access to river (%)	14,4	20	8	r=.149, p=.004	12.0	16.0	n.s.
Access to phone (%)	57,2	57	58.0	n.s.	61.0	55.0	n.s.
Access to road (%)	85,0	89	81.0	–	83.0	86.0	–
Possess a car (%)	16,4	16.73	16.18	n.s.	22.87	9.58	r=.263, p<.001
Access to electricity (%)	44,65	40.82	48.55	r=−.157, p=.002	55.16	34.58	r=.269, p<.001
Access to TV (%)	24,28	21.63	26.97	n.s.	34.08	14.17	r=.291, p<.001
Access to internet (%)	5,35	3,67	7.05	n.s.	8.07	1.25	r=.235, p<.001
Health System							
Nearest health centre by car (in hours)	15.33 (±20.3; R: 1–65)	17.73 (±20.7)	12.64 (±19.5)	r=−.144, p=.005	9.42 (±15.8)	20.5 (±22.3)	r=−.317, p<.001
Type of nearest HC (%) _hospital (H) _clinic (C) _others (O)	H: 20.6 C: 77.4 O: 2.1	H: 23.7 C: 75.5 O: 0.8	H: 17.4 C: 79.3 O: 3.3	χ²(2)= 6.223, p=.045	H: 19.7 C: 77.6 O: 2.7	H: 20.8 C: 77.5 O: 1.7	n.s.

The groups characterized by higher or lower health literacy and higher or lower quality of life vary significantly in sociodemographic data, contextual factors and access to the health system. Although age and education level ($r = -.20$, $p < .001$) are slightly associated, age is neither associated with the level of health literacy ($r = -.059$, $p = .196$) nor with the quality of life ($r = -.043$, $p = .345$) of male heads of the household.

Concerning health literacy, the two groups are largely comparable except for the main source of income. Controlled for education and age, most contextual factors other than health literacy and access to electricity ($p = .009$) are not relevant, except for car, river, telephone, road, TV or Internet. Weak but mixed associations exist between men's health literacy levels and the number of pupils in the household ($r = .109$, $p = .016$), having migrants in the family ($r = .143$, $p = .002$) and the main source of income ($r = .191$, $p = .000$), but the correlation between these three factors and health literacy is statistically mediated by education. Regarding access to the health center, we found a mixed picture, while the group with lower health literacy lives closer to health centers (12,64 h vs. 17.73 h) ($r = .150$, $p = .002$), they are less likely to go to the clinic than are those with a higher level of literacy who live further away.

The level of quality of life correlates with various social determinants of health and access to technology. For example, those people reporting higher quality of life have more access to technical devices such as Internet ($r = .299$, $p < .001$) and TV ($r = .331$, $p < .001$), and also to electricity ($r = .271$, $p = .001$) and a car ($r = .253$, $p < .001$), but not to a phone ($r = .015$, $p = .746$). These people are also more likely to have higher education and not to work as farmers.

5.3 Health Behavior and its Relationship with Education, Health Literacy, and Quality of Life

We explored the relationship between health behavior and education, age, health literacy, quality of life (see Table 3). For the sake of the analysis, the group was divided into higher and lower levels of these indicators.

As Table 3 illustrates, health-promoting behavior is more often associated with education and quality of life but less often with health literacy. In general, there is no clear picture of the relationship between health behavior and the indicators we used to predict individual health behavior.

Help-seeking: In case of sickness, just every second man goes to the doctor (48.8%); one in four men (25.5%) uses traditional treatment while 15.2% go to local experts, and 10.5% to mullahs to seek health advice. When a pregnant

Table 3 Relationship between Health Behavior and Health Literacy and Quality of Life (*source: own depiction*)

Male heads of the household (in villages)	Health Literacy				Quality of Life		
	General (N=486)	High HL (N=245)	Low HL (N=241)	Sig.	High QoL (N=240)	Low QoL (N=223)	Sig.
Sick	68.0	64.0	71.0	n.s.	63.0	76.0	$r=-.159$, $p=.002$
Smoking	47.0	49.0	44.0	n.s.	47.0	50.0	n.s.
Help seeking behavior							
Sickness where to go _doctor/HC (D) _local expert (L) _mullah (M) _traditional treatment (T)	D: 48.4 L: 15.2 M: 10.5 T: 25.5	D: 42.9 L: 15.5 M: 6.1 T: 35.5	D: 54.8 L: 14.9 M: 14.9 T: 15.4	$\chi^2(3)=$ 31.908, $p<.001$	D: 66.8 L: 10.8 M: 9.9 T: 12.6	D: 31.3 L: 19.6 M: 12.1 T: 37.1	$\chi^2(3)=64.124$, $p<.001$
Unconscious pregnant women _doctor/HC (D) _local nurse (N) _mullah (M)	D: 21.4 N: 54.1 M: 24.5	D: 23.3 N: 52.2 M: 24.5	D: 19.5 N: 56.0 M: 24.5	n.s.	D: 28.7 N: 52.5 M: 18.8	D: 13.3 N: 55.0 M: 31.7	$\chi^2(2)=20.771$, $p<.001$
Nutrition							
Tea drinking _cold (C) _warm (W) _hot (H)	C: 3.5 W: 53.3 H: 43.2	C: 4.5 W: 61.6 H: 33.9	C: 2.5 W: 44.8 H: 52.7	$\chi^2(2)=$ 17.797; $p<.001$	C: 2.7 W: 39.5 H: 57.8	C: 3.8 W: 65.4 H: 30.8	$\chi^2(2)=$ 34.356, $p<.001$
Vegetable consumption _daily (D) _weekly (W) _monthly (M) _seasonally (S) _none (Nc)	D: 4.1 W: 8.4 M: 10.5 S: 56.6 Nc: 20.4	D: 5.3 W: 9.0 M: 7.8 S: 57.1 Nc: 20.8	D: 2.9 W: 7.9 M: 13.3 S: 56.0 Nc: 19.9	n.s.	D: 7.6 W: 13.9 M: 17.9 S: 45.3 Nc: 15.2	D: 0.8 W: 2.1 M: 4.2 S: 67.5 Nc: 25.4	$\chi^2(4)=69.912$, $p<.001$

(continued)

Table 3 (continued)

Male heads of the household (in villages)	Health Literacy				Quality of Life		
	General (N=486)	High HL (N=245)	Low HL (N=241)	Sig.	High QoL (N=240)	Low QoL (N=223)	Sig.
Fruit consumption (N=443) _daily _weekly _seasonally _none	D: 0.7 W: 3.4 S: 50.8 Nc: 45.1	D: 0.9 W: 3.2 S: 46.3 Nc: 49.5	D: 0.4 W: 3.6 S: 55.1 Nc: 40.9	n.s.	D: 1.5 W: 6.7 S: 52.3 Nc: 39.5	D: 0.0 W: 0.0 S: 49.3 Nc: 50.7	$\chi^2(3)=21.858$, $p<.001$
Family planning, pregnancy and newborn							
Info preventing unplanned pregnancy (N=464)	15.83	17.0	14.0	n.s.	17.49	13.75	n.s.
Use of contraceptives (N=464)	17.71	16.6	17.5	n.s.	24.22	10.42	$r=.173$, $p=.001$
Contraception as sin yes	24.7	20.00	29.05	n.s.	27.35	23.75	n.s.
First breast feeding after birth (h) (N=449)	16.2 (±23.0; R: 0–100)	19.13 (±24.3)	13.22 (±21.3)	$r=.189$, $p<.001$	9.34 (±17.7)	22.71 (±25.6)	$r=-.360$, $p<.001$
Food given (N=464) _breastfed (B) _oil (oil) _others (oth)	B: 36.2 Oil: 49.6 Oth: 14.2	B: 33.2 Oil: 52.8 Oth: 14.0	B: 39.3 Oil: 46.3 Oth: 14.4	n.s.	B: 46.2 Oil: 39.5 Oth: 14.3	B: 27.1 Oil: 58.8 Oth: 14.2	$\chi^2(2)=20.325$, $p<.001$

Information: Not all 486 interviewees have responded to all questions as indicated in the table.

woman is unconscious, more than half of the men (53.8%) report she should be taken to a local nurse, and only one in 5 (21.5%) recommends the doctor while a high number of 24.7% of men recommend the mullah. A trend in the selection of experts based on the literacy level could not be observed, but for health literacy and quality of life. In case of sickness, people with a higher level of health literacy are less likely to go to the doctor than people with a lower level of health literacy, instead they prefer traditional treatment. Whether this can be explained by the greater distance between doctor and place of living in this group, needs to be investigated. Interestingly, people with a higher level of quality of life are much more likely to seek medical assistance than those with poorer quality of life who prefer traditional treatment.

In terms of nutrition, the majority of the men do not eat vegetables or fruit daily (4.1% vs. 0.7%) but seasonally (56.6% vs. 50.8%). Concerning fruit consumption, a high share of people (almost every second man (45.1%) reports not to consume them at all. Regarding the drinking temperature of tea, a statistically significant association exists between higher level of health literacy and drinking the tea warm (and not hot) $\chi^2(2) = 17.797$; $p < .001$. There is no association between the frequency of consuming vegetables or fruit and health literacy levels, but with educational attainment and quality of life. People with higher educational level and a higher quality of life are less likely to 'not consume' vegetables or fruit but rather consume them more regularly (daily, weekly or monthly). Whether this is explained by the education level or the availability of vegetables and fruits in the very cold and snowy winters could not be clarified here. It is noteworthy that those who live closer to health centers are also more likely to eat vegetables and fruit weekly or daily, while those living far away eat them seasonally or not at all.

Due to the high rates of fertility, under-five mortality and maternal mortality, **family health** issues are vital in Afghanistan: Only a small percentage of Afghan men state they have information on how to prevent unplanned pregnancies (15.5%), less than 1 out of 6 (17.0%) refers to the use of contraceptives and every fourth man states he regards the use of contraception as a sin (24.5%). Statistically significant differences exist in reproductive health and the indicators analyzed, but not concerning the item about information on preventing unplanned pregnancy or on the use of contraceptives (higher for those reporting a higher quality of life). Furthermore, those with a higher level of literacy and health literacy less frequently consider contraception a sin. However, 71.7% of the group of illiterates disagree with the statement that contraception is a sin.

Asked about breastfeeding, a higher health literacy level is positively associated with a supportive opinion on breastfeeding (r = .167, p = .000). Nevertheless, the majority say breastfeeding should start many hours after birth (an average of

16.1 h after delivery). This is not associated with education level, but there are small but statistically significant differences between higher levels of health literacy and the time of first breastfeeding (surprisingly in favor of waiting longer (r = .189, p < .001)). However, the choice of food preferably given (breastfeeding, oil or others) to the new-born child is not associated with health literacy but with education and quality of life. People with higher levels of education and quality of life are far more likely to breastfeed their child than those with lower levels, who prefer oil.

6 Discussion

Today, health literacy can be considered a global Public Health concern (Malik et al. 2017) and is therefore the focus of the latest WHO priorities (WHO 2016). In countries where poverty is rampant and ubiquitous, health literacy can make a contribution to overcoming the cycle of poverty and deprivation. Investing in the assessment of health literacy levels of populations is therefore a real step towards launching strategies to overcome these conditions. To deliver such policy relevant data, this paper looked at an Afghan population from a remote area and their health literacy level. The overarching task of capturing health literacy levels of this population is a challenge as today's health literacy models are still not culturally sensitive (Levin-Zamir et al. 2017).

So far, no specific culturally sensitive Afghan health literacy definition or model has been proposed. Little is known about the social representations of health and well-being in the Afghan society in general and in remote areas of Afghanistan in particular. This is a handicap to be considered in the context of the overall topic of health literacy. Moreover, it justifies why importing definitions and models developed in different social contexts and applying them in Afghanistan will only be a starting point for deeper knowledge to be further developed. Therefore, when exploring the adaptation of the health literacy instrument, the research team had to drop one item of the standardized tool intended for use (the HLS-EU-16).

Conducting Public Health-research in Afghanistan is very rare in its nature. For the majority of the people in Afghanistan, the daily struggle for survival is more important than choosing a healthy lifestyle. Four decades of civil war have affected the country hard. It is very difficult to carry out empirical research because of the security situation, on the one hand, and because of the particular topography of Afghanistan, especially its remote areas, on the other hand. For this reason, research often concentrates primarily on the capital Kabul or other major cities and surrounding areas. It is therefore not surprising that, to the best of our knowledge and belief, there is only one study on health literacy involving Afghan people. It was conducted by Wangdahl et al. in Sweden. In their study, they interviewed refugees in the early stage after their arrival in Sweden, including 33 participants from Afghanistan. They report that 29.9% had inadequate, 40.7% problematic and 29.6% sufficient health literacy, when measured using the HLS-EU-16 Survey (Wångdahl et al. 2014). In comparison, our heads of the households in the Hazarajat-area report much lower health literacy levels than the (young male) Afghans who came to Sweden.

The association between low literacy skills and low level of health literacy has been repeatedly reported in many studies (Jordan and Hoebel 2015). Recent research shows the percentage of people with low literacy skills is higher in low-income countries than in high-income countries (Duong et al. 2017; Pelikan et al. 2012) which points in the direction that health literacy levels in Afghanistan might also be very low.

Our study revealed that health literacy in Afghanistan is indeed very low and the health literacy level of Afghan male heads of the household is – according to our data – lower than any result that has ever been reported. *Despite the basic assumption that a low level of health literacy is associated with a low levels of health behavior, our data presents a different picture.* The patterns of correlations between individual self-reported health literacy and self-reported health behavior are not consistent in our data. There are hardly any positive associations between a higher level of health literacy and health behavior. On the other hand, the available health care infrastructure has an obvious impact on health behavior in terms of health-seeking preferences. There are strong associations between the proximity to the nearest health care center and seeking care from a health professional. If there is a hospital available, our respondents are more willing to seek health there, and less likely to seek help from a mullah or use traditional treatment. These data support a more socio-ecological approach to explain the relationship between health literacy and health behavior.

Concerning the determinants of individual health literacy, we found only minor correlations with literacy and age. Although weakly, this study is nevertheless consistent with other studies that have demonstrated that health literacy is associated with education ($r = -148$, $p = .001$) and education is also associated with quality of life ($r = -.221$, $p < .001$)

There are indirect links between health literacy and education that might help to understand the differences in health literacy between the two groups (of people with some education and people without any formal education). Sociodemographic and contextual factors associated with health literacy in our study: the social status of male heads of the household, as measured by their main source of income, is statistically significantly associated with health literacy levels, revealing a relationship between structural resources and self-reported health literacy. This confirms the general relationship between social inequalities and health inequalities (Pickett and Wilkinson 2015; a.o. Wilkinson 2014; Wilkinson and Pickett 2010).

With regard to e-health literacy, we found a surprising result: We cannot conclude that people in our study with better access to communication devices also have higher health literacy levels because we found no association between access to communication devices and self-reported health literacy levels. This result is noteworthy, as numerous health policy approaches within the framework of development cooperation attempt to strengthen the health literacy of people in remote areas by improving the local technical infrastructure. In our view, which is based on the results of our study, the health policy strategy to improve Internet access in order to improve the health literacy level of people in remote areas is not complex enough. According to studies from industrialized countries, Internet access does not automatically determine health literacy (and e-health literacy) levels as these depend on individual media use and adequate (e-)health literacy tools.

Similar to the vast majority of health literacy studies, there is a positive association between education and health literacy. However, these studies should be considered with caution, as there are hardly any health literacy studies involving illiterate people. Whereas in other studies illiterate people are usually systematically excluded, we have succeeded in assessing the health literacy level of illiterate people through personal interviews. On the basis of the traditional understandings of functional health literacy, illiterate people should have almost no health literacy (Bittlingmayer and Sahrai 2018). Nonetheless, our study revealed that a substantial number of illiterate people did not report inadequate health literacy levels.

There are three possible explanations for this result: The first is that our findings are neither reliable nor valid. In this case, the HLS-EU-Q is not suitable for measuring health literacy in countries with a high number of illiterate people. We cannot easily refer to the validation study for six Asian countries by Duong et al. (2017) because they used the HLS-EU-Q47, which is the original, longer version of the instrument, and excluded illiterates. The second explanation refers to the underlying concept of health literacy as comprehensive, rather than just functional health literacy. The HLS-EU-Q focuses on tasks and interaction between people and societal services. It is therefore understandable that people in countries where oral dissemination of health information is common can report on health literacy without having high literacy rates. Thus, we like to stress that there is no reason to distrust people's responses solely because of their status as illiterates. The third explanation refers to the assumption that particularly in developing countries formal education has hardly the same significance as in industrialized countries for day-to-day practice. We like to emphasize the significance of the social context for health literacy as highlighted in several qualitative health literacy studies (Papen 2009; Samerski 2019).

Our study demonstrates that the role of formal education can affect low-income countries such as Afghanistan, particularly in its remote areas, in ways that are different from those seen in high-income countries. For example, it can be considered that health care systems in low-income countries are absent or very far from the population, often less complex and easier to navigate than in high-income countries, where the health care system is better equipped and can provide more accessible services, as well as more and also better specialized treatment. Yet, this study emphasizes that illiterate people can be, especially in social contexts, as capable in health literacy as scientists and that people cannot be judged by their literacy alone. Some people, even if they have almost no formal education, nevertheless have sufficient competencies to act healthily in everyday life.

If we want to learn more about health literacy and behavior—based on a salutogenetic understanding of people's competencies and resources—we need to focus on people's daily lives (Papen 2009; Samerski 2019). In order to explore the living environments of people with low formal education or illiterate people, quantitative research should be complemented by ethnographic approaches (Bittlingmayer et al. 2020; Bittlingmayer and Sahrai 2010). In our perspective, our quantitative data from developing countries and remote areas suggest that more research is needed to explore the specific relationship between health literacy and health-related practices in everyday life.

Besides inquiring about HL levels in Afghanistan, this paper wanted to explore the level of quality of life and possible relationships with educational level.

There are hardly any studies published looking at health literacy in a sample with such a low formal education, where the number of illiterates (51.6%) surpasses that of those with some education. The younger the participants are the more likely they have been getting more education (due to historical and political events) but nevertheless the levels continue to be much lower than in any other research on health literacy done so far.

Levels of health literacy are found to be satisfactory in only 13% of the respondents, and they do not correlate with age or QoL. It is not surprising that all health literacy items that imply access to health professionals or facilities, score the lowest. In fact, the number of hours to get to the nearest health center or hospital is an average 14.8 h (and it can go up to 65 h). Concurrently, the health services indicator of QoL is the lowest (M = 2.1) of all indicators in the four indexes (social relationships, physical health, environment and psychological) of the QoL construct, as only 5.1% are satisfied with the accessibility to health services. In hardly any study, have respondents reported to take so many hours to gain access to health facilities.

Social relationship is the dimension of the QoL that receives high appraisal (M = 3.1) and (naturally) here health literacy is substantially acquired (44.1% find it easy to understand advice given by a family member, an indicator of the health literacy construct). This is in our perspective very consistent to the importance of the social dimension of health literacy for people with low formal education.

7 Conclusion

The purpose of the study was to provide novel data on health literacy in Afghanistan, thereby contributing to the growing evidence on health literacy in Asia. We found that even compared to other low-income Asian countries, the level of (self-reported) health literacy of male heads of the household in the province of Ghazni in Afghanistan is very low. The most obvious explanation is that Afghanistan in general and Ghazni Province in particular as a remote region has one of the highest illiteracy rates. However, this study clearly shows against the odds that illiterate people are not more susceptible to low levels of health literacy and can demonstrate remarkably healthy behavior.

Bearing in mind literacy levels and the geographical and political situation in Afghanistan and other war-torn countries, we plead for further ethnographic research to explore how health literacy is present in each given context, in interpersonal relationships and the common ways of communicating health messages.

As our study reveals, access to infrastructure and information and communication technology is not in itself automatically linked to a higher level of health literacy, hence the dissemination of new technologies in Afghanistan cannot work as the sole strategy to enhance health literacy.

In view of the poor health status in Afghanistan, more comprehensive strategies are needed, covering everyday family life, health centres, and community meetings in mosques and schools to address health literacy as a complex and urgent public health challenge for the people of Afghanistan.

244   S. Harsch et al.

References

Bittlingmayer, U. H., Islertas, Z., Sahrai, E., Harsch, S., Bertschi, I., & Sahrai, D. (2020). *Health Literacy aus gesundheitsethnologischer Perspektive*. Wiesbaden: Springer VS.

Bittlingmayer, U. H. & Sahrai, D. (2010). Gesundheitliche Ungeichheit: Plädoyer für eine ergänzende ethnologische Perspektive. *Aus Politik Und Zeitgeschichte*. (45/2010), 25–31.

Bittlingmayer, U. H., & Sahrai, D. (2018). Health literacy for all? Inclusion as a serious challenge for health literacy. In U. Bauer, O. Okan, P. Pinheiro, D. Levin-Zamir, & K. Sørensen (Eds.), *International Handbook of Health Literacy: Research, Practice and Policy across the Lifespan* (2019).

Bröder, J., Okan, O., Bauer, U., Bruland, D., Schlupp, S., Bollweg, T. M., ⋯ Pinheiro, P. (2017). Health literacy in childhood and youth: A systematic review of definitions and models. *BMC Public Health, 17*. https://doi.org/10.1186/s12889-017-4267-y.

CIA (2019). World Fact Book Afghanistan. Retrieved from https://www.cia.gov/library/publications/the-world-factbook/geos/af.html.

Duong, T. V., Aringazina, A., Baisunova, G., Nurjanah, Pham, T. V., Pham, K. M., ⋯ Chang, P. W. (2017). Measuring health literacy in Asia: Validation of the HLS-EU-Q47 survey tool in six Asian countries. *Journal of Epidemiology, 27*(2), 80–86. https://doi.org/10.1016/j.je.2016.09.005.

European Commission (2014). European Citizens' Digital Health Literacy. Retrieved from http://ec.europa.eu/commfrontoffice/publicopinion/flash/fl_404_en.pdf.

Ghaddar, S. F., Valerio, M. A., Garcia, C. M., & Hansen, L. (2012). Adolescent health literacy: The importance of credible sources for online health information. *The Journal of School Health, 82*(1), 28–36. https://doi.org/10.1111/j.1746-1561.2011.00664.x.

Haerian, A., Moghaddam, M. H. B., Ehrampoush, M. H., Bazm, S., & Bahsoun, M. H. (2015). Health literacy among adults in Yazd, Iran. *Journal of Education and Health Promotion, 4*(1), 91. https://doi.org/10.4103/2277-9531.171805.

Haghdoost, A. A., Rakhshani, F., Aarabi, M., Montazeri, A., Tavousi, M., Solimanian, A., ⋯ Iranpour, A. (2015). Iranian Health Literacy Questionnaire (IHLQ): An instrument for measuring health literacy in Iran. *Iranian Red Crescent Medical Journal, 17*(6). https://doi.org/10.5812/ircmj.17(5)2015.25831.

Harsch, S., Jawid, A., Jawid, M. E., Saboga-Nunes, L., Bittlingmayer, U. H., Sahrai, D., Sørensen, K. (2020 (submitted)). Health Literacy and Health Behavior among Women in Ghazni, Afghanistan.

Jordan, S., & Hoebel, J. (2015). Gesundheitskompetenz von Erwachsenen in Deutschland: Ergebnisse der Studie "Gesundheit in Deutschland aktuell" (GEDA) [Health literacy of adults in Germany: Findings from the German Health Update (GEDA) study]. *Bundesgesundheitsblatt, Gesundheitsforschung, Gesundheitsschutz, 58*(9), 942–950. https://doi.org/10.1007/s00103-015-2200-z.

Jovanić, M., Zdravković, M., Stanisavljević, D., & Jović Vraneš, A. (2018). Exploring the Importance of Health Literacy for the Quality of Life in Patients with Heart Failure. *International Journal of Environmental Research and Public Health, 15*(8). https://doi.org/10.3390/ijerph15081761.

Levin-Zamir, D., Leung, A. Y. M., Dodson, S., & Rowlands, G. (2017). Health literacy in selected populations: Individuals, families, and communities from the international and cultural perspective. *Information Services and Use, 37*(2), 131–151. https://doi. org/10.3233/ISU-170834.

Malik, M., Zaidi, R. Z., & Hussain, A. (2017). Health Literacy as a Global Public Health Concern: A Systematic Review. *Journal of Pharmacology & Clinical Research, 4*(2), 555632. https://doi.org/10.19080/jpcr.2017.04.555632.

Nutbeam, D. (1998). Health promotion glossary. *Health Promotion International, 13*(4), 349–364. https://doi.org/10.1093/heapro/13.4.349.

Nutbeam D. (2000). Health literacy as a public health goal: a challenge for contemporary health education and communication strategies into the 21st century. *Health Promotion International, 15*(3), 259-267. https://doi.org/10.1093/heapro/15.3.259.

Okan, O., Bröder, J., Pinheiro, P., & Bauer, U. (2017). Gesundheitsförderung und Health Literacy. In A. Lange, C. Steiner, S. Schutter, and H. Reiter (Eds.), *Springer Reference Sozialwissenschaften. Handbuch Kindheits- und Jugendsoziologie* (pp. 1–21). Wiesbaden: Springer. https://doi.org/10.1007/978-3-658-05676-6_48-1.

Papen, U. (2009). Literacy, Learning and Health – A social practices view of health literacy. *Literacy and Numeracy Studies, 16/17*(2/1), 19–34. https://doi.org/10.5130/lns. v0i0.1275.

Parker, R. M., Baker, D. W., Williams, M. V., & Nurss, J. R. (1995). The test of functional health literacy in adults. *Journal of General Internal Medicine, 10*(10), 537–541. https://doi.org/10.1007/BF02640361.

Pelikan, J. (2012). Measurement of health literacy in Europe: HLS-EU-Q47; HLS-EU-Q16; and HLS-EU-Q86: The HLS-EU Consortium 2012.

Pelikan, J., Röthlin, F., & Ganahl, K. (2012). *Comparative report of health literacy in eigth EU member states. The European Health Literacy Survey HLS-EU.* Retrieved from http://ec.europa.eu/chafea/documents/news/Comparative_report_on_health_literacy_in_ eight_EU_member_states.pdf.

Pickett, K. E., & Wilkinson, R. G. (2015). Income inequality and health: A causal review. *Social Science and Medicine, 1982*(128), 316–326. https://doi.org/10.1016/j.socscimed.2014.12.031.

Röthlin, F., Pelikan, J. M., & Ganahl, K. (2013). Die Gesundheitskompetenz von 15-jährigen Jugendlichen in Österreich. Retrieved from http://www.hauptverband.at/cdscontent/load?contentid=10008.597350andversion=1395738807.

Sabzwari, S. R. (2017). Health literacy in Pakistan: Exploring new ways of addressing an old challenge. *JPMA. The Journal of the Pakistan Medical Association, 67*(12), 1901–1904.

Samerski, S. (2019). Health Literacy as a social practice: Social and empirical dimensions of knowledge on health and healthcare. *Social Science and Medicine, 81,* 1–26.

Skevington, S. M., Gunson, K. S., & O'Connell, K. A. (2013). Introducing the WHOQOL-SRPB BREF: Developing a short-form instrument for assessing spiritual, religious and personal beliefs within quality of life. *Quality of Life Research: An International Journal of Quality of Life Aspects of Treatment, Care and Rehabilitation, 22*(5), 1073–1083. https://doi.org/10.1007/s11136-012-0237-0.

Sørensen, K., Pelikan, J. M., Röthlin, F., Ganahl, K., Slonska, Z., Doyle, G., et al. (2015). Health literacy in Europe: Comparative results of the European health literacy survey (HLS-EU). *The European Journal of Public Health, 25*(6), 1053–1058. https://doi. org/10.1093/eurpub/ckv043.

Stahl, H. C., Ahmadi, F., Schleicher, U., Sauerborn, R., Bermejo, J. L., Amirih, M. L., Stahl, K. W. (2014). A randomized controlled phase IIb wound healing trial of cutaneous leishmaniasis ulcers with 0.045% pharmaceutical chlorite (DAC N-055) with and without bipolar high frequency electro-cauterization versus intralesional antimony in Afghanistan. *BMC Infectious Diseases, 14,* 619. https://doi.org/10.1186/s12879-014-0619-8.

UNDP (2019). *Human Development Report: Afghanistan.* Retrieved from http://hdr.undp.org/en/countries/profiles/AFG.

Ünver, Ö., & Atzori, W. (2013). Questionnaire for Patient Empowerment Measurement: Document D3.2 Version 1.0. Retrieved from https://docplayer.net/23278255-Support-users-to-access-information-and-services-document-d3-2-questionnaire-for-patient-empowerment-measurement-version-1-0.html.

Wångdahl, J. (2017). *Health literacy among newly arrived refugees in Sweden and implications for health and healthcare.* (Doctoral dissertation, Acta Universitatis Upsaliensis). Retrieved from http://urn.kb.se/resolve?urn=urn:nbn:se:uu:diva-333427.

Wångdahl, J., Lytsy, P., Mårtensson, L., & Westerling, R. (2014). Health literacy among refugees in Sweden - a cross-sectional study. *BMC Public Health, 14,* 1030. https://doi.org/10.1186/1471-2458-14-1030.

WHO (1996). WHOQOL-BREF. Introduction, administration, scoring and generic version of the assessment. Retrieved from https://www.who.int/mental_health/media/en/76.pdf.

WHO (2015). Country Cooperation Strategy at a glance. Retrieved from http://applications.emro.who.int/docs/CCS_Afgh_2015_EN_16725.pdf?ua=1.

WHO (2016). Shanghai Declaration on promoting health in the 2030 Agenda for Sustainable Development. Retrieved from https://www.who.int/healthpromotion/conferences/9gchp/shanghai-declaration.pdf?ua=1.

Wilkinson, R. (2014). *The Impact of Inequality: How to Make Sick Societies Healthier.* New York: The New Press. https://ebookcentral.proquest.com/lib/gbv/detail.action?docID=579087.

Wilkinson, R. G. & Pickett, K. (2010). *The spirit level: Why equality is better for everyone* (Publ. with rev). *Pinguin sociology.* London: Penguin Books.

Reflections on Health Literacy in the European and Colombian Context

Isabella C. Bertschi and Lilliana Villa-Vélez

1 Introduction

Health literacy is a concept that is gaining importance in public health. Strengthening the health literacy levels of citizens is seen as a key strategy to foster equal opportunities and to reduce inequalities within health systems and societies that witness a constant rise in complexity (DeWalt et al. 2004; Kickbusch and Maag 2008; Nutbeam 2000; U.S. Department of Health and Human Services 2010). The European Commission (2007b) and also the US government (National Center for Health Statistics 2012) identify the promotion of health literacy as a priority in health policy. This is consistent with research findings stating that health literacy is a critical competence for active participation in health systems and relevant in the development of health behaviour and healthy lifestyles (Kickbusch and Maag 2008; Nutbeam and Kickbusch 2000; Sørensen et al. 2012). Low health literacy is linked to a variety of negative health outcomes, e.g. reduced life expectancy, lower self-reported health status, lower participation rates in preventive health offers and higher rates of hospitalization (Canadian Council on Learning 2007; DeWalt et al. 2004; HLS-EU Consortium 2012; Kindig et al. 2004; Statistics Canada and OECD 2005; Weiss 2005).

I. C. Bertschi (✉)
Department of Psychology, University of Zurich, Zurich, Switzerland
e-mail: isabella.bertschi@psychologie.uzh.ch

L. Villa-Vélez
National Faculty of Public Health, University of Antioquia, Medellín, Colombia
e-mail: liliana.villa@udea.edu.co

© The Editor(s) (if applicable) and The Author(s), under exclusive license to
Springer Fachmedien Wiesbaden GmbH, part of Springer Nature 2021
L. A. Saboga-Nunes et al. (eds.), *New Approaches to Health Literacy*,
Gesundheit und Gesellschaft, https://doi.org/10.1007/978-3-658-30909-1_13

Health literacy is also conceptualised as an outcome of health promotion and especially health education activities (Nutbeam 2000). As such, it is closely linked to reflections on the meaning and conceptualisation of education in the area of health.

There is no doubt about the importance of education for public health; however, in practice we can observe many occasions in which education is reduced to a merely instrumental matter (Nutbeam 2000). It is reduced to a summation of 'educational activities' where the goal of public health—to foster people's capacities to stay healthy, increase their well-being and prevent the deterioration of their health—is lost sight of. Therefore, it is necessary to think of education in the scope of health as a subject that allows for capacity-building based on the recognition of the individual.

Hereafter, we present some reflections that emerged during the Health Literacy Summer School organized by HLCA consortium in Freiburg, Germany in September 2016. We focus on differences regarding the understanding of the concepts of health literacy and health education and stress their importance when discussing experiences from diverse political and cultural contexts. These reflections are essential to advance reflection on health literacy and to strengthen research and educational practice in health.

2 The Definition and Conceptualisation of Health Literacy

Health literacy is a concept that has gained attention both in academia and on the Western political agenda in recent years. Although there has been a rapid increase in publications and policies on the topic (Heijmans et al. 2015), to date there is no generally accepted definition of the term. Rather, there are different approaches to conceptualizing and defining health literacy (Abel 2008; Berkman et al. 2010; Frisch et al. 2012; Vogt et al. 2016; Wills 2009). Mancuso (2009) summarises this observation: "The concept of health literacy is not entirely straightforward and the term is defined broadly and in a variety of ways in the literature" (p. 88). One main reason for differences in the understanding of health literacy seems to be rooted in the adoption of the concept in two differing contexts: in clinical care and in public health (Nutbeam 2008).

In clinical care, the focus has largely been on the difficulties low literacy skills of patients can cause when those patients navigate the health system. Definitions of health literacy in this context consequently stress functional competences, defining health literacy as "the degree to which individuals have the capacity to obtain, process, and understand basic health information and services" (Parker et al. 2003, p. 147). Examples for this school of thought include research into reduced adherence to medication in people with low (health) literacy (Geboers et al. 2015) or lower rates of participation in preventive screening efforts that seem to be linked to limited understanding of oral and written health information (Bennett et al. 2009; Cho et al. 2008). It is therefore not surprising that this line of research is said to reflect a concept of health literacy as a "clinical risk" by Nutbeam (2008). The measurement tools for assessing health literacy levels of individuals that have been developed under this perspective include the Test of Functional Health Literacy in Adults (TOFHLA) (Parker et al. 1995) and its short version S-TOFHLA (Baker et al. 1999). TOFHLA consists of text passages with related text comprehension exercises and numeracy tasks taken from medical contexts. It is used to screen patients for limited literacy skills and ideally, health care professionals adapt their language complexity and communication strategies as well as health information materials to the patients' supposed (health) literacy level. This measurement approach "places health literacy as a risk factor that needs to be identified and appropriately managed in clinical care" (Nutbeam 2008, p. 2074).

Public health – and in particular health promotion – approaches to health literacy focus on the role the concept can play in "enabling individuals to exert greater control over their health and the range of personal, social and environmental determinants of health" (Nutbeam 2008, p. 2074). Health literacy is conceptualized as an asset and linked to empowerment (Kickbusch 2004; Nutbeam 2000; Nutbeam and Kickbusch 2000; World Health Organization 1998). From this line of research stems the definition of health literacy that is widely used in Europe today and was developed by the team of the European Health Literacy Survey (HLS-EU):

Health literacy (...) entails people's knowledge, motivation and competences to access, understand, appraise, and apply health information in order to make judgments and take decisions in everyday life concerning healthcare, disease prevention and health promotion to maintain or improve quality of life during the life course. (Sørensen et al. 2012, p. 3)

The conceptual model developed in accordance with this definition aims to broaden the context in which health literacy matters away from the health care system only to include the population level, i.e., a public health perspective. The related questionnaire (HLS-EU-Q; Sørensen et al. 2013) relies on self-reported difficulties with accessing, understanding, appraising and applying health information in different contexts.

The European Health Literacy Survey was conducted in eight member states of the European Union to determine their populations' health literacy (HLS-EU Consortium 2012; Sørensen et al. 2015). Its questionnaire has since been used in several population-based studies from other European countries, e.g. Malta (Office of the Commissioner for Mental Health 2015) and Switzerland (gfs.bern 2016). Across all countries, almost every second person has limited health literacy. This finding has refuelled efforts to bring health literacy to European policy agendas. A brief overview of these efforts is provided in the following section.

3   Health Literacy in European Policy

In 2004, Ilona Kickbusch organized a workshop on health literacy during the European Health Forum Gastein (EHFG), a main platform for exchange on health policy in Europe. The background paper for this workshop (Kickbusch 2004) summarized research on health literacy and suggested that Europe take on international leadership in implementing the concept into health policies. The topic was taken up during EHFG 2005, and health literacy was prominently mentioned in Gastein Health Declaration (2005) stating that "[e]veryone has the right to (…) access to health literacy" (p. 6). In the European Commission's (2007b) framework for a new health strategy for the European Union health literacy was explicitly included and linked to empowerment and the participation of citizens. Likewise, competences fostering citizens' "understanding of how individuals can ensure optimum physical and mental health" (European Commission 2007a, p. 9) were included in the European reference framework 'Key competences for lifelong learning'. Also the European Patients' Forum (2009) and some time later the World Health Organization (WHO) Regional Office for Europe (2013) demanded that health literacy be established as a concept at EU and national level and that governments invest in programs to strengthen health literacy. Subsequently, health literacy was mentioned in the Vilnius Declaration (2013) and the Riga Roadmap (2015) until finally in 2016, the consensus paper 'Making health literacy a priority in EU health policy' was launched. The authors are the Standing Committee of European Doctors (CPME), the European Patients' Forum (EPF), Health Literacy Europe, Maastricht University (UM), and Merck-Sharp & Dohme (MSD). They emphasize that strengthening the health literacy level of citizens helps fight some of the most important challenges outlined in Europe

2020 strategy, e.g. a rise in chronic diseases and demographic change. They ask the European Commission to develop a European strategy on health literacy and to establish a monitoring system of health literacy levels across the European Union. To date, a shared European understanding and policy framework on health literacy has not been established yet. Still, some countries have adopted the concept and incorporated it into national public health policies with great variation in the degree of formalization (Health Literacy Centre Europe 2015; Heijmans et al. 2015).

4   Health Literacy, Its Translation(s) and Health Education

As was outlined above, health literacy has been taken up by policy makers in Europe in several forms. When trying to investigate whether the concept has been used in Colombian policies, the difficulty of translation arises. As Sørensen and Brand (2014) have noted "health literacy cannot yet be considered a mainstream notion" (p. 640). Therefore, "translation may act as an influential factor with regard to health literacy valorisation" (p. 635) and should be carefully considered when working on the topic in different linguistic contexts. There are several translations of 'health literacy' to the Spanish language, e.g. 'instrucción sanitaria' and 'alfabetización en salud'. The latter is used most frequently (Falcón Romero and Luna Ruiz-Cabello 2012; Sørensen and Brand 2014) and will therefore be used in this article.

In the process of abstracting meaning from one language to another, this meaning can be altered. The interpretation of 'alfabetización en salud' can be problematic as 'alfabetización' can refer to the process of 'alphabetization', but it can also be translated to 'literacy'. This difficulty is taken up by Falcón Romero and Luna Ruiz-Cabello (2012) who were part of the Spanish research group of HLS-EU. Given that the word 'alfabetización' in Spanish can refer to very instrumental skills limited to reading and writing, Falcón Romero and Luna Ruiz-Cabello (2012) make it clear that

'[a]lfabetización en salud' goes beyond general literacy. It means not only to be able to read a leaflet or understand information on a treatment provided by a health professional, but it involves knowing how to access appropriate information,

to understand and appraise it, and to apply it in order to take informed decisions regarding our own health and the health of our community.[1] *(Falcón Romero and Luna Ruiz-Cabello 2012, p. 92)*

We found that the concept of health literacy has not been adopted in Colombian policies (yet). Still, many policies in the country can be said to aim at improving the health literacy levels of citizens. They stress the importance of education to achieve and maintain good health. Following Nutbeam's (2000) conceptualization of health literacy as an outcome of health education, these policies therefore do include a notion of health literacy although the term itself may not be explicitly mentioned. Programs and activities in health education are referred to in Spanish mainly by the term 'educación para la salud'.[2]

5 Public Policies on Educación Para La Salud in Colombia

In Colombia, education in the area of health is a topic that has received increasing attention during the last years. Nevertheless, it continues to be a marginal topic in national research, public policy, public health and clinical practice. Policies that include 'educación para la salud' take a public health perspective following WHO's suggested definition: "Health education comprises consciously constructed opportunities for learning involving some form of communication designed to improve health literacy, including improving knowledge, and

---

[1]For the sake of uniformity of language, the quote was translated into English by the authors. To avoid the pitfalls associated with translation we mention in the article, we provide also the Spanish original quote: "La AES [alfabetización en salud] va más allá de la alfabetización general, significa no solo saber leer el prospecto de un medicamento o entender la información que nos facilita el profesional sanitario respecto a un tratamiento, sino que implica saber cómo acceder a la información adecuada, interpretarla, juzgarla y aprovecharla para tomar decisiones bien fundamentadas sobre nuestra propia salud y la de nuestra comunidad".

[2]In some publications, the term 'educación en salud' is used as well. To our knowledge, there is no consistent pattern of using either 'educación en salud' or 'educación para la salud'. Similarly, in English we can mainly observe the use of 'health education' while some authors use the term 'education for health'. In this article we used the term in Spanish to avoid confusion.

developing life skills which are conducive to individual and community health" (Nutbeam 1998, p. 353). Nevertheless, it has to be made clear that the definition and conceptualization of 'educación para la salud' are vague and unclear. Some authors even state that the term lacks identity. This is partly due to the tension between health education and health promotion and the fact that in some occasions, the meaning of health education is reduced to be understood as a mere instrument serving the purpose of health promotion (Diaz-Valencia 2012, pp. 381–382).

Many local Colombian experiences give an account of educational processes in health, especially in nursing where the topic has traditionally been developed. Although there is no single national policy on 'educación para la salud', we have been able to identify the topic in public policies from different areas. For example, the 1) Plan Decenal de Salud Pública 2012–2021 [10-Year Public Health Plan 2012-2021] suggests realizing educación para la salud applying the strategy information-education-communication across various programmes. 2) The Ley 1164 de 2007 [Law 1164 of 2007] on the formation of human capital in the health sector explicitly states that educación para la salud is part of the responsibilities of health professionals. Likewise, 3) the Resolución 412 de 2000 [Resolution 412 of 2000] on the 'technical norms and treatment guidelines for the development of specific protective actions and treatment of diseases of interest' in its Article 5 posits education of the affiliated population as a responsibility of health institutions across the country. To conclude the overview, 4) the Ley General de Educación [General Law on Education] adopted already in 1994 proclaims health to be a transversal issue embedded in the overall objectives of education: "Education will be developed serving the following goals: (…) Education for promotion and preservation of health and hygiene, the integral prevention of socially relevant problems, physical education, leisure, sports and appropriate use of free time"[3] (p. 1 f.).

Public Colombian policy does include educación para la salud in a wide range of political areas. Nevertheless, there is much work to do as the topic of education is treated as very general and transversal, but it is not developed in detail.

---

[3]The Spanish original reads as follows: "[L]a educación se desarrollará atendiendo a los siguientes fines: (…) La formación para la promoción y preservación de la salud y la higiene, la prevención integral de problemas socialmente relevantes, la educación física, la recreación, el deporte y la utilización adecuada del tiempo libre".

6   The Meaning of 'Educación Para La Salud'

Although in the literature there is a willingness to consider educación para la salud according to the goal of achieving healthier and more equitable societies, in practice we can observe that there is a tendency to instrumentalize educación para la salud for the purposes of health promotion and mere lifestyle changes in many cases without acknowledging the importance of working *with* people.

> *Disappointingly, the potential of education as a tool for social change, and for political action has been somewhat lost in contemporary health promotion. Close attention to the impact of public policy decisions on health, and the need to create supportive environments for health may have had the unintended consequence of leading to structural interventions 'on behalf' of people - health promotion which is done 'on' or 'to' people, rather than 'by' or 'with' people. (Nutbeam 2000, p. 265)*

From this observation stems a very important issue when articulating theory and practice of educación para la salud. According to Whitehead (2003), the theory of health education and new strategies in health promotion are associated with empowerment and socio-political interventions which seek liberation and autonomy of the individual. Nevertheless, in the practice of educación para la salud one frequently observes that these requests are not met. It is therefore fundamental to advance the pedagogical reflection on alternative suggestions such as Educación Popular that allow to understand learning processes in more depth.

> *[A]n individual 'learns' when it incorporates in its being something that goes beyond experience; there is learning when there is modification of the ways of understanding and behaving, when the previous knowledge structure is influenced.[4] (Torres Carrillo 2011, p. 54)*

From this we can derive key issues for reflection and practice in educación para la salud: 1) Training of health professionals oftentimes does not include the learning process as a central aspect in its outcomes, and educación para la salud is considered an instrumental and unspecific tool that is based in traditional education with a biomedical focus (Peñaranda et al. 2014). 2) The educational methodologies

---

[4]The Spanish original quote reads as follows: "[U]n individuo 'aprende' cuando se incorpora a su ser algo que va más allá de la experiencia; hay aprendizaje cuando hay modificación de las formas de comprender y actuar de los sujetos, cuando se afecta su estructura previa de saberes".

are not well aligned with traditional or alternative models of education although there is great potential in aligning them (e.g. health education based on Freire's Empowerment Education, see Wallerstein and Bernstein, 1988). 3) There is often an important contradiction and mismatch between the education that is suggested and the one that is realized in projects and programs (Alzate Yepes 2006, p. 21). 4) Political, economic and cultural issues greatly affect the practice of educación para la salud and should be carefully considered (e.g. Glanz and Bishop 2010). 5) Above all, a profound reflection is required as to exactly what health and what education is to be promoted and how they can be achieved with the people under the given circumstances. Tones et al. (1990) summarize these reflections: "Those who seek to educate about health are subject not only to the intrinsic controversies of education but have also to address the problem of defining the nebulous notion of health" (p. 1).

7 Conclusion and Closing Remarks

The topic of health literacy as part of educación para la salud is of crucial importance. In Europe we have witnessed an effort to formulate public policies that contribute to the development and implementation of health literacy and some countries have even adopted centralized national policies on health literacy. However, a consensus regarding the definition and conceptualization of the concept has not been reached. Additionally, the translation of the term 'health literacy' into other languages has turned out to be a source of misunderstandings and changes in the interpretation that need to be reduced considerably in order to allow for coordinated international action. In the Colombian context there is no public policy on health literacy per se. Yet, following Nutbeam's (2000) conceptualisation of health literacy as an outcome of health education, we can identify Colombian public policies that aim to promote population health through education and the improvement of people's capacities to take care of their health. We found that the conceptualizations of health literacy and health education are diverse and that education in the field of health is not understood in one single way in different contexts.

In the area of public health, health education and health literacy have traditionally been thought of in terms of interventions. However, when it comes to the educational process in the first place, thorough reflections are required as to exactly what health and what education is to be promoted and how these can be achieved under the given circumstances with the people concerned. We therefore conclude that interventions in health education and health literacy should be developed and implemented taking into account the particularities of any given context. Consequently, the current debate on health literacy is of high priority and needs to be continued in order to promote healthier and more equitable societies.

References

Abel, T. (2008). Measuring health literacy: Moving towards a health-promotion perspective. *International Journal of Public Health, 53*(4), 169–170. https://doi.org/10.1007/s00038-008-0242-9.

Alzate Yepes, T. (2006). Desde la educación para la salud: Hacia la pedagogía de la educación alimentaria y nutricional. *Perspectivas en Nutrición Humana, 16,* 21–40.

Baker, D. W., Williams, M. V., Parker, R. M., Gazmararian, J. A., & Nurss, J. (1999). Development of a brief test to measure functional health literacy. *Patient Education and Counseling, 38*(1), 33–42. https://doi.org/10.1016/S0738-3991(98)00116-5.

Bennett, I. M., Chen, J., Soroui, J. S., & White, S. (2009). The contribution of health literacy to disparities in self-rated health status and preventive health behaviors in older adults. *Annals of Family Medicine, 7*(3), 204–211. https://doi.org/10.1370/afm.940.

Berkman, N. D., Davis, T. C., & McCormack, L. (2010). Health literacy: What is it? *Journal of Health Communication, 15*(Suppl. 2), 9–19. https://doi.org/10.1080/10810730.20 10.499985.

Canadian Council on Learning. (2007). *Health literacy in Canada: Initial results from the International Adult Literacy and Skills Survey.*

Cho, Y. I., Lee, S.-Y. D., Arozullah, A. M., & Crittenden, K. S. (2008). Effects of health literacy on health status and health service utilization amongst the elderly. *Social Science and Medicine, 66*(8), 1809–1816. https://doi.org/10.1016/j.socscimed.2008.01.003.

DeWalt, D. A., Berkman, N. D., Sheridan, S. L., Lohr, K. N., & Pignone, M. P. (2004). Literacy and health outcomes – A systematic review of the literature. *Journal of General Internal Medicine, 19*(12), 1228–1239. https://doi.org/10.1111/j.1525-1497.2004.40153.x.

Diaz-Valencia, P. A. (2012). Theoretical conceptions on the theory on health education. Systematic review. *Investigación y Educación en Enfermería, 30*(3), 378–389.

European Commission. (2007a). *Key competences for lifelong learning: European reference framework.* https://eur-lex.europa.eu/legal-content/EN/TXT/PDF/?uri=CELEX:52 018SC0014&from=EN.

European Commission. (2007b). *Together for health: A strategic approach for the EU 2008–2013.* https://ec.europa.eu/commission/presscorner/detail/en/IP_07_1571.

European Health Forum. (2005). *Gastein Health Declaration. Partnerships for Health.* Retrieved from Gastein

European Patients' Forum. (2009). *150 million reasons to act. EPF's Patients' Manifesto for the European Parliament and Commission 2009.* https://www.eu-patient.eu/library/EPF-Manifesto-150-Million-Reasons-to-Act/.

Falcón Romero, M., & Luna Ruiz-Cabello, A. (2012). Alfabetización en salud; concepto y dimensiones. Proyecto europeo de alfabetización en salud. *Revista de Comunicación y Salud 2*(2), 91–98.

Frisch, A.-L., Camerini, L., Diviani, N., & Schulz, P. J. (2012). Defining and measuring health literacy: How can we profit from other literacy domains? *Health Promotion International, 27*(1), 117–126. https://doi.org/10.1093/heapro/dar043.

Geboers, B., Brainard, J. S., Loke, Y. K., Jansen, C. J. M., Salter, C., Reijneveld, S. A., et al. (2015). The association of health literacy with adherence in older adults, and its role in interventions: A systematic meta-review. *BMC Public Health, 15,* 903. https://doi.org/10.1186/s12889-015-2251-y.

gfs.bern. (2016). *Bevölkerungsbefragung "Erhebung Gesundheitskompetenz 2015". Schlussbericht.* https://www.obsan.admin.ch/sites/default/files/uploads/152131_geskomp_sb_def.pdf.

Glanz, K., & Bishop, D. B. (2010). The role of behavioral science theory in development and implementation of public health interventions. *Annual Review of Public Health, 31*(1), 399–418. https://doi.org/doi:10.1146/annurev.publhealth.012809.103604.

Health Literacy Centre Europe. (2015). National Health Literacy policies and what we can learn from them. http://healthliteracycentre.eu/national-health-literacy-policies/.

Heijmans, M., Uiters, E., Rose, T., Hofstede, J., Devillé, W., Van der Heide, I., et al. Rademakers, J. (2015). *Study on sound evidence for a better understanding of health literacy in the European Union.* https://ec.europa.eu/health/sites/health/files/health_policies/docs/2015_health_literacy_en.pdf.

HLS-EU Consortium. (2012). *Comparative report of health literacy in eight EU member states.* https://cdn1.sph.harvard.edu/wp-content/uploads/sites/135/2015/09/neu_rev_hls-eu_report_2015_05_13_lit.pdf.

Kickbusch, I. (2004). *Improving health literacy – A key priority for enabling good health in Europe. Background paper.* https://www.infosihat.gov.my/images/Bahan_Rujukan/He_Ict/Improving_Health_literacy.pdf.

Kickbusch, I., & Maag, D. (2008). Health literacy. In K. Heggenhougen & S. Quah (Eds.), *International encyclopedia of public health* (Vol. 3, pp. 204–211). San Diego: Academic Press.

Kindig, D. A., Panzer, A. M., Nielsen-Bohlman, L., Committee on Health Literacy, Board on Neuroscience and Behavioral Health, & Institute of Medicine (Eds.). (2004). *Health literacy: A prescription to end confusion.* Washington, DC: National Academies Press.

Mancuso, J. M. (2009). Assessment and measurement of health literacy: An integrative review of the literature. *Nursing & Health Sciences, 11*(1), 77–89. https://doi.org/10.1111/j.1442-2018.2008.00408.x.

Ministerio de Salud y Protección Social. (2007). *Ley 1164 de 2007.* https://www.minsalud.gov.co/Normatividad_Nuevo/LEY%201164%20DE%202007.pdf.

National Center for Health Statistics. (2012). *Healthy People 2010 Final Review.* https://www.cdc.gov/nchs/data/hpdata2010/hp2010_final_review.pdf.

Nutbeam, D. (1998). Health promotion glossary. *Health Promotion International, 13*(4), 349–364. https://doi.org/10.1093/heapro/13.4.349.

Nutbeam, D. (2000). Health literacy as a public health goal: a challenge for contemporary health education and communication strategies into the 21st century. *Health Promotion International, 15*(3), 259–267.

Nutbeam, D. (2008). The evolving concept of health literacy. *Social Science and Medicine, 67*(12), 2072–2078. https://doi.org/10.1016/j.socscimed.2008.09.050.

Nutbeam, D., & Kickbusch, I. (2000). Advancing health literacy: A global challenge for the 21st century. *Health Promotion International, 15*(3), 183–184. https://doi.org/10.1093/heapro/15.3.183.

Office of the Commissioner for Mental Health. (2015). *Health Literacy Survey Malta 2014.* https://deputyprimeminister.gov.mt/en/CommMentalHealth/Pages/health-literacy-survey.aspx.

Parker, R. M., Baker, D. W., Williams, M. V., & Nurss, J. R. (1995). The test of functional health literacy in adults. *Journal of General Internal Medicine, 10*(10), 537–541. https://doi.org/10.1007/BF02640361.

Parker, R. M., Ratzan, S. C., & Lurie, N. (2003). Health literacy: A policy challenge for advancing high-quality health care. *Health Affairs, 22*(4), 147–153.

Peñaranda, F., Giraldo, L., Barrera, L. H., & Castro, E. (2014). Significados de la educación para la salud en la Facultad Nacional de Salud Pública de la Universidad de Antioquia (2011-2012). *Revista Facultad Nacional de Salud Pública, 32*(3), 364–372.

Sørensen, K., & Brand, H. (2014). Health literacy lost in translations? Introducing the European Health Literacy Glossary. *Health Promotion International, 29*(4), 634–644. https://doi.org/10.1093/heapro/dat013.

Sørensen, K., Pelikan, J. M., Röthlin, F., Ganahl, K., Slonska, Z., Doyle, G., et al. (2015). Health literacy in Europe: comparative results of the European health literacy survey (HLS-EU). *The European Journal of Public Health, 25*(6), 1053–1058. https://doi.org/10.1093/eurpub/ckv043.

Sørensen, K., Van den Broucke, S., Fullam, J., Doyle, G., Pelikan, J. M., Slonska, Z., et al. (2012). Health literacy and public health: A systematic review and integration of definitions and models. *BMC Public Health, 12,* 80. https://doi.org/10.1186/1471-2458-12-80.

Sørensen, K., Van den Broucke, S., Pelikan, J. M., Fullam, J., Doyle, G., Slonska, Z., et al. HLS-EU Consortium. (2013). Measuring health literacy in populations: illuminating the design and development process of the European Health Literacy Survey Questionnaire (HLS-EU-Q). *BMC Public Health, 13,* 948. https://doi.org/10.1186/1471-2458-13-948

Standing Committee of European Doctors, European Patients' Forum, Health Literacy Europe, Maastricht University, & Merck-Sharp & Dohme. (2016). *Consensus paper: making health literacy a priority in EU health policy.* https://www.eu-patient.eu/globalassets/policy/healthliteracy/health-literacy-consensus-paper_2016.pdf.

Statistics Canada, & OECD. (2005). *Learning a living: First results of the Adult Literacy and Life Skills Survey.* https://www.oecd-ilibrary.org/education/learning-a-living_9789264010390-en.

The Riga Roadmap. (2015). *Investing in health and wellbeing for all.* http://rigahealthconference2015.eu/the-riga-roadmap/.

Tones, K., Tilford, S., & Robinson, Y. K. (1990). *Health education. Effectiveness and efficiency.* Dordrecht: Springer.

Torres Carrillo, A. (2011). *Educación popular. Trayectoria y actualidad.* Caracas: Universidad Bolivariana de Venezuela.

U.S. Department of Health and Human Services. (2010). *National action plan to improve health literacy.* Washington, DC: Office of Disease Prevention and Health Promotion.

Vilnius Declaration. (2013). *Sustainable health systems for inclusive growth in Europe.* http://www.euro.who.int/en/health-topics/Health-systems/pages/news/news/2013/11/sustainable-health-systems-for-inclusive-growth-in-europe.

Vogt, D., Messer, M., Quenzel, G., & Schaeffer, D. (2016). „Health Literacy" – ein in Deutschland vernachlässigtes Konzept? [Health literacy – a neglected concept in Germany?]. *Prävention und Gesundheitsförderung, 11*(1), 46–52. https://doi.org/10.1007/s11553-015-0519-9.

Wallerstein, N., & Bernstein, E. (1988). Empowerment education: Freire's ideas adapted to health education. *Health Education & Behavior, 15*(4), 379–394. https://doi.org/10.1177/109019818801500402.

Weiss, B. D. (2005). The epidemiology of low health literacy. In J. G. Schwartzberg, J. VanGeest, & C. Wang (Eds.), *Understanding health literacy: Implications for medicine and public health* (pp. 65–81). Washington, DC: American Medical Association.

Whitehead, D. (2003). Health promotion and health education viewed as symbiotic paradigms: Bridging the theory and practice gap between them. *Journal of Clinical Nursing, 12*(6), 796–805. https://doi.org/10.1046/j.1365-2702.2003.00804.x.

WHO Regional Office for Europe. (2013). *Health 2020 – A European policy framework and strategy for the 21st century.* https://apps.who.int/iris/bitstream/handle/10665/131303/Health2020Long.pdf?sequence=1&isAllowed=y.

Wills, J. (2009). Health literacy: New packaging for health education or radical movement? *International Journal of Public Health, 54*(1), 3–4. https://doi.org/10.1007/s00038-008-8141-7.

World Health Organization. (1998). *Health Promotion Glossary.* https://www.who.int/healthpromotion/about/HPR%20Glossary%201998.pdf.

Health Literacy in Afghanistan – Astonishing Insights Provoke a Re-Consideration of the Common Concept and Measures of Health Literacy

Asadullah Jawid, Stefanie Harsch and M. Ebrahim Jawid

1 Introduction: Health Literacy Around the World – a Plea for a Fresh Perspective

The concept of health literacy (HL) plays a pivotal role in modern public health discussions around the world (WHO 2016). Practitioners and researchers consider health literacy a key concept in health, an outcome of health education and a prerequisite for health behavior and a healthy lifestyle (Kickbusch 2013). A promising new concept, health literacy helps identify national health systems' shortcomings, compare competencies in health across groups and countries, and serve as the empirical basis for policy decisions (Sørensen 2016). Although an impressive body of literature on health literacy is available in Western countries,

A. Jawid (✉)
American University of Afghanistan, Institute of Mathematics and Statistics, Kabul, Afghanistan

S. Harsch
University of Education Freiburg, Institute of Sociology, Freiburg, Germany
e-mail: stefanie.harsch@ph-freiburg.de

M. Ebrahim Jawid
Director Shuda Hospital, Shuhada Organization, Ghazny, Afghanistan
e-mail: ebrahim.jawid@shuhada.org

© The Editor(s) (if applicable) and The Author(s), under exclusive license to
Springer Fachmedien Wiesbaden GmbH, part of Springer Nature 2021
L. A. Saboga-Nunes et al. (eds.), *New Approaches to Health Literacy*,
Gesundheit und Gesellschaft, https://doi.org/10.1007/978-3-658-30909-1_14

multiple open questions remain: What is the level of health literacy in other countries, e.g. in the Middle East and South Asia, or in low-income and crisis- and conflict-ridden states; why do some countries score very poorly as a whole; why do some groups perform worse than others within the same country, and what are the relevant health literacy skills in a particular context. Apart from some noteworthy studies (The Asia Foundation 2018; UNDP 2019), only limited data on these countries, including Afghanistan, are available to date. Particularly in Afghanistan, where most diseases and mortality rates are caused by communicable and preventable diseases, improving health literacy and thus health behavior could lead to remarkable health gains (Burhani 2009). Empirical evidence on health literacy in Afghanistan could lead to prioritizing related interventions and increasing financial resources aimed at improving health literacy through education, which in their turn could lead to more healthy behaviors and better health in the long run. This article contributes to the growing volume of research on health literacy by qualitatively exploring the concept of health literacy and its application to a previously neglected country: Afghanistan. The literature provides various definitions of health literacy: functional, interactive, comprehensive and critical readings. For this study, however, we use the definition proposed by Sorensen et al. (2012) as the starting point:

"Health literacy is linked to literacy and entails people's knowledge, motivation and competences to access, understand, appraise, and apply health information in order to make judgments and take decisions in everyday life concerning healthcare, disease prevention and health promotion to maintain or improve quality of life during the life course." (Sørensen et al. 2012, p. 3)

Based on a narrow understanding of health literacy, it is described as the interplay (the equation) of two (de)nominators: the health system requirements and the individual's capacity (Kickbusch 2013, p. 1). So health literacy is not exclusively defined by the individual's skill but also considers the context, the situation and even the interaction of all agents involved not only in the health system but also in everyday life (Sabzwari 2017). Comparing European countries with low-income countries, it becomes apparent that the situations vary substantially. For this reason, using the same questionnaire to assess health literacy in both groups of countries could lead to an average level of health literacy in one, but a low level of health literacy in the other country statistically. Thus might lead to misinterpretations of the findings and consequently misdirect the development of interventions because it does not tell anything about the practical relevance of these findings. For instance, if a person/a population in a country scores poorly in a health literacy instrument, then the reason might be that the person/the population has inadequate health literacy (which is the most obvious explanation).

However, another possible explanation for the low level could be that the questionnaire may not be adequate for the country, because, firstly, the questions are not easily comprehensible or, secondly, the questions are irrelevant or, thirdly, the activities described in the items are very difficult for all people to perform in this context.

We therefore advocate exploring the context and (the severity of) diseases and comparing and adapting existing HL instruments to reflect the living conditions of the population in each country adequately. Our main research questions are: (a) what health literacy skills are relevant in Afghanistan, in what context are health literacy skills used and how a standard questionnaire – the HLS-EU questionnaire – can be used or adapted to measure health literacy there.

This chapter is structured as follows: After this brief introduction, we provide information on the procedure developed and proposed. In section three, we describe the findings on health and health literacy in Afghanistan using data of reports and qualitative studies. In section four, we seek to compare the concept and measurement of health literacy operationalized in the EU-HLS-Q47 (Sørensen et al. 2016; Pelikan 2012) with our empirical findings. In section five, we will discuss our findings and the lessons learned. Finally, we summarize the application of health literacy measures in a new country and give an outlook on future research activities.

2   Methods: Suggestions for Adaptation

By way of a roadmap, we have developed and utilized the strategy in Fig. 1 to assess health literacy systematically in any given country.

To answer our research questions, we compiled and analyzed data from these sources. The Table 1 displays the steps of the analysis, the sources of information, and the samples.

3   The Process of Applying Health Literacy to Afghanistan

3.1   Health Literacy in Afghanistan

The first step was to identify any document on health literacy in the country of interest, i.e. Afghanistan. In an extensive desk research conducted in July 2016, we identified only two documents on Afghan health literacy: a presentation given by the former Deputy Minister at the Afghan Ministry of Public Health, Dr. N. H.

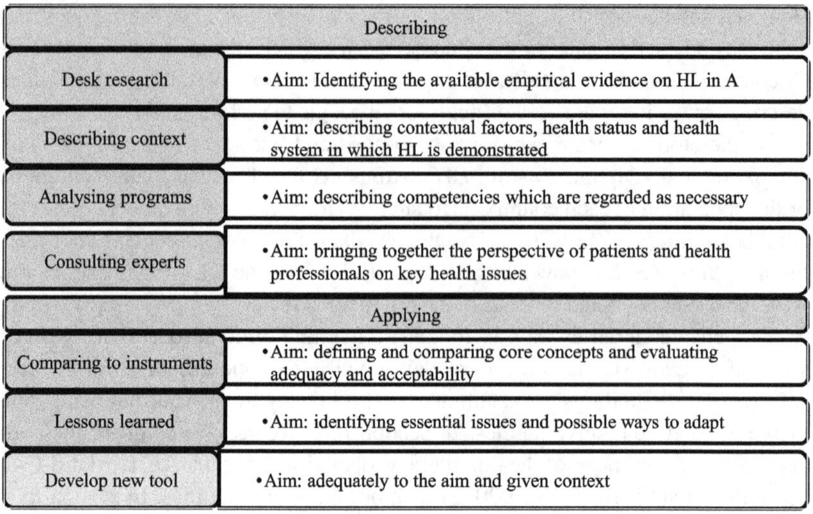

Describing	
Desk research	• Aim: Identifying the available empirical evidence on HL in A
Describing context	• Aim: describing contextual factors, health status and health system in which HL is demonstrated
Analysing programs	• Aim: describing competencies which are regarded as necessary
Consulting experts	• Aim: bringing together the perspective of patients and health professionals on key health issues
Applying	
Comparing to instruments	• Aim: defining and comparing core concepts and evaluating adequacy and acceptability
Lessons learned	• Aim: identifying essential issues and possible ways to adapt
Develop new tool	• Aim: adequately to the aim and given context

Fig. 1 Process of exploring and applying HL to a new country *(source: own depiction)*

Table 1 Steps of analysis and sources *(source: own depiction)*

Step	Source	Sample
HL research in the country	Academic databases Grey literature research	N = 2, Survey on HL of Afghan refugees in Sweden; presentation by a former Minister of Health
General data	WHO, World bank, Ministry of Public Health Grey literature review	UNDP WHO global exploratory World bank Ministry of Public Health Afghan Central Statistic Organization
Programmatic data	Health interventions of the government of NGOs	Programs (N = 4): BPHS & EPHS Community health workers Family health action groups
Experts	Focus group discussion Expert interviews	Focus group: (N = 5 participants), Afghanistan, health & HL experts Expert interviews: health professionals and NGO workers in Afghanistan (N = 29)

Burhani, at the Regional Ministerial Meeting for Asia and the Pacific on "Promoting Health Literacy" in 2009 in Beijing (Burhani 2009); and a study on health literacy of Afghan migrants in Sweden (Wångdahl et al. 2014). Although the latter study used the global health literacy instrument (the HLS-EU-Q), the results are of secondary importance as the sample of 33 young Afghan male refugees does not represent Afghanistan's general population and focuses on the health literacy of Afghans in the context of the new country and not in their country of origin. Conversely, Burhani's speech provides ideas on the understanding of health literacy in Afghanistan. Without defining health literacy, she reports on visible achievements in improving health literacy since 2001 mainly due to community health workers in the villages; communication and vaccination campaigns; improving the quality of health facilities and establishing the Healthy School initiative. To address the remaining challenges, Burhani suggests that Afghanistan should establish and strengthen telemedicine, media, cooperation (expertise, standards/norms, protocols, plans) and improve pictorial language and interpersonal communication of health workers (Burhani 2009). However, she fails to define a viable definition of the term health literacy: Is it a skill based on reading and writing or rather on verbally shared health knowledge, what is the content, and when and where is it used?

3.2 Overview of Health, Health System and Determinants of Health

In the second step, we argue that for the application of the health literacy concept to Afghanistan, it is essential to know about the general context of the country: determinants of health; health status; and to profoundly understand the complexity and demands of the health system as well as the skills and competencies of individuals (see the two components of the health literacy equation (Kickbusch 2013)).

Afghanistan is a mountainous landlocked country in the South of Central Asia and shares borders with six countries: Pakistan, Iran, Tajikistan, Uzbekistan, Turkmenistan and China. The population of Afghanistan (estimated between 30 and 37 million, e.g. 34.9 M (CIA 2019)) faces many drastic man-made disasters (war, conflict, corruption, brain drain, migration) and natural disasters (droughts, landslides, floods, severe winters, hot summers, food shortage exacerbated by climate change) (WHO 2010; The Asia Foundation 2018). Although the whole of Afghanistan is affected by one or multiple of these challenges, the situation is very divers and varies between geographical locations, between rural and urban places, ethnic or religious groups, people of different socio-economic status and educational attainment. Furthermore, the availability and accessibility of infrastructure and (health) services is also very important. For instance, people in rural and remote areas have (almost) no access to health services and in many cases health facilities are poorly equipped or out of work, so that only a small number of services are available. However, the situation in urban areas is different, with a high density of medical professionals and mostly well-equipped health centers.

Overall, Afghanistan is one of the most disadvantaged countries in terms of human development indicators (UNDP 2018) and *determinants of health*, such as age distribution, household economy and literacy to name but a few, which also play an important role in terms of health literacy. Afghanistan population is very young (with an average age of 18.6 years, others point to 15 years) and a high fertility rate of 5.3 children per woman (CIA 2019). Nearly half of all Afghans are food insecure or borderline food insecure and only 54% of the total population use improved drinking water, the unemployment rate is 23.9% (CIA 2019) and approximately 56.1% live in multidimensional poverty (UNDP 2019). One consequence of the high poverty rate, for instance, is that households are unable to bear the costs of health services. Despite the fact of Article 52 of the Afghan Constitution stating that preventive health care should be free for all, the latest evidence suggests about 73.6% (others even say up to 90%) of health financing is out-of-pocket expenditure and many people may not be able to afford it and therefore forego health care in clinics or hospitals. The overall literacy rate in Afghanistan is very low: approximately 31% are considered literary, (with an enormous gender gap; about 45% among men and 17% among women). If one considers literacy skills such as reading and writing as prerequisites for health (literacy), a large number of people lack these skills and consequently may have a low level of health literacy based on common measurements.

Combining the data on the prerequisites and determinants of health, it comes as no surprise that the overall *health status* of Afghans is generally poor. The maternal mortality rate is very high at 372/100.000; the under-5-mortality rate is approximately 83/1000 (AMS 2011[1]) and 4 to 84% of the children are stunted and 5 to 66% underweight, depending on the area (Akseer et al. 2018). Similar to most low-income countries, the rate of communicable diseases is high (the most

---

[1]This estimation is based on a nationwide census published in 2011, reporting that the data was 91/1000 (AMS 2011) This is the last one available; since then all estimations have been based on these data and try to take changes into account.

frequent diseases in 2015 were cough and colds (20%, 28% for<5 year old children), diarrhea (10.4%, 18.7% for<5 year old children) and pneumonia (3.6%; 7%) (Afghan Central Statistics Organization 2017). Additionally, other communicable diseases (polio and leishmaniasis) are also widespread in Afghanistan. The reported number of patients with non-communicable diseases (e.g. diabetes) has increased substantially in recent years. Many of the most prevalent diseases are either preventable or influenceable by a healthy lifestyle and an adequate health system, so that health literacy skills are highly relevant.

When describing the still inadequate *health system*, it is worth noting that Afghanistan has already achieved remarkable success since 2001 which are attributable to the establishment and operation of a very unique structure (Waldman and Newbrander 2014; Newbrander et al. 2014). In 2002, after more than two decades of war, the Afghan health system was almost completely destroyed and the health indicators of most Afghans were extremely bad (e.g. life expectancy was about 44 years, the maternal mortality rate was 1,600/100,000 women and under-five mortality rate was 257 per 1,000 (Viswanathan et al. 2010) one of the highest ever recorded). Furthermore, resources (finances, health professionals, facilities, equipment, medicine...) were vastly lacking and a pressing need arose to reach the entire population in the urban, rural and remote areas of Afghanistan. To accomplish this task, the Ministry of Public Health (MoPH) and international donors identified urgent needs, prioritized areas for action and developed a comprehensive concept comprising 4 core strategies. The main objectives were mother and child health (including vaccination), communicable diseases, nutrition, mental health and disability. First, they installed a hierarchical system of health facilities: The system starts with a regional hospital, followed by provincial hospitals, district hospitals, comprehensive and basic health centers, health posts, and concludes with community volunteer health workers. Next, they defined services, skills and materials relevant to each of the different levels of the health system. They are well described in the strategy of the Essential Packages for Health Services (EPHS), which address the regional and district levels; and the Basic Packages for Health Services (BPHS), which describe interventions at the village and community levels (MoPH 2005a, b). As many of the health issues are preventable, addressing the needs on the local level became a priority. Therefore, part of this global strategy was the idea of not only equipping health professionals, but also building capacity at the local level by installing and training Community Health Workers (CHW) and lay women, who gathered in so called Family Health Action Groups (FHAG) (see description below). Setting up and maintaining such a health infrastructure and maintaining it is a costly venture, for which reason the MoPH received annual funding from three main donors (the World Bank, USAID, and the European Commission) and contracted the services to NGOs. By 2008 about 60 to 85%[2] of all districts in Afghanistan had access to BPHS, according to the MoPH (Frost et al. 2016).

To obtain a complete picture of *health care* in Afghanistan, emphasis must be placed on the existence of numerous private health care providers, traditional healers, traditional health attendants, elders and mullahs. These last four are key players in the delivery of health services, especially in remote areas without available health facilities. Besides final dependency on international donors, various other weaknesses characterize the Afghan health system such as lacking or poor regulation, poor monitoring and surveillance systems, and poor civil registration (WHO 2015). Furthermore, no regulation exists that allows only certified doctors to work as medical doctors in Afghanistan. All these aspects must be taken into account when studying the concept of health literacy in Afghanistan.

3.3 Defining Basic Health Competencies Conceptually

As described above, the living situation, health status and capacity of the health system in Afghanistan differ widely from high-income countries. Therefore, the nature and content of health literacy might be different from what it is in Europe. By arguing that health literacy is a context-specific social practice (Santos et al. 2014), it is essential to define, prior to analysis, a set of adequate, important health-related competencies and knowledge that everyone in Afghanistan should acquire. This was the question faced by a group of MoPH experts and international donors who in 2001/2002, after the Taliban regime, were confronted with severe health issues. The answers and strategies found by them helped define the feasible requirements for health knowledge and skills. The proposed measures are considered feasible if they are relevant and applicable to low-income communities with less formal education. Furthermore, due to the lack of health facilities, these measures should be implemented at local level and entail quick impacts on the health status because of high needs. Hence, the government developed two approaches in the villages: The Community Health Workers (CHW) and the Family Health Action Group (FHAG). A group of experts developed manuals with

---

[2] At this point an important comment has to be made concerning the accuracy of the data. Many authors explain that the objectivity, reliability and validity of the data has to be questioned, and the comparison of the results of several studies encourages a cautious interpretation of these data (SIGAR 2017).

a range of topics that symbolize the least set of knowledge and health behavior that should be known in the village even by non-medical professionals. We believe these manuals are the best source as they summarize the basic requirements that most Afghans should know in order to be health literate in the rural context of Afghanistan.

Strategy 1: Community Health Workers (CHW). The CHWs are responsible for 1000–1500 people and it is proposed that a group of two CHW (preferably a man and a woman) work together. Their task is to help the local population with minor diseases, to refer them to hospital in severe cases and to educate them on several health issues. Furthermore, the CHWs of one region meet regularly and receive further training, e.g. on health topics, communication, training for members of the Family Health Action Group, but also on tackling rumors, mapping the village and checking for signs and giving medication. The CHW training guide covers three main areas: (1) communicable diseases and a clean and healthy environment, (2) the promotion of maternal and child health and family planning, and (3) childhood illnesses (see Table 2). The manuals contain easy-to-understand instructions in simple language and many pictures. They address aspects such as knowledge, behavior and even attitudes (…). The ability to read and write is not a prerequisite for the household to be able to use the manuals.

Strategy 2: The Family Health Action Group (FHAG). A FHAG consists of 10-15 young women, each representing a household, with small children who first receive training on basic health issues, and then each woman is asked to share her new knowledge with 10-15 houses. The FHAG curriculum covers six topics related to hygiene; family planning and pregnancy, newborn nutrition; childhood and communicable diseases. Moreover, the FHAG members learn how to convey the messages supported by pictures.

Table 2 summarizes the various aspects and organizes them along the three most important fields of action.

In line with the activities specified for CHW and FHAG, two issues were treated as priorities: healthy and clean housing and thus the prevention of communicable diseases and mother and child health.

This community-based health promotion program helps individuals find nearby information. The flipside is that people are restricted to the knowledge of CHW or FHAG members and the topics discussed, but rarely have access to information on other health issues. Although the program is concerned with individual health behavior, it does not promote health advocacy. Learning more about inhibiting and enabling factors such as the decision maker in the family (household leader or the mother-in-law) is not an objective of the program either. Apart from the total number of Community Health Workers in Afghanistan (Najafi-

Table 2 Content of community-based health programs *(source: own depiction)*

	FHAG	CHW
A healthy community through preventing infectious diseases	Health Promotion Hygiene and cleanliness Nutrition Clean drinkable water Disease Prevention Tuberculosis Diseases caused by mosquito bites (influenza H1N1, Hepatitis C, Malaria)	Prevention Personal and home hygiene Safe food Safe water Immunization Health care Communicable diseases Control of diseases spread by insect-bites Diarrhea Common skin and eye diseases
Promoting maternal, child health, and family planning	Method of lactation amenorrhea and its characteristics Birth spacing methods Antenatal care Danger signs during pregnancy Labor plan and control of possible dangers Postnatal care New-born care New-born danger signs Importance of breast feeding Breast feeding methods	Promoting birth spacing Providing certain contraceptives in the village HIV/Aids Pregnancy and antenatal care Getting ready for birth Care of mother and newborn after birth Breast feeding Feeding young children: starting additional foods Eating for good health Structure & function of the human body
Childhood illnesses	Prevention Vaccination Involvement of the community in the evaluation of child growth Health Care Diarrhea identification and treatment	Check for general danger signs Cough or difficult breathing Fever Ear problems Tuberculosis Malnutrition and nutrient deficiencies Intestinal parasites First aid Drug abuse Mental health

zada 2016), we could not find any further quantitative and qualitative data on the acceptance or implementation of the practices. Since practitioners can provide more insights and the applicability of the concepts to Afghanistan, we consulted and interviewed them individually and conducted focus group discussions with them.

4 Local Experts: Exploring Health Literacy from the Point of View of Practitioners

To investigate the concept of health literacy from the practitioners' point of view, we interviewed 29 local health professionals and had a group discussion with four Afghans, among them two medical doctors. We cannot present all the rich and comprehensive qualitative data here, therefore we center on three topics which we consider crucial for understanding health literacy in Afghanistan: understanding of health, treatment of diseases and common health behavior, promising health interventions.

Understanding of health: A doctor's comment in the focus group discussion helps frame the discussion: *"First of all there has to be a health care sector, then we can start to promote health"* (Participant 2 2016). This quote indicates the different perceptions of health and how this has an impact on health behavior and the assessment of the health literacy in Afghanistan. Since health practices and health literacy are closely linked to knowledge of the understanding, causes, development and appropriate treatment of health, we provide empirical insights on the concept of health first. The following example illustrates the general functional and social understanding of health shared among Afghans: *"As long as you don't feel severe pain and can help your family, Afghans think that they are healthy"* (Interviewee 14 2016). Hence, most Afghans predominantly do not talk about health, but about physical diseases linked to environmental factors, such as the lack of safe and clean water, weather and season (summer/winter), factors that affect the functionality of the individual in his or her social context. Some Afghans also integrate a mental dimension into their physiological understanding of health (depressed/burdened) and say that their mental health is also affected by hearing good/bad news about family members. Others, mainly healthcare professionals, expand the understanding and also add the socio-economic component ('wealth'/'income'), such as having the financial resources to seek help from the medical doctor. Overall, a variety of different opinions exists on the topic health, partly depending on the location (urban/rural), the education level and the (non-) medical background. The focus on diseases can also shape health-related behavior and the breadth or narrowness of an individual's understanding of health literacy. One example is the very popular and widespread belief that mental illness is given by God, hence the responses to a mental illness can be passivity, and even acceptance/recognition of the disease as a way to remove sins.

Treatment and seeking medical care: Concerning treatment, seeking health care is the first stumbling block and it is made up of structural, social and cultural factors and barriers. Health professionals can provide thousands of stories about common health-related behaviors in a country with a shortage of health workers, uneven distribution, and the important role played by private and traditional health professionals in treating diseases. But often, even before the patient is able to seek health care, the decision-makers or moral power holder within the family defines whether and where the patient can seek help. A further barrier for women is that they must be accompanied by a male relative. Due to the lack of health professionals and health centers, it is very likely that people will treat themselves with homemade remedies or seek advice first from family, neighbors, mullahs, traditional healers, and/or elderly women because they are easily accessible, respected and well-known. Besides, a common habit is to ignore the disease until it has drastically progressed, as a result of which people with very severe diseases show up in the health facility. The doctor-patient-interactions are characterized by the patients' perception of a good doctors: *"The more medicine prescribed, the better the doctor is"* (I14). Thus, patients often ignore doctors' advice on lifestyle behavior. Moreover, people perceive doctors as being responsible and competent for certain diseases, primarily infectious diseases treatable with drugs. But when it comes to a broken leg or a broken hand, people often go to a traditional healer; and in case of mental illness, they often consult mullahs. Likewise, it is not uncommon for the patient to follow the instruction of the family elders/mullahs to take the medication or to plan the diet beyond the doctors' instructions: *"while doctors tell the patient to eat bread and meat, the Mullah tells them to only consume fluids which will not strengthen them"* (I9).

Table 3 provides further information and details on the key issues – as specified by the doctors and interviewees.

Health intervention approaches: In the qualitative interview study, the participants mentioned several health intervention approaches on five levels. Such as A) nation-wide levels (campaigns to raise awareness of certain issues), B) facility level (instruction and health education, also specific technical (e.g. neurological problems)), C) on the community level C.1) *health workers* in the community: for example through *timed and targeted counselling;* C.2) *groups:* Family Health

Action Groups, health shuras, self-support groups, C.3) *ambassadors/heroes:* mullah, teachers, students, <u>religious leaders' wives</u>, police officers, peers, governmental officials; C.4) *mobile health teams:* herd immunization, Expanded Program on Immunization (EPI). Moreover, interventions in institutions on the D) school level <u>e.g. school-based health</u> education or through E) media & health. In addition, other approaches such as drop-in centers, health-promotion in orphanages, through "cultural containers", books for healthy reading or projects like the establishment of kitchen gardens or rearing of chickens in some cities. In general, they stated: *"community-based health promotion should be strengthened because CBHC is something that works with people and strengths and empowers them. Once the people are empowered, particularly the women, they take care of their health, especially for the prevention aspect of their health"....* (I6)

Apart from the health issues addressed by the two community-based strategies, the medical professionals added various issues related to the health system, such as knowing about services and specialists and when to seek help, communication and misconceptions.[3]

---

5   Applying Health Literacy Survey Items and Empirical Findings

5.1   Summarizing the Findings N Health Literacy in Afghanistan

In the following subchapter, we summarize the key findings along the three dimensions of health literacy and the four steps of health literacy

The *healthcare seeking behavior* is influenced not just by a lack of knowledge, but also by many barriers such as lack of availability (of health services nearby), accessibility (location and transportation), acceptability (gender concordance treatment) and affordability (including the treatment and the travel costs) (Qarani and Kanji 2015; Frost et al. 2016). Furthermore, moral barriers exist, such as shame-related health concerns, or the mullah prohibits certain health behavior (e.g. use of contraceptives). Understanding these barriers and the many explana-

---

[3]Some of the misconception are: breastfeeding is bad, children's immunization makes some of them sick, giving liquids in case of diarrhoea increases it, oral contraceptive pills cause cancer, injectable contraceptive depot-medroxyprogesterone acetate are perceived as a tool to dominate Afghans (USAID 2008).

Table 3 Common health behavior in Afghanistan *(source: own depiction)*

Health care	Disease prevention	Health promotion
(i) Common *health behavior in the village*		
Ignoring → treatment at home → in the village → at the health facility Treatment *at home:* consulting mother-in-law; home-made remedies, lack of trust in modern medicine *Village* → asking elders about health behavior; consulting mullah e.g. on mental health issues (common practice: Duah, Damm, Tavis); *Traditional healer* → e.g. for fractures	Family health practices: Rarely/no family planning (in rural areas) Delivery: mostly at home, some even in the stable Seldom/no breastfeeding in the first few days	Hygiene & nutrition education
(ii) Common in *Health System Services*		
First: Services have to be available, acceptable, accessible and affordable Second: need for reliable, committed staff and good quality Lack of knowledge about services and specialists and when to seek help Limited ability to describe symptoms, body function etc. *Perception:* Doctor can heal everything; Perception: the more drugs, the better Behavior: Consume only water/tea/bread after a surgery *Mental health* issues are rarely seen as a necessity to be treated and rather as common traits, others are highly stigmatized or induced by a 'jinn' (epilepsy) *Medicine:* adequate intake	Focus on vaccination and awareness-raising activities *Communicable diseases* Vaccination, bed-net, ORS *Non-communicable diseases* In cities it is increasingly important to address the negative effects of sedentary lifestyle and diabetes	(not applicable)
(iii) Barely *covered issues*		
Non-communicable diseases, environmental health, occupational health, pharmaceutical affairs *Health system issues*: more difficult diseases can rarely be cured		

tory patterns behind certain health-related activities is relevant to address health literacy holistically.

Disease prevention is a key strategy of the government and it receives much financial support from international donors committed to it. The main activities are the nationwide vaccination campaigns (e.g. polio, measles) and awareness-raising interventions on communicable diseases like malaria and tuberculosis. However, other disease prevention activities are untypical such as visiting the doctor for regular check-ups or health screenings. Looking more holistically at disease prevention and the setting, it becomes obvious that the community-based health education is primarily directed towards preventing diseases through individual behavior. However, awareness of the risk factors is seldom raised and health interventions rarely target the setting and its environment. The provision of water and supply of food is within the competence of other sectors, not the health sector.

Health promotion: When asked about health promotion in Afghanistan, local health experts usually give two answers: first, they state that there is no health promotion; and second it is a part of the BPHS and they refer to hygiene education that could serve health protection rather than health promotion. Additionally, many doctors provide mainly primary health care rather than health promotion. An interviewee asked critically whether health promotion is meaningful, feasible or a major concern in a country where the majority of the population is concerned about survival. Another important aspect deserves to be highlighted. Despite these difficulties and harsh conditions, the interviewees and medical doctors repeatedly report the astonishing resilience that many Afghans demonstrate.

For further analysis of the level of health literacy, discussing the availability and the process of dealing with health information is important. According to doctors, many of their patients have little access to health information and low levels of health literacy. Therefore, learning more about the process of finding, understanding, appraising and applying health information will help to analyze and develop appropriate assessment tools and interventions (see Fig. 2).

Finding: As health services are not available nearby and information through media is rarely available, the main sources for finding and transmitting health information are locally available people such as CHW and FHAG, health professionals, religious leaders/mullahs, elders, family members, neighbors, and, in urban areas, media. Mostly this information is only sought when a disease has already progressed dramatically, but rarely for prevention or health promotion purposes. Therefore, exposing people to health information through active outreach from mobile health teams or FHAG members, or in hospitals through education and videos in the waiting room is essential to stimulate thinking about new ideas and to demonstrate and learn practical ways to apply it. In addition, the interviewees indicated that other channels of disseminating news on health issues (websites, magazines, trainings, info in the health center etc.) should be supported as well.

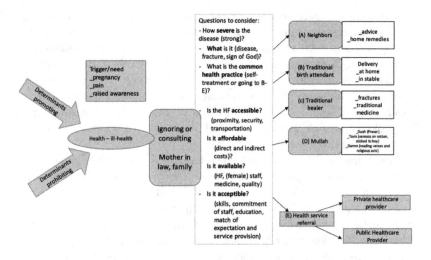

Fig. 2 Ways of responding to health issues *(source: own depiction)*

In the interviews, health professionals have given many examples of challenges associated with patients such as the difficulties patients have in describing their pain or that the patients keep secrets often and that they are influenced by misconceptions. All this could therefore affect people's (dis)ability to understand and appraise health information.

Understanding: To facilitate understanding, it is recommended to reduce the complexity of the message by mostly presenting one message in plain language with pictures or videos and focusing on teaching relevant health behavior that is easily transferrable by people into the community.[4]

Appraising: In Afghanistan, the perception of others (e.g. family members, elders, mullahs, etc.) is often given more weight than one's own perception of what is appropriate. To increase the acceptance of health information, each lesson in the FHAG manual starts with some corresponding religious teachings. Generally, most health education materials focus only one preferred way of health-promoting/-protecting behavior presented with each topic, and not several

---

[4]This might be very useful because this way the content is wrapped in words that are easily understood by people but it may also happen that interpersonal issues might interfere in accepting the message of the sender.

behaviors which would stimulate the need to compare and evaluate. Besides, we could not find any evidence on how the people are assisted in appraising the information or how they define the credibility or accuracy of the information received. Without empirical data, however, it is not possible to say anything about the process of application.

Applying: This step is easier to observe in everyday behavior than the more cognitive steps of understanding and appraising. Based on their own experiences, the doctors repeatedly named three of the most important behavioral issues such as the lack of health-related behavior (see following doctor's instruction); the need to use medication appropriately; and the individual's ability to make health-related decisions (which is influenced and/or limited by his or her social context). Comparable to the "appraising" step, it is the family members and elders who decide rather than the affected person herself/himself how to apply information. Therefore, low competency in appraising might be due to a deficiency of the individual person or to the high complexity of the information or the non-existence of the system. We try to expand this list by adding two other issues (influencing health literacy): the difficulty of the health issue and the barriers people face.

6   Summarizing Findings on Health Literacy in Afghanistan

In this section, we utilize the widely used health literacy instrument, EU-QS-47 (Pelikan et al. 2012), and review it gradually item by item, domain by domain and dimension by dimension to examine its applicability and relevance to Afghanistan. Although many questions (items) are formulated in a very generic manner and are therefore adequate for many contexts, two aspects became very important: the underlying assumptions about the availability and accessibility of structural issues such health information in general (and through the media) and specific health services and treatment; and second personal issues such as the opportunity that allow an individual to shape his/her health behavior or influence his/her context/environment. These are not available everywhere in Afghanistan, so, when using the HLS-EU questionnaire in Afghanistan, the application and answering of these questions should be considered with caution (Table 4).

Healthcare: Apart from the need to take care of diseases of affluence and communicable diseases, in a country where medications are not always available, and if they are available, their quality can vary (Harper and Strote 2011), relying on the instructions given by doctors or pharmacists can be difficult and will not achieve the same results as it does in a country with high standards for

Table 4 Comparison between HLS-EU and Afghanistan *(source: own depiction)*

	Assumption	Afghanistan
HC	Information on symptoms/treatment is available Health care support in case of medical emergency and ambulance exist Professionals (doctors and pharmacists) exist Communication between doctors and patients Instructions are provided by doctors and pharmacists Medicines and leaflets are available Info in the media	Information limited in rural areas Barely any medical emergency services exist Professionals are not available Hierarchical interaction between patient (more passive) and doctor Limited time for giving instruction (large number of patients) No medical leaflets or patients cannot read it Little/no info in media exist Influenced by availability, accessibility, acceptability and affordability
DP	Manage mental health/depression Availability of vaccination and health Screening (also flu vaccine) Info on (sedentary) lifestyle Warnings about lifestyle factors Info in media Advice of friends	Most people suffer from depression Basic vaccine is not available everywhere (see policy) Changes in lifestyle might be limited No devices or little/no info in media Often advised by friends etc. Primarily with regard to communicable diseases, no screening
HP	Info about a healthy lifestyle (and mental health) Info about healthy environment Political changes that are effective Health in the workplace Nutrition labels info in the media Sports clubs Opportunity to impact health in environment and community	Limited impact on most environmental/life conditions Lucky to have any kind of work Little info available No sports club in rural areas Little addressing of determinants or prerequisites for health (which have a strong impact on health)

HC: Health Care; DP: Disease Prevention, HP: Health Promotion

medication. Contrary to the items of HLS-EU-Q47, the treatment of certain health problems such as diarrhea and the adherence to a high standard of hygiene is essential in Afghanistan. Moreover, health care varies between rural and urban areas. While people in the rural areas still suffer from diseases driven by poverty, in urban areas, with many health care professionals, these diseases are treated easily. Therefore, in urban areas, diseases of affluence, chronic diseases and sedentary lifestyle factors are increasingly common – which is also the case in Europe and should be addressed in the questionnaire.

Disease prevention: In this dimension, the central issues are the type of diseases, information dissemination, available services and health behavior. Disease prevention is of great importance both in Europe and Afghanistan. However, health problems, their consequences and the common ways of responding to them vary. In rich countries, health issues such as smoking, low physical activity, alcohol, stress and depression, as well as vaccination and screenings are relevant to prevent or reduce the severity of diseases of affluence. But in the rural areas of Afghanistan, communicable diseases and malnutrition are more common, and so is the need for preventive measures in hygiene and nutrition. Furthermore, not all disease prevention services are available. Whilst Afghanistan has made considerable progress in vaccination, screening is still rare. The items in the questionnaire tackle health issues more common in rich countries and need to be adapted for Afghanistan. In addition, the channels of dissemination and search for information are different: Not only health professionals, but also family members, mullahs, community elders, and (in urban areas) media provide such information. While disease prevention is critical in a country like Afghanistan, these 'channels' convey information mainly about health care and health promotion. apart from adequate health behavior (see paragraph 2.2) it is also essential to address disease prevention and health protection within the setting now and, in view of forthcoming changes, it is becoming increasingly important to enhance the ability to adapt to climate change. Hence, in the dimension "disease prevention", it is recommended to address issues such as hygiene, sleeping under the mosquito net, the use of latrines, vaccine, danger signs of pregnancies and delivery in hospital, and breastfeeding. So, it is crucial to educate people about current and future risk factors of climate change and adaptation strategies.

Health promotion: Whilst most items are formulated in general terms, some deserve special attention. For example, some of the questions appear to be less relevant in a country with a high number of illiterates, limited access to media and low-standard consumer information (e.g. items related to the understanding the food packages). Furthermore, participating in community activities requires the time to do so and not to be too occupied with other obligations. It is questionable whether the people can perform their tasks or succeed in fulfilling their desire to create a more health-promoting environment and whether this is on their agenda at all. In a country with immense security, protection and poverty issues, priority could be given to providing sufficient nutrition and working towards a healthy environment (i.e. health protection).

Table 5 Main topics in each dimension of HL *(source: own depiction)*

Domain	Specified
Health care	Assumptions about availability and other healthcare providers, quality of medicines, most common diseases, existing services, barriers, treatment at home (hygiene!)
Disease prevention	Type of disease, dissemination of information, available health services, behavior
Health promotion	Relevance, available time, understanding of health, possibility to influence the environment, cultural impacts
4 steps	Role of message providers and decision maker

The Table 5 provides an overview of the main topics in each dimension to be observed.

7   Discussion

7.1   Key Aspects of Interest

Up until now, no analysis on health literacy in Afghanistan has existed and researchers have rarely explored the process of applying an HL instrument developed in Western countries to a low-income and crisis-ridden country such as Afghanistan. In this article, we have systematically described the context, identified crucial needs and interventions and compared the findings with the HLS-EU questionnaire. In the process, several questions emerged related to the relevance of the concept, the need for conceptualization, the underlying model of change and types of adaptation. These questions are not exclusive to Afghanistan, but can also arise in the application of health literacy to other countries. The key lessons learned from these questions are presented in the next sections to support developers in critically evaluating and adapting the concept of HLS-EU to other contexts.

Translation of 'health literacy' and the relevance of the concept: A key challenge for all translators is to find an equivalent or the most adequate word for 'health literacy' in the other language covering the complex concept of 'literacy" either as a reading and writing skill or as a broader competence to effectively engage with health information. By definition, the population of Afghanistan, with its high illiteracy rate would be perceived as possessing low levels of health literacy – if health literacy is understood as the competence to read and write. But in Afghanistan, written health information is rare (including leaflets on treatment options or medication leaflets, nutrition labels), instead health information is mostly shared orally. Hence, knowing people one can consult, their credibility and the accuracy of the information they share is of great importance. For these reasons, we argue that health literacy should be understood as an everyday competency that manifests itself in the decisions made by people in their day-to-day lives (see setting approach) regarding the main health concerns as opposed to narrowing the concept of health literacy down to an understanding that exclusively focusses on the health system.

Contextualization: The findings presented in this article indicate that it is relevant to conceptualize health literacy by embracing an ecological perspective of health, and acknowledging the impact of the prerequisites and determinants of health. This appears to be more illuminating than the narrowly defined understanding of health literacy (see REALM).

Relevant health issues and characteristics of health literacy: Apart from the necessity to understand the context, it is important to adapt the items to the most common health concerns (such as communicable diseases, pregnancy, injuries etc.). Otherwise, if the content of an item is irrelevant, then the item can be difficult to understand or misinterpreted.

Model of changing health literacy in Afghanistan: The linear model of health literacy is often used to explain the relationship between various health issues. It suggests that health education results in health literacy which improves behavior and ultimately health. However, this linear, causal model is criticized for a number of reasons. First, the model reduces the high complexity of the family, social, educational and health system environment in which health literacy is developed (Levin-Zamir et al. 2017). Second, it assumes that improved health literacy (a cognitive change) leads directly to improved health behavior. In Afghanistan, however, not only difficulties in understanding the health information exist but also moral obligations as well as good reasons for not following some health instructions. Third, the model assumes that improved behavior leads to improved health which ignores the multitude of environmental and social determinants that play an extremely crucial role in the individual's health. This applies, for instance, to the role of the household decision-makers and the oldest women in the house which is often very powerful in Afghanistan and so, even if a young woman knows about family planning and she (and her husband) want(s) to practice it, the mother-in-law often has the final word.

Necessity of improved health literacy for a healthy lifestyle? Furthermore, we want to raise the question whether well-developed cognitive skills (finding, understanding, judging and applying) are needed to lead a healthy life. In fact, it can be argued that imitating a person who models a healthy lifestyle can also result in a healthy lifestyle, even without understanding the various processes. In this section, we have not touched on the role of the community which can also interfere heavily in making one's own health decisions, because each individual tries to avoid losing face. If the objective is to improve health through improving individual health behavior, then it might be useful to explore how people learn health promotion and disease preventing behavior: e.g. do they learn by modelling, by doing, by observing, by instruction or by listening? This will also reveal more about the nature of the concept of health literacy in Afghanistan.

7.2   Approaches to Assess Health Literacy

Assessing health literacy or what can be learned from the process? If health literacy and its assessment are to be relevant, it must consider the different local contexts (countries, health systems, key health issues and health inequalities) and the available structural conditions (available, accessible and affordable health professionals and services), but also topics acceptable (to the individual, the family, and the community) as well as upcoming future issues (preparedness for and adaptation to future natural events due to climate change). Furthermore, the manner of posing the questions should receive attention in a country with a high illiteracy rate (written, orally, closed questions, open ended, narrative questions). The assessment of health literacy should also consider the appropriateness of the content of the questions based on the relevance and availability of the issues included in the questionnaire. These are predominantly: How are the determinants of health, the environment, and the health system described? What are the main health and morbidity problems and common and/or accepted treatment and prevention methods? What is the common, accepted and preferred way of transmitting information and who/what is the most suitable source of information?

So how to deal with a questionnaire like the HLS-EU-Q47, developed in Western countries and utilized worldwide. We can think of at least five possible ways (use of the original version, addition of new questions, adaptation the questions and exclusion of questions, development of a new tool) which vary in terms of comparability, relevance and feasible length.

First of all, the questionnaire can be used in its original form, so the data and findings collected are comparable to other studies worldwide. This might be interesting not only for researchers but also for politicians or organizations who want to acquire more funding for programs targeting health literacy. One main disadvantage is that these data are of limited importance to the practitioners in the particular country because it might use the 'wrong' i.e. less relevant items and participants might face difficulties understanding the questions.

Secondly, it is plausible to use the questionnaire in its original form and to add further questions that might help assess the relevance of the items in the questionnaire (e.g. Is a doctor available? Can you go to the doctor in case of …?). Therefore, the data would still be internationally comparable but also locally relevant. However, this could increase the length of the questionnaire, possibly making it less feasible.

Third, it is possible to use the questionnaire and change the words within the items e.g. health promotion targeting communicable diseases, and additionally differentiate between the source of information and the help the interviewees request, also addressing barriers hampering the way to the health services. In this case, the challenge is to determine how much change can be made so that the items are still comparable internationally, yet relevant to the local context (see Table 6).

Fourth, it is an option to adapt the wording and add new questions, thereby increasing the relevance but reducing the feasibility at a low level of comparison. Fifth, it is also appropriate to exchange all items and develop a new questionnaire that exclusively asks relevant questions, which might increase its relevance and feasibility albeit diminishing its comparability to international studies.

There is not a single best way to apply health literacy. We must decide which purpose to serve: scientific research or practical use, so that the concept meets the demands of either comparability, relevance, or feasible length.

Table 6 Options to adapt HL tool (*source: own depiction*)	Strategy	Comparison	Relevance	Feasible length
	Original	x	–	x
	Original + add	x	x	–
	Adaptation	–	x	x
	Adaptation + add	–	x	?
	New questionnaire	–	x	x

8   Summary and Recommendations

Multiple health issues exist in Afghanistan, some of which are beyond the control and influence of individuals or health system actors, while others can be addressed, such as health literacy. To prevent diseases and to save lives, targeting and improving the low level of health literacy is very important. This paper presented findings on health literacy in a crisis-ridden, low-income country, Afghanistan. We argued that when focusing on the concept of health literacy, particular needs, priorities, and the social context should be considered. A variety of contextual factors were presented which have a direct and indirect influence on health (literacy). Then, the basic health literacy skills of lay people in the village were presented with a focus on cleanliness, mother and child health and various issues related to the interactions in the health system. Furthermore, we discussed the relevance and applicability of HLS-EU-Q47 to Afghanistan. We argued that it is necessary to integrate questions related to the context, diseases of poverty and common channels for transferring health information. In the last section, four key aspects encountered in the process of applying health literacy to other countries were introduced: issues related to the concept of health literacy, contextualization, relevant health issues, models of change and also questions regarding the assumed necessity of health literacy for a healthy lifestyle and adaptation strategies.

Our findings suggest that overall health literacy in Afghanistan is poor and improving it is urgently recommended. However, the way of doing so may differ from Western countries. In the course of exploring and applying the concept with qualitative data, we could not cover all aspects related to health literacy, and various ideas arose concerning factors related to health literacy, but the authors could not clarify them in this study. Therefore, the authors wanted to take one step forward and planned to conduct a health literacy survey in Afghanistan to gain a better understanding of the level of health literacy, its distribution among different groups, and the factors associated with it. In applying the health literacy instrument, we recommend using the original survey instrument and adding further questions to meet local needs. To keep the length of the survey feasible, the authors suggest using the HLS-EU-Q16 short version (Wångdahl et al. 2015; Röthlin et al. 2013) and translating it into the local languages, Dari and Pashtu. The results could reveal a need to modify the instrument, which will then be tested in advance and followed by a larger study e.g. "Measurement of Afghans' Health Literacy in Afghanistan" (MAHLA). More information on the survey on health literacy in Afghanistan can be found in chapter 12.

This present study helps to define the core competencies and their operationalization within the HL instrument. Furthermore, it increases the awareness on health literacy and the results can support politicians, organizations and donors in prioritizing health literacy as a field of action. Moreover, this study can help identify several target groups, on the one hand those, who are particularly vulnerable and, on the other hand those who have a major impact on many others (such as health professionals, traditional healers, mullahs, community health workers or mothers-in-law, ...) and to develop strategies to address them.

Bringing together the context of health, basic health skills, and the experiences of health professionals, we critically analyzed the applicability of the HLS-EU-Q47 questionnaire. The five steps utilized in this article can serve as a blue print for other researchers to adapt existing questionnaires to their own situation and inspire other researchers in the process of modifying health literacy research instruments to other countries. The ultimate goal should be not only to develop instruments measuring health literacy, but also to promote health literacy worldwide; so that people will be able to make good health-related decisions, maintain and improve their health as well as a healthy environment and contribute to achieving the sustainable development goals and peace.

References

Afghan Central Statistics Organization (2017). Health indicators. Retrieved from http://cso.gov.af/en.

Akseer, N., Bhatti, Z., Mashal, T., Soofi, S., Moineddin, R., Black, R. E., et al. (2018). Geospatial inequalities and determinants of nutritional status among women and children in Afghanistan: An observational study. *The Lancet Global Health, 6*(4), e447–e459. https://doi.org/10.1016/s2214-109x(18)30025-1.

Burhani, N. H. (2009). Health Literacy in Afghanistan Achievements and Way forward. Retrieved from http://www.un.org/en/ecosoc/newfunct/pdf/burhani.ppt.

CIA (2019). World Fact Book Afghanistan. Retrieved from https://www.cia.gov/library/publications/the-world-factbook/geos/af.html.

Frost, A., Wilkinson, M., Boyle, P., Patel, P., & Sullivan, R. (2016). An assessment of the barriers to accessing the Basic Package of Health Services (BPHS) in Afghanistan: was the BPHS a success? *Globalization and health, 12*(1), 71. https://doi.org/10.1186/s12992-016-0212-6.

Harper, J. R., & Strote, G. (2011). Afghanistan pharmaceutical sector development. problems and prospects. *Southern Med Review, 4* (1). https://doi.org/10.5655/smr.v4i1.75.

Interviewee 14 (2016). Interview on health promotion in Afghanistan. With assistance of Stefanie Harsch. University of Education Freiburg.

Kickbusch, I. (2013). *Health literacy. The solid facts.* Geneva: World Health Organization. Retrieved from http://www.euro.who.int/data/assets/pdf_file/0008/190655/e96854.pdf.

Levin-Zamir, D., Leung, A. Y. M., Dodson, S., & Rowlands, G. (2017). Health literacy in selected populations: Individuals, families, and communities from the international and cultural perspective. *ISU, 37*(2), 131–151. https://doi.org/10.3233/isu-170834.

MoPH (2005a). BPHS 2005/1384. Retrieved from http://apps.who.int/medicinedocs/documents/s21746en/s21746en.pdf.

MoPH (2005b). *The Essential Package of Hospital Services for Afghanistan.* Retrieved from https://apps.who.int/medicinedocs/documents/s16169e/s16169e.pdf.

Najafizada, S. A. M. (2016). *The Afghan Community Health Worker Program: A Health Systems Analysis of a Population Health Intervention.* Université d'Ottawa/ University of Ottawa. Retrieved from https://pdfs.semanticscholar.org/ab1b/850c583ffa3839e8ca0f 499e482ce4a99d99.pdf.

Newbrander, W., Ickx, P., Feroz, F., & Stanekzai, H. (2014). Afghanistan's basic package of health services: Its development and effects on rebuilding the health system. *Global Public Health, 9*(Suppl 1), S6–S28. https://doi.org/10.1080/17441692.2014.916735.

Participant 2 (2016). *Focusgroup discussion on HL in Afghanistan - Workshop during the summer school on HL.* Freiburg: University of Education.

Pelikan, J. (2012). Measurement of health literacy in Europe: HLS-EU-Q47; HLS-EU-Q16; and HLS-EU-Q86. The HLS-EU Consortium 2012.

Pelikan, J., Röthlin, F., & Ganahl, K. (2012). Comparative report of health literacy in eigth EU member states. The European Health Literacy Survey HLS-EU. Retrieved from http://ec.europa.eu/chafea/documents/news/Comparative_report_on_health_literacy_in_ eight_EU_member_states.pdf.

Qarani, W. M., & Kanji, S. I. (2015). *Health system analysis: Pakistan and Afghanistan.* http://oaji.net/articles/2015/1909-1448230343.pdf. Accessed on 8. Feb. 2016.

Röthlin, F., Pelikan, J., & Ganahl, K. (2013). Die Gesundheitskompetenz von 15-jährigen Jugendlichen in Österreich. Retrieved from http://www.hauptverband.at/cdscontent/load ?contentid=10008.597350&version=1395738807.

Sabzwari, S. R. (2017). Health literacy in Pakistan: Exploring new ways of addressing an old challenge. In *JPMA. The Journal of the Pakistan Medical Association* 67 (12), pp. 1901–1904.

Santos, M., Handley, M., Omark, K., & Schillinger, D. (2014). ESL Participation as a mechanism for advancing health literacy in immigrant communities. *Journal of health communication, 19* (2), pp. 89–105. https://doi.org/10.1080/10810730.2014.934935.

SIGAR (2017). Afghanistan's Health Care Sector: USAID's use of unreliable data presents challenges in assessing program performance and the extent of progress. Retrieved from https://www.sigar.mil/pdf/audits/SIGAR-17-22-AR.pdf.

Sørensen, K. (2016). Health literacy is a political choice. https://www.researchgate.net/publication/311455482_Health_literacy_is_a_political_choice_A_health_literacy_guide_for_politicians.

Sørensen, K., van den Broucke, St., Fullam, J., Doyle, G., Pelikan, J., Slonska, Z., & Brand, H. (2012). Health literacy and public health: A systematic review and integration of definitions and models. *BMC Public Health, 12*, p. 80. https://doi.org/10.1186/1471-2458-12-80.

The Asia Foundation (2018). A Survey of the Afghan People. Afghanistan in 2018. Retrieved from https://asiafoundation.org/wp-content/uploads/2018/12/2018_Afghan-Survey_fullReport-12.4.18.pdf.

UNDP (2018). *Human development indices and indicators. 2018 statistical update.* Retrieved from http://hdr.undp.org/sites/default/files/2018_human_development_statistical_update.pdf.

UNDP (2019). *Human Development Report.* Afghanistan. Retrieved from http://hdr.undp.org/en/countries/profiles/AFG.

Viswanathan, K., Becker, S., Hansen, P. M., Kumar, Dh, Kumar, B., Niayesh, H., et al. (2010). Infant and under-five mortality in Afghanistan: current estimates and limitations. *Bulletin of the World Health Organization, 88*(8), 576–583. https://doi.org/10.2471/blt.09.068957.

Waldman, R. J., & Newbrander, W. (2014). Afghanistan's health system: Moving forward in challenging circumstances 2002–2013. *Global Public Health, 9*(Suppl 1), S1–5. https://doi.org/10.1080/17441692.2014.924188.

Wångdahl, J., Lytsy, P., Mårtensson, L., & Westerling, R. (2014). Health literacy among refugees in Sweden – a cross-sectional study. *BMC Public Health, 14*(1), 1030. https://doi.org/10.1186/1471-2458-14-1030.

Wångdahl, J., Lytsy, P., Mårtensson, L., & Westerling, R. (2015). Health literacy and refugees' experiences of the health examination for asylum seekers – a Swedish cross-sectional study. *BMC Public Health, 15,* 1162. https://doi.org/10.1186/s12889-015-2513-8.

WHO (2010). Country Cooperation Strategy for WHO and Afghanistan. 2009–2013. Retrieved from http://apps.who.int/iris/bitstream/10665/113236/1/CCS_Afghanistan_2010_EN_14480.pdf?ua=1.

WHO (2015). Afghanistan: Health system profile. Retrieved from http://applications.emro.who.int/docs/Country_profile_2015_EN_16722.pdf?ua=1.

WHO (2016). *Shanghai Declaration on promoting health in the 2030 Agenda for Sustainable Development.* Retrieved from https://www.who.int/healthpromotion/conferences/9gchp/shanghai-declaration.pdf?ua=1.

Future Perspectives

Health Literacy Champions

Kristine Sørensen

1   Introduction

From being an educational and clinical challenge acknowledged by few, health literacy is now on the brink of becoming a global social movement developed by many. The mounting mobilization of activities, networks and organizations involved in the promotion of health literacy worldwide indicate the rise of a global health literacy movement which is predominantly driven by professionals aiming to improve the capacity of patients and citizens as well as inducing a change in organizations and systems to become health literacy responsive (Sørensen et al. 2018).

Historically, social movements were developed to impact health for different purposes: 1. Bring about change in the experience and delivery of healthcare, 2. Improve people's experience of disease, disability, or illness, 3. Promote healthy lifestyles, 4. Address socioeconomic and political determinants of health, 5. Democratize the production and dissemination of knowledge, 6. Change cultural and societal norms, and 7. Propose new health innovation and policymaking processes (del Castillo et al. 2016). Interestingly, the areas of change concerning the advancement of health literacy towards empowerment and health equity relates to all the seven reasons listed for social movements which in turn, emphasizes its importance and impact regarding policy development, research, education and practice (Sørensen et al. 2018).

K. Sørensen (✉)
Global Health Literacy Academy, Risskov, Denmark
e-mail: contact@globalhealthliteracyacademy.org

Since the first mentioning of health literacy in the 1970s by Simonds (1974) as part of educational policy in the United States of America, the interest has grown exponentially among scholars, practitioners and decision-makers. The transformation of health literacy towards the mainstream has especially been pushed by change agents who took it upon themselves to advocate for its dissemination, change agents whom we often call health literacy champions. They choose to be front runners in a disruptive process of change for better health because they believe in the cause. They get engaged because among various reasons they reckon that health literacy is evident, measurable, feasible and for the public good (Sørensen 2016).

Traditionally, the term champion referred to a knight who fought in single combat on behalf of the monarch (Google Dictionary 2018). The term can be dated back to early 13c., 'a doughty fighting man, a valorous combatant' and 'one who fights on behalf of another or others, one who undertakes to defend a cause'. From Old French the word 'champion' can be related to 'combatant, a champion in single combat (12.c)' and Late Latin 'campionem, campio', a gladiator, fighter, combatant in the field (Online Etymology Dictionary 2018). In contemporary times, a champion is someone who has won the first prize in a competition, contest, or enthusiastically fights for a person, a cause, or a principle whom or which the champion supports or defends (Cambridge English Dictionary 2018). Synonyms include advocate, proponent, promoter, proposer, supporter, standard-bearer, torch-bearer, defender, protector, upholder, backer, exponent, patron, sponsor, prime mover; booster and a pleader for, campaigner for, propagandist for, lobbyist for, fighter for, battler for, crusader for, or apologist for a certain cause (Google Dictionary 2018). Within the field of health literacy, the terms heroes and trailblazers also apply (Health Literacy Media 2018; Osborne 2000).

Recognizing the important role of health literacy champions for re-designing and re-orienting health systems towards people-centeredness, as suggested by the World Health Organization (World Health Organization Regional Office for Europe 2016), this chapter aims to explore health literacy championship and how health literacy champions are characterized and nurtured as change-agents for the development of health literate organizations, settings and societies.

2   Health Literacy Champion Awards

There are several examples of identifying and rewarding health literacy champions by handing out awards. Health Literacy Media, previously Health Literacy Missouri, established the Cecilia and Leonard Doak Health Literacy Champion

Award to honor individuals and organizations who make outstanding contributions in health literacy and whose work focuses on bridging the gap between the skills of people and the demands of the health care system. The award, named after the founders of the health literacy movement in the U.S., is presented to a single individual or organization each year and recognizes those who exhibit the highest standards of excellence, dedication and accomplishment over a sustained period of time, and who are creative and highly skilled pioneers in the health literacy field. The award recognizes rigorous work and celebrates collaborative efforts to shape a path to good health (Health Literacy Media 2018).

The Crystal Clear Award in Ireland is a partnership between MSD and NALA, the National Adult Literacy Agency, with representation on the judging panel from the Health Service Executive (HSE), the Health Information and Quality Authority (HIQA), University College Dublin (UCD), a General Practitioner, NALA, and Trinity College, Dublin (MSD 2012). The award is handed out to projects helping patients to take a more active role in the management of their own lifestyle, condition or illness and to make informed decisions about their own health. Four out of ten people in Ireland have trouble with health literacy and can have difficulty understanding health information. The many initiatives that have been lined up for the awards help patients to have a better understanding of their health.

Similarly, in Belgium the Well Done MSD Health Literacy Awards competition aims to stimulate best practice-sharing in order to empower patients, optimize the communication between healthcare professionals and patients and ultimately to safeguard the sustainability of the healthcare system. Health care professionals and associations are encouraged to submit their disease management projects with real impact on patients' lives. The initiative was established in 2012 and builds on a collaboration entailing partners from 12 main healthcare organizations with a jury chaired by the country's health literacy expert (MSD 2016).

3   The Role of Champions in Developing Health Literacy Policies

Health literacy is about rights, access and transparency. It is about a new form of health citizenship, in which citizens take both personal responsibility for health and become involved as citizens in social and political processes that address the root causes of health inequalities as well as inequalities in access to care (Kickbusch 2004). Subsequently, health literacy is a political choice which requires informed decision-makers and politicians. Essentially, health literacy advocacy and policy making is a process of supporting and enabling people to:

- express their views and concerns regarding health and quality of life,
- access health information and services,
- defend and promote their rights and responsibilities in terms of health,
- explore choices and options relevant for healthcare, disease prevention and health promotion,
- create health literate organizations to facilitate better services,
- support the development of health literate settings such as schools, work places, and communities,
- educate the health-related work force on health literacy,
- ensure monitoring of health literacy, and
- develop health literacy action plans to accommodate the needs (Sørensen 2016).

When studying health literacy policies, it becomes clear that often single individuals play significant roles in their development. For example, the United States of America was in the leading role regarding the launch of a national action plan on health literacy in 2010 (U.S. Department of Health and Human Services 2010). The plan was developed with strong support of Surgeon General Admiral Moritsugu who served as an example of a policy champion in the area of health literacy. Furthermore, Cynthia Baur from the Centre of Disease Control has played a key role in the development of the national action plan. She is recognized as a champion when it comes to the strategic development of health literacy policy in the U.S. (Centers for Disease Control and Prevention. 2011)

In Europe, the consortium leading the European Health Literacy Project (2009–2012) was vital for the manifestation of health literacy in the wider European region. They received the European Health Award in 2012 for their societal impact (Sørensen and Brand 2017). In Scotland, Graham Kramer was the personification of the health literacy action plan launched by the National Health System in 2014 (NHS Scotland 2014), while Jürgen Pelikan, Christina Dietscher and Peter Nowak were instrumental for the inclusion of health literacy as one of ten national health targets in Austria in 2013 (Bundesministerium für Gesundheit 2013). In Germany, the health literacy evidence vitally contributed to the development of a national action plan (Nationaler Aktionsplan Gesundheitskompetenz Geschäftsstelle 2018) building on the work of Doris Schaeffer, Ullrich Bauer, Klaus Hurrelmann and Kai Kolpatzik. Similarly, Ilona Kickbusch and Don Nutbeam have relentlessly advocated for the inclusion of health literacy in global policies exemplified by the Shanghai Declaration on Health Promotion where health literacy is one of three pillars to achieve the sustainable development goals (World Health Organization 2016). While these champions are mentioned by name, it should be emphasized that the policies would not have been possible without the push from the many health literacy stakeholders who demanded their realization through decades of work.

Hence, worldwide, individuals as well as organizations play a vital role in highlighting health literacy as an important topic related to human development and health and notably, change agents are required to push the evolutionary developments to the next levels. It is recognized that the process may be longwinded and requiring patience and endurance. As health literacy champion Graham Kramer from Scotland describes it in a Tweet:

"...Transformational system change is slow, complex and evolutionary and requires long term vision and patience. Revolutionary reform whilst politically attractive, usually creates disruption and unintended consequences" (Kramer 2018)

4   The Role of Champions in Developing He Alth Literate Organizations

Organizational health literacy, described as an organization-wide effort to make it easier for people to navigate, understand, and use information and services to take care of their health, is an emerging topic for healthcare systems to address (Brach 2017). Research reveals that health systems remain less responsive than needed to the public health challenge of low levels of health literacy in populations. Lack of involvement of patients in decision-making; unintentional non-adherence to treatments and medications; difficulties with informed consent; patient-provider communication, discharge instructions, and increasing rates of emergency care, hospitalizations, and re-admissions have been reported for patients with limited health literacy. The vicious cycle of negative health outcomes and limited health literacy is perpetuated by impossible to navigate healthcare systems and difficult to understand communication (Farmanova et al. 2018). Becoming a health literate organization requires multiple, simultaneous, and radical changes. A literature review of organizational health literacy by Farmanova and colleagues (2018) identified thirteen key barriers to organizational health literacy which is illustrated in Table 1, including the lack of change champions in an organization.

The literature study refers to three overarching themes: organizational and institution culture and leadership, design and planning of interventions, and human resources. Few organizations have pursued a systemic approach in their

Table 1 Key barriers to organizational health literacy (Farmanova et al. 2018)

Organizational and institution culture and leadership	1. Low priority of health literacy and related activities 2. Lack of commitment to health literacy 3. Limited or no buy-in from leadership 4. Becoming health literate is not perceived as advantageous
Design and planning of interventions	5. Lack of culture of change and innovation 6. **No change champions in the organization** 7. Not having procedures, policies, protocols supporting health-literate practice 8. Not having enough time 9. Lack of resources 10. Complexity of health literacy tools and guides
Human resources	11. Ambiguity of roles among staff 12. Lack of training in health literacy 13. Lack of awareness about health literacy

attempts to develop their health literacy. Specifically, organizational commitment toward health literacy is weak and efforts to enhance organizational health literacy via policies, planning, and programmes are insufficient. A lack of awareness about health literacy and its impacts on health outcomes and sustainability of the health system means that health literacy is most often not an integral part of organizations' mission, vision and strategic planning. In turn, some health literacy practices may be implemented by frontline staff but may not be recognized as such due to lack of familiarity with the concept. In case health literacy is recognized, there may not be workforce training in place to roll-out health literacy as part of organizational services and culture. The presence of advocates for organizational change is critical, however, their impact depends highly on support from leadership, while a management structure and culture that supports innovation and quality improvement is regarded as essential (Farmanova et al. 2018).

Organizational health literacy aims to help build person-centered, evidence-based, and quality-driven healthcare, however, it requires a substantial change and reform of the organizational thinking. To stimulate the process organizations are encouraged to identify change agents, health literacy champions, who can induce the process and develop it according to the organizations' focus and context. The health literacy champions can move the agenda forward and explain the necessity to perform a change of practice. This may be met with resistance, but mostly, the immediate impact of more contented clients and patients also creates more contented employees. Staff that helps to make it easier for clients and patients to access, understand, appraise and apply information to manage their health may also find it rewarding to see how an empowered patient will become more active and engaged and take control regarding self-care and needed actions for better outcomes. When patients and providers work in partnerships, this can undoubtedly enhance the success of the patient journey (Kickbusch 2013). Health literacy commitment needs to come from champions positioned at the highest levels of the organization to ensure a substantial impact (Brach et al. 2012).

5 Practical Examples of How to Nurture Health Literacy Championship

The following three examples illustrate how the idea of health literacy championship can be incorporated into practice.

5.1 The Centers for Disease Control and Prevention (CDC)

The first case story stem from the CDC in the United States. According to the CDC, every organization involved in health information and services needs its own health literacy plan. Without an action plan, organizational improvements to address health literacy will likely be uncoordinated and not sustainable. Everyone has limited time and resources, and having a plan helps the organization to know what to do first. The organizational plan may start because of one person's interest, but it can't be developed by one person alone. Therefore, it is a good idea to begin by identifying advocates. While planning, it is recommended to think broadly about whom the advocates may be and not to count people out until they have been asked. Notably, strong advocates are needed within the organization, but one can also benefit from identifying advocates who are external to the organization and can be partners and/or facilitators. A broad group of advocates is needed for successful planning and implementation of organizational change. The CDC distinguishes between:

- *Champions:* These individuals are typically leaders and/or decision-makers in the organization who have the influence needed to approve or put the plan into action. These Champions may or may not be familiar with the issue but should be people who would be open to learning and being a powerful voice for the issue.

- *Allies:* These individuals and/or organizational components are those who can provide support to the plan and the vision for health literacy in the organization. Allies are critical as they may have slightly different perspectives and needs that will be invaluable in the planning process.
- *Workgroup Members:* Whether or not a formal workgroup is needed will depend on the organization. While Champions and Allies are essential to planning, they may not be involved in day-to-day planning, organization and coordination. Therefore, you need commitments from individuals with diverse perspectives from across your organization as core work group members could be needed. This does not have to be a large group, but it needs to include people who are willing to roll up their sleeves and work (Centers for Disease Control and Prevention 2011).

5.2 The Nebraska Association of Local Health Directors' Health Literacy Champion

5.2.1 Designation

The second case story is derived from the Nebraska Association of Local Health Directors who is known for health literacy expertise and excellence (Nebraska Association of Local Health Directors 2018). In order to provide ongoing health literacy quality improvement support to their members and community partners, they created the Health Literacy Champion process with the aim to award 2-year Health Literacy Champion designations based upon health literacy check-ups and action plans. They encourage their members to become Health Literacy Champions to

- *Implement* accreditation *standards and goals.* The Health Literacy Champion process addresses strategies for meeting the Public Health Accreditation Board (PHAB) Standards and The Joint Commission (TJC) Safety Goals.
- *Improve the organization's reach and effectiveness.* The Health Literacy Champion process helps your organization identify specific programs and projects affected by low health literacy and to make a plan to address health literacy to improve the effectiveness of these initiatives.
- *Target key opinion leaders with health literacy information.* The Health Literacy Champion process poises your organization to brief policy makers, legislators, stakeholders, and other key decision makers on the importance of health literacy with the aim to explain how health literacy relates to the organization's mission, goals, and strategic plan and how it can be incorporated into existing programs.

- *Increase your organization's credibility.* The importance of health literacy is gaining recognition nationally. Through the Health Literacy Champion process, you will establish accountability for your health literacy activities.
- *Become a* technical *assistance provider in your community.* The Nebraska Association of Local Health Directors supports Health Literacy Champions with local technical assistance providers.

To be considered for a Health Literacy Champion designation, the applying organization must comply and incorporate health literacy into their performance management system, their policies and procedures and their collaboration with community partners as well as commit to a health literacy action plan (Nebraska Association of Local Health Directors 2018).

5.3   Sydney Local Health District

The third case concerns the Sydney Local Health District (2016) which is committed to improving health literacy by using a coordinated and collaborative approach that includes: embedding health literacy in organizational policies, practices and systems and ensuring that health information is clear, focused and useable and that interpersonal communication is effective as well as integrating health literacy into education for healthcare providers and the community (Australian Commission on Safety and Quality in Health Care). The health literacy framework developed by the Sydney Local Health district builds on the ten attributes of health literate organizations derived from the Institute of Medicine (Brach et al. 2012) including organizational commitment, a well-trained workforce, and policies and procedures. Evidence shows that there is not just one path to a health literate organization and many departments within the Sydney Local Health District have addressed or are addressing different attributes according to the need of the populations they serve. The aim of the health literacy framework is to assist departments in assessing what they have in place and also to identify attributes that require action to ensure that everyone gets the greatest benefit possible from their health care information and services. All departments are encouraged to evaluate how well their strategies work and to share the results of their efforts with others. Approaching health literacy at both the local departmental and the organizational level ensures that the Sydney Local Health Department is an organization that makes it easier for all people to navigate, understand and use information and services (Sydney Local Health District 2016).

6   Concluding remarks

This chapter aimed to explore health literacy championship and how health literacy champions can be characterized and nurtured as change-agents for the development of health literate organizations, settings and societies. Synthesizing the scope of their characteristics, the following definition is proposed:

> A health literacy champion is a person or an organization that enthusiastically and relentlessly defends and fights for the cause of health literacy to the benefit of people and societies at large.

The examples from practice highlighted the role of health literacy champions in inducing the necessary change and transformation of organizations and settings for them to become health literate. While the paths may differ with regard to how the organizations pursue the health literacy-related attributes, the significance of change agents still stands. Pushing health literacy from the margin to the mainstream could not have happened without health literacy champions. The challenge in the future is to keep identifying people who can undertake the role of pushing health literacy to the next frontier.

References

Australian Commission on Safety and Quality in Health Care. (2014). Health Literacy. Taking action to improve safety and quality. https://www.safetyandquality.gov.au/sites/default/files/migrated/Health-Literacy-Taking-action-to-improve-safety-and-quality.pdf. Accessed 28 May 2020.

Brach, C. (2017). The journey to become a health literate organization: A snapshot of health system improvement. *Studies in Health Technology and Informatics, 240*, 203–237.

Brach, C. Keller, D., Hernandez, L., Baur, C., Parker, R., Dreyer, B., et al. (2012). Ten attributes of health literate health care organizations. *NAM Perspectives, 02*(6). https://doi.org/10.31478/201206a.

Bundesministerium für Gesundheit. (2013). Rahmen-Gesundheitsziele Richtungsweisende Vorschläge für ein gesünderes Österreich. Wien. http://www.gesundheitsziele-oesterreich.at.

Cambridge English Dictionary. (2018). Champion. https://dictionary.cambridge.org/dictionary/english/champion. Accessed 8 Nov 2018.

Centers for Disease Control and Prevention. (2011). Health literacy. Identify advocates. https://www.cdc.gov/healthliteracy/planact/develop/IdentifyAdvocates.html. Accessed 8 Nov 2018.

del Castillo, J., Khan, H., Nicholas, L., & Finnis, A. (2016). Health as a social movement: The power of people in movements. Nesta. https://media.nesta.org.uk/documents/health_as_a_social_movement-sept.pdf. Accessed 28 May 2020.

Farmanova, E., Bonneville, L., & Bouchard, L. (2018). Organizational health literacy: Review of theories, frameworks, guides, and implementation issues. *Inquiry: A Journal of Medical Care Organization, Provision and Financing, 55,* 46958018757848. https://doi.org/10.1177/0046958018757848.

Google Dictionary. (2018). Champion. Google. https://www.google.com/search?q=Diction ary#dobs=Champion. Accessed 8 Nov 2018.

Health Literacy Media. (2018). Missouri health literacy trailblazers lead the way. https://www.healthliteracy.media/blog/missouri-health-literacy-trailblazers-lead-the-way. Accessed 8 Nov 2018.

Kickbusch, I. (2013). *Health literacy. The solid facts.* Copenhagen: World Health Organization Regional Office for Europe (The solid facts). http://www.euro.who.int/__data/assets/pdf_file/0008/190655/e96854.pdf. Accessed 28 May 2020.

Kickbusch, I. (2004). Health and citizenship: The characteristics of 21st century health. *World Hospitals and Health services, 40*(4), 12–14.

Kramer, G. (2018). Tweet. https://twitter.com/KramerGraham/status/105732913690410188 9?s=20.

MSD (2012). Announcing the shortlist for the Crystal Clear MSD Health Literacy Awards 2012. Press release. MSD. http://msd-ireland.com/resources/files/Crystal-Clear-2012-General-Shortlist-release-120412.pdf. Accessed 13 Feb 2016.

MSD. (2016). Well Done Awards. http://www.welldoneawards.be/nl/. Accessed 13 Dec 2016.

Nationaler Aktionsplan Gesundheitskompetenz Geschäftsstelle. (2018). *Der Nationale Aktionsplan Gesundheitskompetenz.* Berlin: Nationaler Aktionsplan Gesundheitskompetenz Geschäftsstelle. Hertie School. http://www.nap-gesundheitskompetenz.de/. Accessed 24 June 2018.

Nebraska Association of Local Health Directors. (2018). Health literacy champions. http://nalhd.org/our-work/hl-champions.html. Accessed 8 Dec 2018.

NHS Scotland. (2014). Making It Easy - A National Action Plan on Health Literacy for Scotland. http://www.gov.scot/Resource/0045/00451263.pdf. Accessed 28 May 2020.

Online Etymology Dictionary. (2018). Champion. Origin and meaning of champion. https://www.etymonline.com/word/champion. Accessed 8 Dec 2018.

Osborne, H. (2000). Take action: Be a health literacy hero. https://healthliteracy.com/2000/01/26/take-action-be-a-health-literacy-hero/. Accessed 8 Dec 2018.

Simonds, S. (1974). Health education as social policy. *Health Education Monograph, 2,* 1–25.

Sørensen, K. (2016). *Making health literacy the political choice. A health literacy guide for politicians.* Urmond: Global Health Literacy Academy. https://www.researchgate.net/publication/311455482_Health_literacy_is_a_political_choice_A_health_literacy_guide_for_politicians. Accessed 28 May 2020.

Sørensen, K., & Brand, H. (2017). Developments and perspectives of health literacy in Europe. *Public Health Forum, 25*(1), 10–12. https://doi.org/10.1515/pubhef-2016-2175.

Sørensen, K., Karuranga, S., Denysiuk, E., & McLernon, L. (2018). Health literacy and social change: Exploring networks and interests groups shaping the rising global health literacy movement. *Global health promotion, 25*(4), 89–92. https://doi.org/10.1177/1757975918798366.

Sydney Local Health District. (2016). Health Literacy Framework 2016–2020. Sydney. https://www.slhd.nsw.gov.au/pdfs/SLHD_HLF.pdf. Accessed 28 May 2020.

U.S. Department of Health and Human Services. (2010). Action Plan to Improve Health Literacy. Washington DC. https://health.gov/communication/initiatives/health-literacy-action-plan.asp. Accessed 28 May 2020.

World Health Organization. (2016). Shanghai Declaration on Health Promotion in the 2030 Agenda for Sustainable Development. World Health Organization. Geneva. http://www.who.int/entity/healthpromotion/conferences/9gchp/shanghai-declaration.pdf. Accessed 28 May 2020.

World Health Organization Regional Office for Europe. (2016). Strengthening people-centred health systems in the WHO European Region: framework for action on integrated health services delivery (No. EUR/RC66/Conf.Doc./11). Copenhagen. http://www.euro.who.int/en/who-we-are/governance. Accessed 28 May 2020.

Health Literacy as a Key Concept for a Healthy Life? I Think There Is a Bigger Picture Here

Paulo Pinheiro and Ullrich Bauer

1 Introduction

Health literacy has recently become a topic of relevance among researchers, practitioners and policy-makers who work on issues related to health and education. It has increasingly been portrayed as a social innovation which can make a significant contribution to improving the health of populations and to understanding and tackling social inequalities in health (WHO 2013; Schaeffer et al. 2018). Various empirical studies such as the European Health Literacy Project have supported such a perspective with a range of findings suggesting the need for action (e.g. Berkman et al. 2011; Sørensen et al. 2015).

In a very basic sense, health literacy embodies a number of perspectives that are concerned with the use of print or screen based information with health-related content and, thus, addresses multiple actions associated with written language to communicate health-related issues. Perspectives on health literacy are not only restricted to written texts—which has traditionally been the central mode of language representation,—but increasingly concerned with the use of imagery or the reading of sound and image which have become more prevalent modes of digital communication in almost every society.

P. Pinheiro (✉) · U. Bauer
Faculty of Educational Sciences, Bielefeld University, Bielefeld, Germany
e-mail: paulo.pinheiro@uni-bielefeld.de

U. Bauer
e-mail: ullrich.bauer@uni-bielefeld.de

The growing recognition of health literacy as a guiding concept for action in the fields of health and education, however, should not obscure the fact that a number of key questions still remain open. This includes, for example, issues related to the conceptualisation and the determinants of health literacy, the positioning of health literacy within causal pathways and the web of causation, and the research-to-practice or research-to-policy translation. This is not surprising, since research on health literacy has gained momentum only since the turn of the millennium and the process of establishing a scientific evidence-base is still ongoing. What seems more surprising here and worth subjecting to a critical reflection is that health literacy has increasingly been promoted as a response to a number of central challenges in education- and health-related policy and practice despite a fragmented or even poor scientific underpinning. The apparent discrepancy suggests that the issue of health literacy has been advanced by different stimuli and with different intensities in research and policy. It, thus, raises questions about how the discourses on health literacy in research and policy have been evolving and interacting with each other and how the power to define and the prerogative of interpretation have been distributed within the fields that have been addressing health literacy.

This paper is based on the premise that there is a bigger picture in which health literacy is embedded, but which has not yet been embraced by the scientific discourse. The overall objective of this paper is, therefore, to approach and outline in a first approximation some contexts of health literacy that hold the potential to advance and contribute significantly to the understanding of the issue, but have so far hardly been considered by mainstream discourse. This implies that the paper critically reviews the current conceptualizations of health literacy, identifies open questions and responds to the gaps with an outline of perspectives that provide new opportunities for the ongoing development of the concept of health literacy.

The paper, thus, begins with a retrospective on how health literacy has been addressed in different fields and disciplines in the past. This provides an initial framing that allows to outline and map the diversity of possible interpretations and approaches to health literacy. The reasoning is then tailored to the discourses within which the recent conceptualizations of health literacy have been shaped. It evolves from a descriptive portrayal of currently dominant notions of health literacy that is informed by research literature and includes the illustration of widely recognized core characteristics of the concept. The reconstruction of conceptual constituents will then be subjected to a critical analysis aiming at the identification of shortcomings and gaps, whose elaboration holds promise for the advancement of the conceptual understanding. New avenues for the discussion of what health literacy is are then opened up through making reference to major perspectives used in literacy research. With this contextualisation of health literacy, the paper progresses to broader frameworks, addresses and discusses the associations between health literacy and key themes such as decision-making, self-management and health lifestyles, taking into account theoretical orientations that shape these key themes. By addressing the agency/structure issue, the paper then presents and discusses a wider framework that can prove helpful for the ongoing conceptual elaboration of health literacy. The agency structure issue also serves as a bridge to finally outline and discuss the associations between health literacy and broader social issues such as the digital transformation and population health transitions.

2 Health Literacy: A Bunch of Disciplines, but Little Interdisciplinary Concertation

A glance at the research literature reveals that the topic of health literacy has been addressed and studied in the past by different disciplines or fields of work. This is well documented, for instance, by the results of a bibliometric analysis which highlight a sharp increase in the number of published articles about health literacy that are indexed not only in health-related databases such as PubMed, but also in bibliographic databases on education, library and information sciences, nursing, pharmacy, communication or sociology (Bankson 2009). The large interest in health literacy and its international uptake are also well documented on the policy level. In its recent Shanghai Declaration on promoting health in the 2030 Agenda for Sustainable Development, the World Health Organization WHO has defined health literacy as one major key driver for health promotion and as a priority in education (McDaid 2016). In 2018, the WHO and the United Nations Children's Fund UNICEF presented the Astana Declaration, highlighting the significance of health literacy for primary health care and health policy-making (WHO and UNICEF 2018). Similar, the United Nations' Economic and Social Affairs Council ECOSOC released a declaration in 2010 to strengthen health literacy on the policy level (United Nations Economic and Social Council ECOSOC 2010). Most recently, the Organisation for Economic Co-operation and Development OECD included health literacy into their strategy for people-centred care (Moreira 2018). Health literacy has also been included in various other public policies, such as strategic and action plans in several countries (e.g. Rowlands et al. 2018; Weishaar et al. 2018; Trezona et al. 2018; Heijmans et al. 2015). Beyond health policies, health literacy has also become part of educational policies, placing health literacy at the core curriculum of teaching and learning (Bauer et al. 2018).

A screening of the topic's evolution over time also reveals that health literacy has been addressed with different emphases and discussed using various conceptual approaches in different disciplines (Okan 2019). Health literacy has been viewed, for example, as a learning outcome of school-based health education. In adult education, on the other hand, it has been involved in literacy teaching and basic education programmes rather as a domain-specific task of literacy learning. In clinical health care, health literacy has attracted attention as a target dimension for the analysis of physician-patient interactions and has found its way into discussions on strategies for improving therapy adherence and compliance. Another apparent trend has been in the field of public health, where health literacy has, for instance, been integrated into health promotion research and policy. Here, health literacy is understood as a measure that enables empowerment and the participation in health-related decision-making processes. Given the proximity of literacy to fields related to language and education, it is worth noting that the recent debate on health literacy has been significantly shaped—and to a certain extent narrowed—by stimuli that have emerged predominantly in disciplines and fields of action related to health care and public health.

The multidisciplinary and multi-sectoral uptake of health literacy suggests that the subject has been appealing in different manifestations for a wide range of purposes and adaptable to different schools of thought or theories of reference. The review of the literature also reveals that the topic has occasionally been discussed outside disciplinary boundaries but has not yet been integrated consistently and systematically into interdisciplinary contexts. Overall, the research discourse on health literacy refers—on the one hand—to a range of topics such as communication, health, learning, knowledge processing, or language and language acquisition, but is—on the other hand—characterised by segregation, inconsistencies, fragmentations and blurred discursive lines in which programmatic, descriptive, and analytical purposes are mixed. This apparently underlines the need for researchers to seek information about health literacy in a wider range of sources and to familiarize with different vocabularies and concepts. The findings also imply that there is a need for more collaborative scholarship on health literacy if a more comprehensive and integrative view is to be envisaged and the bias in approaches to health literacy is to be kept to a minimum.

3 Current Conceptions of Health Literacy: Health Literacy as a Set of Skills

The question of how health literacy is currently defined by the research discourse can be answered quite accurately by looking at a series of systematic literature reviews in which definitions, models and measurement methods of health literacy underwent analysis. This collection of papers helps identify and get an overview of commonalities and differences that have shaped the dominant notions of health literacy.

The understanding of health literacy in the European region (including Germany) has been coined by the results of a systematic review of literature presented by the European Health Literacy Project (HLS-EU). This study followed the objectives (a) to identify core characteristics of definitions and concepts of health literacy and, building on that, (b) to develop an integrated definition as well as a conceptual model of health literacy (Sørensen et al. 2012). The review revealed 17 definitions and 12 conceptual frameworks of health literacy. A content analysis of the definitions allowed to group the terms and notions used in the definitions into six clusters: (1) competence, skills, abilities; (2) actions; (3) information and resources; (4) objective; (5) context; and (6) time. These results were used to subsequently develop a new and integrated definition of health literacy that has since then become a key reference in the field of health literacy. According to the HLS-EU definition, health literacy "is linked to literacy and entails people's knowledge, motivation and competences to access, understand, appraise, and apply health information in order to make judgments and take decisions in everyday life concerning healthcare, disease prevention and health promotion to maintain or improve quality of life during the life course" (Sørensen et al. 2012, p. 3). The analysis of the twelve conceptual models showed various shortcomings such as the lack of theoretical foundation, empirical validation, or pathways outlining the causes and effects of health literacy. Based on the findings from the content analysis of the conceptual models, the authors proposed, in addition to the integrated definition, their own model of health literacy (Sørensen et al. 2012). The health literacy model claims to be an integrated model and confirms this by combining main dimensions of health literacy with proximal and distal determinants of health literacy and by outlining pathways that link health literacy with health outcomes. The main dimensions of health literacy are represented by a matrix in which knowledge, motivation, and competencies to carry out tasks related to the use of health information (namely access, understand, appraise, and apply health-related information) are combined with the three domains healthcare, disease prevention, and health promotion (Sørensen et al. 2012). The authors conclude that the integrated model can be used as a conceptual basis for the development and validation of measurement tools as well as for developing of interventions promoting health literacy.

It is worthwhile to refer to another recently published systematic literature review that addressed the theoretical foundations of health literacy. Malloy-Weir et al. (2016) performed a systematic review of definitions of health literacy published between 2007 and 2013 in journals indexed in MEDLINE. This study used the same methodological approach, however, unlike the study of the EU-HLS group, the objective was not to harmonize and standardize the range of definitions, but to get an overview of commonalities and differences, and to critically analyse the wording of and the assumptions underlying commonly used definitions. The study was able to find 250 different definitions of health literacy, six of which were identified as the most commonly used. 133 definitions were modified versions of these six definitions, and another 111 definitions of health literacy were classified as "other" because they differed in wording. The analysis of similarities and differences across definitions showed that "each of the most commonly used definitions treated a person's abilities (or skills) as central to the concept of health literacy" (Malloy-Weir et al. 2016, p. 338). Differences across definitions were reported to be in terms of the "number and types of abilities (or skills) and/or actions believed to comprise health literacy; the context and/or time frames in which the various abilities and/or actions are believed to be important; and thus, what each implies a health literate person is" (Malloy-Weir et al. 2016, p. 338). The term knowledge appeared—with different types of knowledge mentioned—in some of the definitions of which the wording was not related to the six most commonly used definitions. The critical analysis of the most commonly used definitions of health literacy revealed that these six definitions are open to multiple interpretations and incorporate basic assumptions that are not always justifiable. Malloy-Weir et al. voice several concerns about the scope for interpretation allowed by the definitions of health literacy due to the wording and/or underlying assumptions. They highlight that the most common definitions implicitly include the assumption that information or health information on its own can be used to promote or maintain health, or to reduce health risks and increase quality of life. The emphasis on health information tends to disregard other well-known determinants of health such as structural features of society. The authors further point out that some definitions incorporate the assumption that there are relationships between (a) the health literacy or the capacity to use health information and (b) the making of appropriate or sound health decisions in the context of everyday life. They question this assumption by arguing that health-related decision-making is influenced by a much broader set of factors, such as personal values and beliefs, or life context. In addition, they argue that the terms sound and appropriate when used to describe decision-making are open to assessments based on different criteria. Some definitions e.g. do not rule out the possibility that assessments of health literacy could be based on normative judgements about the appropriateness of people's choices. Finally, the critical analysis showed that the wording used in the most common definitions does not preclude the interpretation that the burden of responsibility of achieving health literacy falls on the individual. The authors highlight that this can turn out to be a pitfall because such a wording "leaves scope for the neglect of non-modifiable individual-level factors ..., structural features of society ... as well as features of health care provisions" (Malloy-Weir et al. 2016, p. 342). They further argue that although the importance of social considerations beyond individuals is recognised in the contemporary discourse on health literacy, this has not been reflected by definitions that seem to promote more individualistic ideas and obfuscate barriers that individuals may face.

Both studies clearly show that the social construct that currently defines health literacy relies on a set of shared characteristics in which personal skills play a major role. The studies also highlight that health literacy in its present form can be subjected to a critical review. The focus of health literacy on domain-specific abilities has, for instance, been questioned in another recently published article by Reeve and Basalik (2014). The authors evaluated the conceptual and empirical distinctiveness of health literacy and did not find any evidence of a health literacy factor in their analysis. The critical discussion of these results questions the uniqueness of the health literacy construct, argues in favour of construct redundancy and construct proliferation, and concludes that measures of health literacy rather reflect domain-specific contextualized measures of basic cognitive abilities (Reeve and Basalik 2014).

Another open point that can make a significant contribution to a better understanding of the topic is the question of how health literacy emerges over time. Knowledge about this is poor or unspecific because research perspectives have preponderantly focused on adult populations and operated with a more static idea of health literacy. A tailored view on the target groups of children and adolescents seems, therefore, to be a promising approach to address issues related to health literacy learning. Children and adolescents can be distinguished from adults by several characteristics (see e.g. Rothman et al. 2009): They differ, for instance, in their developmental potentials, have different disease, risk, and disability profiles, as well as a higher vulnerability to unfavourable sociodemographic factors. Further, their dependency on adults for social and health care is significant and highlights a particular relevance of issues such as intergenerational and power relationships which are unequally distributed between children and adults. It is thus to be expected that social contexts, interactions, and agency are more pronounced within views of health literacy when children are explicitly targeted.

To approach issues related to health literacy learning, two recently published systematic reviews of literature on definitions and on measurement methods of health literacy in childhood and adolescence (Bröder et al. 2017; Okan et al. 2018) can be consulted. The findings of these studies reveal a strong focus on personal attributes such as skills that are considered important to respond to predefined requirements for the use of health information. The conceptualisation of health literacy in childhood and adolescence, therefore, appears to be fairly similar to the majority of definitions for adults (Bröder et al. 2017). The importance of social and cultural conditions or environments is widely acknowledged and seems to be considered more than in the definitions for adults. The social context in which health literacy is embedded, however, is mostly shaped by a relational perspective in which the context defines the demands on a child or an adolescent to use information for the purpose of health. The systematic reviews, in addition, indicate that childhood and adolescence are distinguished from adulthood usually through reference to developmental issues and tasks (e.g. Borzekowski 2009). Most of the articles draw on traditional concepts from developmental psychology rather than on sociological approaches, which might contribute to the promotion of individualistic ideas of health literacy (Bröder et al. 2017).

The review of the measurements of health literacy in childhood and adolescence additionally pointed out that the assessments of health literacy in children and adolescents usually rate personal attributes and involve distinctions between high and low or adequate and inadequate levels of health literacy (Okan et al. 2018). The dominance of rating systems for health literacy in childhood and adolescence reflects that there is—on the one hand—a trend to make the subject commensurable and—on the other hand—a normative notion inherent in conceptualizations of health literacy that calls for the identification of populations at risk. A clear predominance of quantitative approaches is discernible at the moment. If no alternative non-hierarchical approaches that are able to describe rather than count the phenomenology of health literacy are added to the quantitative armamentarium in the future, then any manifestation of health literacy to which quantified ratings cannot be applied—including notions that put emphasis on social practice—remains disregarded.

With the proliferation of health literacy research and policy measures, it has become clear that there is no unanimously accepted definition but rather a coexistence of different views on health literacy. However, the analysis also illustrates that the theoretical-conceptual approaches to health literacy share some considerable commonalities and, thus, permits of a pattern to be traced that reflects some preferences within the current discourse.

First, it is quite evident that the reference to skills is very central when defining health literacy. In this way, the perspective focuses more on the personal prerequisites for action and treats the actual actions with subordinate priority. The variance can first of all be explained with the fact that the specifications of skills that are considered to be important constituents of health literacy can draw on many options.

Second, the skill-based approaches are guided by a rational choice logic and assume informed decision-making to be the link between skills and actions in health matters. Here, there is an underlying assumption that there is a range of choices as well as unrestricted freedom of choice in the context of health information, and that within the range of choices there are offers of different value, thus enabling a categorisation and hierarchisation of the choices on offer. Consequently, rational choice becomes the preferred perspective on action.

Third, activities based on health information or even health information itself are ascribed the potential to contribute to improving health status. This permeates most definitions by way of a general assumption and suggests that analogies can be drawn between health information and medication. To put it pointedly: the assumption is that if the right information is selected and internalised correctly, this contributes to improving health.

4 Health Literacy and Its Social Embeddedness: Health Literacy as a Relational Concept

In a nutshell, the health literacy discourse revolves around the abilities of a person or a system and uses global concepts such as education, lifelong learning, knowledge and skills. It follows the premises of a methodological individualism, which claims to explain social phenomena of varying complexity through the analysis of individual behaviour. Health literacy concepts define their topic as a result of learning processes and put this result in a functional context. They make the topic commensurable, and thus accessible to quantitative empirical research and open to a shift from an empirical-descriptive to a normative level.

As indicated before, the currently dominant views of health literacy have mainly been nurtured by perspectives from healthcare and public health that started to evolve three decades ago. During this time, the topic of health literacy has undergone a metamorphosis. It initially focused on functional skills such as reading, writing and numeracy, and was then complemented with communicative and critical skills in order to improve adherence, compliance or navigation in the context of health care systems. The public health approach then extended the focus to people's everyday life settings, and associated health literacy more closely with health promotion and empowerment goals. Advocates of the public health perspective argue that this shift towards the social determinants of health, participation in society and health agency has created a social justice approach and they conclude that health literacy has become a major influence on the capacity of the individual to make sound health decisions in everyday life.

Recent research activities have responded to the call for considering social, cultural, economic and political contexts by developing approaches that are guided by a system perspective. As an example, there is growing work on concepts for health-literate healthcare organisations that aim at the physical and social infrastructure of a system in order to facilitate the development of health literacy-friendly settings and to improve the system's responsiveness (Brach 2017). Considerations of context are shaped by a perspective that views health literacy as a relational concept (Parker and Ratzan 2010). The focus on health literacy as a relational concept can be regarded as a principle rather than a comprehensive approach. It calls for a perspective in which the abilities of a person who is expected to act as a user of health information are to be juxtaposed with the demands posed by a system (which can be on a meso or meta level) that is expected to act as a provider of health information. The relational principle implies and also aims at achieving a fit between the two parties through measures that strengthen the skills on the user's side and the responsiveness on the provider's side. It is, therefore, based on the idea that the use of health-related information can be targeted in order to adequately meet requirements arising from or within different social contexts in which the user is embedded. How adequacy is classified remains unclear, but results most likely from the comparison of the action with standards defined and established for the management of diseases and risk factors as well as for health lifestyles or quality of life. Presumably, such a framework is gaining momentum within health literacy research because it matches well with notions of empowerment in which self-control and self-management are emphasized.

Perspectives beyond a relational approach, i.e. ones which, for instance, are centred around the social embeddedness of a person, have so far hardly found their way into the research discourse revolving around health literacy (e.g. Parikh et al. 1996; Fairbrother et al. 2016; Sentell et al. 2017; Bauer 2019) and have not yet been translated into a definition of health literacy.

The social environments of health literacy are mainly addressed within a skill-based approach that integrates perspectives on health literacy as a relational concept. The analysis, however, also shows that health literacy as a relational concept fail to do justice to the issue of social contexts as it neither takes social structures and backgrounds in which individuals are embedded into account nor have they got much to say about the impact of social determinants such as living conditions and structures on the agency associated with health literacy.

5   Learning from Literacy and Literacy Learning: Approaching Health Literacy as a Social Practice

One of the most commonly used definitions of health literacy claims that "health literacy is linked to literacy" (Sørensen et al. 2012). However, the review of literature shows that most definitions and models do not address this link with literacy. Explicit references to literacy or a broader discussion and integration of core perspectives addressed in literacy research are scarce within the debate on health literacy. It is likely that the lack of communication between the research discourses on literacy—on the one hand—and health literacy—on the other hand—results from the different disciplines in which the two discourses have been embedded (literacy: affiliated to linguistics and education, health literacy: affiliated to public health and healthcare). Provided that literacy and health literacy have a thematic proximity to each other, it seems promising and imperative to address and examine the research discourse on the topic of literacy, and to contrast key perspectives on literacy with the on-going discussions about health literacy.

Perspectives of literacy embrace activities revolving around reading, writing and calculating and are concerned with the acquisition and implementation of these activities. Depending on purpose, literacy can be viewed in different ways: (a) as a set of functional skills, helping people to meet demands made by the society on them, (b) as a civilising tool, allowing people to access a literary culture, or (c) as a means of emancipation, enabling people to control their lives and to become autonomous citizens in a democracy (Hamilton 2010). The subject of literacy has been underpinned by a broad range of theoretical perspectives which have evolved over time, shaped the understanding and teaching of literacy and informed education policy making. Currently, the discourse on literacy is mainly shaped by cognitive and sociocultural perspectives (Kennedy et al. 2012; Gaffney and Anderson 2000).

Cognitive perspectives on literacy are concerned with mental processes that take place while the words, structures and grammar of a text are recognised, information or meaning are retrieved from text, processed during the reading process and stored in the memory for future retrieval (Lyytinen 1985). A cognitive theory of reading development can be exemplified by the work of Chall (1983) who postulated that all individuals progress through stages of reading acquisition in characteristic ways, within certain age limits, and following the same sequence. Based on this, Chall developed stages of reading and recommended norm-referenced tests to diagnose reading problems. From a cognitive perspective, acting is determined by mental processes rather than by external conditions or stimuli. Development is seen as an active process of a subject equipped with cognitive functions such as recognition and awareness. Davidson (2010) highlights that cognitive researchers are interested in normative behaviour, believe that literacy is largely taught and learned, and, thus, stages of reading or writing development are necessary to guide teaching.

Critical literacy theory positions have questioned such views and argue that a focus on cognitive processes implies that individuals outside prescribed stages or standard norms are deficient in their literacy skills (Davidson 2010). They claim that adherence to cognitive views systematically disadvantages children from non-mainstream backgrounds who have poor access to education in the home and, therefore, out-of-school literacy practices that conflict with predefined reading and writing stages of development (Tracey and Morrow 2006). Others have raised concerns that cognitive views of literacy are limited in understanding how individuals learn to read and write because they fall short in considering the impact of social and cultural environments on the individual's literacy development (e.g. Street 1984).

Scholars endorsing literacy as a social practice aim to respond to the call for a sociocultural perspective in which the social embeddedness of literacy is represented by emphasising that literacy is "what people do with reading, writing, and texts in real world contexts and why they do it" (Perry 2012) and that "in the simplest sense literacy practices are what people do with literacy" (Barton and Hamilton 2000). According to this line of thought, practices involve more than interactions with texts. They connect to, and are shaped by values, attitudes, feelings, and social relationships. The notion of literacy as a social practice has been coined by the work of Brian Street and then promoted by the New Literacy Studies NLS. Views on literacy as a social practice question the premise that texts have meanings independent of their context of use. As the NLS locate reading and writing in the social and linguistic practices that give them meaning, they claim that literacy is more than acquiring content (Street 2005) and that texts do not have uses independent of the social meanings and purposes people construct

(Barton and Hamilton 1998). Hence, such perspectives aim to describe how literacy is practiced in everyday life, recognising that this practice is not neutral, but dependent upon the context in which it takes place and is embedded in social relationships and power relations hidden in the nature of this context (Barton and Hamilton 2000). Literacy as a social practice draws on two ideas that are interdependent: Literacy events and literacy practices (e.g. Barton and Hamilton 2000). According to Street (1984), a literacy event is "any occasion in which a piece of writing is integral to the nature of the participants' interactions and their interpretative processes". The idea of literacy practices is broader and incorporates not only literacy events but also the ways in which people understand, feel and talk about those events (Hamilton 2010). Perry (2012) highlights the distinction between literacy events and literacy practices when she argues that literacy events are observable and thus allow an observer to see what people do with texts while literacy practices must be inferred because they connect to unobservable beliefs, values, attitudes, and social structures.

Dominant views of health literacy show a proximity to cognitive perspectives on literacy as both are more or less characterised by a focus on skills and the premise that individual skills are developed in a context-independent way. As outlined above, the research discourse on literacy has systematically responded to concerns about the neglect of the learning environments with the development of the so-called New Literacy Studies NLS. The NLS view literacy as something people do inside society and argue that literacy is a sociocultural rather than a mental phenomenon which needs to be understood and studied in its full range of contexts. They address the impact of contexts and structures on the acquisition and application of literacy and suggest that literacy is understood as a set of social practices rather than as a set of skills.

If one agrees that health literacy is linked to literacy, it is obvious to suggest that the current debates about health literacy should take up and systematically explore the sociocultural approaches to literacy. There are certainly analogies between health literacy and literacy when we refer to health literacy as those dimensions of literacy that address health information or messages. Although the definition of health literacy to which reference is made in many European countries highlights that "health literacy is linked to literacy", a systematic exploration of core perspectives in literacy research has not been carried out yet. If we further contrast the currently dominant notions of health literacy with those perspectives of literacy which take a sociocultural view, then the obvious first step is to question that health literacy is basically the individual processing of health information. Current health literacy definitions and models tend to focus on personal skills, abilities and competencies, while they disregard perspectives in which social practices and sociocultural structures are addressed. The bias towards skills and cognitive perspectives gives behavioural determinants priority over contextual factors, whose relevance for health and educational outcomes, however, has largely been demonstrated in the past. Such a bias can therefore lead to misinterpretations in both research and transfer (e.g. policy and programme developments). Following a sociocultural approach would call for shifting the focus from a skill-based view to perspectives focusing on the doing or in other words the practice of health literacy. Shifting the focus of health literacy towards sociocultural approaches would also have implications for the methodological approaches used within health literacy research, including alterations in the unit of observation. In line with the NLS, health literacy could benefit from a framework that is shaped by the notion of literacy events and practices. Accordingly, the unit of observation would shift from personal attributes of a person—which is the current mode in health literacy research—to health literacy events and practices that a person is involved in.

6   Choices, Informed Decision Making, and Self-Management

Another input for reflection resulting from the systematic reviews outlined before is the finding that health literacy is guided by the premise that health information is strongly linked with decision making that is beneficial to health (Malloy-Weir et al. 2016). Informed decision making is based on the assumption that there are choices and that choices are made through rational mental processes. It seems appropriate to critically pursue this line of thought, as the link between health information and decision making has diffused widely into the health sector, but has been viewed not without significant controversy.

The endorsement of "choice" has become a key goal of healthcare and public health and has been supported by the widespread reorganisation of health and welfare systems in Western societies. According to Collyer et al. (2015), the current interpretations of the idea of choice are encapsulated within rational choice theory, which sees health consumers as rational actors who act purposively to maximise individual outcomes. Collyer et al. describe that the theory of rational choice is based on several assumptions about human behaviour. People act intentionally and independently of their social context, they are stable and consistent in their decisions when faced with risks and uncertainties and they prefer more choices to fewer, having an unlimited desire for choice (Collyer et al. 2015). They, however, argue that these assumptions underlying rational choice theory are contested when applied to health issues where choice is embedded in the complexity of interrelationships, vulnerabilities and interdependencies. Health consumers differ from the ideal model of the consumer because they might experience a situation of higher vulnerability and threat and, thus, are affected by this in making rational choices. Further, the asymmetry in knowledge about medical matters between healthcare professionals and laypeople is still an important determinant of help-seeking in that a layperson tends to trust and rely on the judgement of experts. As suggested by a plethora of studies, there is little predictability concerning the making of health-related choices because they are influenced by how the choice is offered, how information is framed, and the context in which choices are made (Collyer et al. 2015).

Pescosolido (1992) voices concerns about the rational choice framework with a number of further arguments that are based on the significance of social life and the relative place in society for help-seeking and decision-making in health issues. Accordingly, she considers the process of interaction to be the mechanism through which social phenomena occur and thus suggests the individual in interaction and the structure of interactional events to be the most basic unit of analysis in decision making (Pescosolido 1992). She further argues that problems as well as solutions and choices are socially organized and thus embedded in social networks. This premise matches poorly with the conceptualization frequently made in rational choice that defines actions of other people as exogenous factors or another utility in the individual cost-benefit analysis. A further limitation according to Pescosolido is that rational choice models focus on one action at a time and ignore how sequences of events are patterned, contingent, and emergent. Her rationale finally questions the use of rational choice as a general orientation to social action, highlighting the importance of habits and routines for social action and the difficulties to address this with rational choice models that imply that action is guided by reflective weighing. There is thus limited plausibility in using the rational actor framework for social actions that proceed through habit and routines because it neglects these forms of social action (Pescosolido 1992).

The centrality of choice and the shift towards a more consumerist conception of health services and health information in public or health policy is well reflected by studies in which discourse analysis was applied to the policy debate (e.g. Teghtsoonian 2009; Nordgren 2010). The studies reveal the ways in which choice, responsibility and empowerment are identified as manifestations of the consumerist orientation of professional organisations and cultures. The proliferation of choice in the policy discourse is viewed as a response to the call for better meeting the citizen's demands for efficiency, responsiveness, and flexibility of health services and goods. It implies an emancipatory momentum that calls for re-adjusting the balance of responsibility between the public and the citizens. This can be associated with the empowering of individuals to make informed choices, but is not without challenges as indicated by the results of a discourse analysis (Nordgren 2010) in which an oversimplification of the language used in health policy discourses and the neglect of issues such as patient vulnerability, lack of knowledge, dependency, and need for care were identified. Besides, the issue of responsibility connects strongly with, or shows significant overlap with notions or conceptions of the self. Self-management of chronic diseases or self-optimization of everyday life represent not only the primary form of task solution but are at the same time conceptual representations of the imagery of an entre-preneurial self that follows the idea of thinking of oneself and acting in private and professional spheres as a set of skills that are in need of constantly building, improving, or adapting.

Self-management has become ubiquitous in health-related policies and strate-gies, health promotion campaigns and intervention programs across most of the Western societies. The emphasis on the self can be regarded as a response to the ageing of populations and the rise of the burden of chronic and mental diseases, and is driven by the idea of an empowered citizen who is enabled to control his/her own health and initiate positive change. However, as Greenhalgh (2009) argues, the evidence for the efficacy of self-management based on the expert patient model is weak as it has been shown that the majority of self-management programs have been unsuccessful for reasons such as lack of attention to cultural norms and the need for support (Greenhalgh 2009). Other studies focusing on the shift of responsibility for social risks to individuals and on the processes by which the idea of self-management is internalised and naturalised by individuals even highlight the risk for adverse effects on health and quality of life. Peacock et al. (2014) e.g. concluded from a series of biographical-narrative interviews conducted with women living in the United Kingdom to explore shame and social comparison that the multi-stranded narratives were guided by a motif which they termed "no legitimate dependency". It describes that "almost everything about participants' lives were deemed to be the responsibility of the individual, who alone should be able to manage whatever was happening to them and where turn-ing to others, or even acknowledging the need for help, was seen as weak and unacceptable" and that "taking a socially contextualised perspective was inter-preted as a self-serving attempt to rationalise or justify either failure or personal inadequacy" (Peacock et al. 2014).

The analysis of Brijnath and Antoniades (2016) on practices of self-management of depressed patients provides another exemplification of risks for adverse health effects caused by inconsistencies between the policy rhetoric of self-management, its implementation in care systems and practices of self-management. The results from in-depth interviews with participants from Australia who are in need for mental health care highlight that, on the one hand, participants actively looked for solutions, made their own decisions, or valued being in control. On the other hand, the participants also reported that the success of self-management was connected with the disengagement from, and non-utilisation of health services, as well as with self-medication and self-labour. They did not feel entitled to make use of public services and felt that changes had to occur only within them for their depression to improve. The authors conclude that the participants "had absorbed, enacted and responded to the current rationalities and techniques of care within community psychiatry by emphasising personal responsibility, self-directing their help-seeking and treatments and blaming themselves when they failed to achieve their desired outcome" (Brijnath and Antoniades 2016).

Health literacy is consistently defined in self-descriptions as a determinant for decision-making. This connection appears to be plausible at first glance, but is to be discussed in a more differentiated way when looking more carefully at the state of research on choice, decision-making and self-management in health-related matters. Making reference to these topics and their theoretical underpinnings, evokes an analysis of a consumerist orientation that gives priority to rationality and self-responsibility in decision-making. For health-related purposes of seeking help and information, however, such a framework can be affirmed only to a limited extent, since the vulnerabilities and uncertainties associated with the event need to be given greater consideration. The definition of empowerment as a programmatic goal should be subjected to critical reflection, too.

7 Health Lifestyles and the Agency-Structure Issue

The discourse on health literacy addresses a wide range of outcomes in which health is represented not just as the absence of disease but, more pronouncedly, as an asset for well-being or quality of life (Malloy-Weir et al. 2016). The effects of health literacy are thus rooted not only in health care but predominantly in many daily lifestyle practices. There is therefore a significant overlap between the debates on health literacy and the discourse on health lifestyles. Both approaches view health rather as an achievement and, therefore, as something that people are supposed to work on. Health literacy focuses on health information as the means to achieve health, whereas health lifestyle approaches comprehensively encompass any human activity in that they claim that any decision has become a decision about health (Clarke et al. 2003).

Cockerham (2005) argues similarly, asserting that many daily lifestyle practices involve considerations of health outcomes, but concludes that there is no health lifestyle theory. He substantiates the need for such a theory by indicating that concepts of health lifestyles have been guided by individualist paradigms, neglected structural dimensions and been poorly applicable to empirics. His approach to the development of a health lifestyle theory is then framed and informed by the agency-structure debate (Cockerham 2005). Cockerham does not contest that theoretical perspectives on health lifestyles disregard either the capacity of individuals to act or the power of structural conditions in contouring individual dispositions and actions, but underscores that the interplay and mutual influence between agency and structure remain either unclear or in favour of one perspective. He defines agency e.g. as "a process in which individuals, influenced by their past but also oriented toward the future (as a capacity to imagine alternative possibilities) and the present (as a capacity to consider both past habits and future situations within the contingencies of the moment), critically evaluate and choose their course of action" and social structures as "sets of mutually sustaining schemas and resources that empower or constrain social action and tend to be reproduced by that social action" (Cockerham 2005).

The debate concerning the primacy of agency or structure in shaping human behaviour has long been pivotal in social sciences and, in particular, in issues that help to understand whether individuals act as a free agents or determined by social structures (autonomy vs socialisation) (Hurrelmann and Bauer 2018). Illuminating contributions that help get an overview of the agency structure debate and its significance in the context of health are presented by Bittlingmayer (2016) and Sperlich (2016). Bittlingmayer addresses structural perspectives on health and disease, whereas Sperlich discusses agency perspectives and then considers how the agency and structure perspectives can be related to each other in a mutually appropriate way.

Bittlingmayer (2016) first explains why it can be useful to study sociological perspectives on social structures under the heading of health. He argues that knowledge about this can create a good sense of the power of social structures but without at the same time transfiguring these structures into "powers of destiny". Furthermore, structural perspectives instill a sense of power relationships in society, in which health and illness are also integrated, and are able to promote a reflexive comprehension of one's own positions and options for action. He then clarifies, among other things, that there is a need for an up-to-date definition of structure. He emphasizes that the notion of structure is not to be formulated deterministically because social structures represent social relations and thus specific probabilities. He discusses this by arguing that social structures are something that is created by people themselves, and thus something that can in principle be changed and hence transformed. He also highlights that the idea of social structures has been interpreted differently over history. He follows this up with the conclusion that an analysis of social structures should be able to address two diametrically opposed scenarios: The inertia inherent in processes of structural social change and the possibility that social structures—though exercising power over a person—can in principle cease to exist. According to Bittlingmayer, there are three important variants of sociological theories of structure with regard to the topic of health: structural functionalism according to Parsons, the genealogical-archaeological approach according to Foucault, and the neo-Marxist perspective of the Frankfurt School (Bittlingmayer 2016).

Sperlich (2016) explains that all theories of agency have in common the assumption that agency is the deliberate act of a person. This includes rational as well as habitual or value-oriented action. The various theories of agency mainly differ with regard to the question of how purposeful, controlled, rational and reflexive agency is to be defined (Sperlich 2016). Sperlich identifies three approaches within the theories of agency: a normative, an individualistic and an interpretative paradigm. Proponents of the normative paradigm (e.g. theory of structural functionalism) postulate that agency can be derived from social order, i.e. from superordinate norms, institutions and rules. The individualistic paradigm encompasses different approaches (such as the theory of rational decision according to Esser and Coleman) that share the idea that social phenomena such as institutions, norms and social structures can be explained by individual behaviour. Unlike the normative paradigm, social phenomena are therefore viewed from the angle of deliberate action by individuals. Approaches representing an interpretative paradigm (such as symbolic interactionism according to Mead and Blumer) are guided by the idea that social order does not emerge through the internalisation of values and norms, but as the result of actions, interactions and interpretations. Social reality is therefore not to be justified normatively but is continually constructed by the actors through social interaction and interpretation (Sperlich 2016).

The second part of Sperlich's paper responds to the critical voices raised against a narrow subjectivist focus of health-related agency and explores theoretical approaches to health and disease that aim to link agency and structure. Here, she recognizes—like Cockerham (2005) and Collyer et al. (2015)—the importance of Bourdieu's habitus theory. Habitus can be viewed as a socially acquired system of mental dispositions that structures a person's perception, thinking and feeling. Cockerham quotes Bourdieu who defines habitus as "systems of durable, transposable dispositions, structured structures predisposed to operate as structuring structures, that is, as principles which generate and organize practices and representations that can be objectively adapted to their outcomes without presupposing a conscious aiming at ends or an express mastery of the operations necessary in order to attain them" (Cockerham 2005). Cockerham's own interpretation of the habitus highlights that "the habitus serves as a cognitive map or set of perceptions that routinely guides and evaluates a person's choices and options. It provides enduring dispositions toward acting deemed appropriate by a person in particular social situations and settings. Included are dispositions that can be carried out even without giving them a great deal of thought in advance. They are simply habitual ways of acting when performing routine tasks. The influence of exterior social structures and conditions are incorporated into the habitus, as well as the individual's own inclinations, preferences, and interpretations" (Cockerham 2005). Collyer et al. (2015) focus on the interrelated concepts of habitus, capital and field, and conclude that health choices can be understood in a Bourdieusian approach as the processes of agency in action. They argue that health choices are structured within the habitus and that "this occurs through the interplay and interaction of the various forms of capital where individual practices are aligned with those of one's social group". The habitus and its dispositions are "in turn structured by the dynamics of the field", which is "the mechanism through which the various capitals are produced and socially distributed" (Collyer et al. 2015). Accordingly, it is the field that structures "the capacities of actors, differentially enabling or suppressing the realisation of various forms of power, and giving shape to the kind of choices that can be made" (Collyer et al. 2015).

In what way could health literacy research benefit from the agency structure debate? Studying the causal pathways linking health literacy with the promotion of health lifestyles and outcomes against the backdrop of the discussions on the relationship between agency and social structure appears highly insightful for several reasons: It helps to define more precisely the mutual interplay between social structures and the autonomy of individuals to act and thus might contribute to a revision of the current ideas about what health literacy is and what it is capable of. It also helps to better understand what determinants on the personal and social levels have an impact on actions involving health-related information, so that implications for effective promotion strategies can be identified and issues of health inequalities can be considered more appropriately.

8　Health Information and the Digital Transformation

One broader social context in which health literacy is entangled is the so-called digital transformation; a term that makes reference to the processes of change in society triggered by the rise of digital technologies such as the Internet, the World Wide Web and the Web 2.0. Digital transformation describes the effects of digitalization on various dimensions of social life in—mainly but not exclusively—Western societies and addresses pervasive changes of, e.g., consumption patterns, organizational patterns and business models, socio-economic structures and cultural lifestyles. One common manifestation of the ongoing digital transformation is the move towards a situation in which most of the information—including significant professional and scientific information—is available in digital rather than printed form. The rise of digital technologies has been associated with both a tremendous increase in the multimodal availability of, and a simplified access to information and data. These technical advances have led to a much more rich and complex information environment, with a greater amount of information available, in a greater variety of formats and sources, and accessible through a greater variety of media and communication channels.

People are challenged by these transformations in various ways. The provision is typically delivered through digital devices such as computers, tablets or mobile phones. There are thus minimum requirements if one wants to participate and benefit from digital offers. The equipment needs to be affordable and the use of the technology needs to be learned. The raise of digital resources has also led to a shift in the provision of information, with screen-based media increasingly taking precedence over print-based media. This process has not been without discussions in which scenarios of a cultural devaluation of text-based written language have been addressed and possible negative effects on the acquisition and use of reading and writing have been pointed out.

The communication and sharing of information, and specifically web-based information, has become more embedded in everyday life, rather than being restricted to scholarly and professional domains. This was made possible and promoted, among other things, by the fact that knowledge has increasingly been transformed into a commodity and used as such. At the same time, the widespread diffusion of knowledge from professionals to laypersons and the massive amplification of laypersons' knowledge as a manifestation of Web 2.0 has been coinciding with a reorientation of the role-relationships between experts and laypersons. These changes in sensibilities and attitudes have called into question the traditional asymmetry of power relations in the production, evaluation and dissemination of knowledge. As a result of the call for less paternalistic and more equalised relationships, we see the decline in the status and professional authority of experts, whose control over the production and release of knowledge has lessened, and a redefinition of self-conceptions on the part of both the producers and consumers of information that revolves around motifs such as democratization and empowerment, and moves towards mutual participation models of the expert-layperson relationship.

As the Internet has grown, so too have health-related purposes. Consumers are now afforded low threshold access to a vaster array of health information than ever before. Research on consumers' health information-seeking behaviours indicates that health information is typically sought for the purposes of, e.g., self-empowerment, emotional reassurance, acquisition of knowledge, and decision-making (Cline and Haynes 2001; Lee et al. 2015). Health information may have its own significance in the spectrum of information, because of vulnerabilities associated with the reasons for information-seeking.

The health-related sector including domains such as health care, health education or health promotion is similarly concerned with the challenges as outlined above. Concepts such as shared or informed decision making highlight the growing awareness of the need to equalise relationships between health professionals and laypeople and reflect a decline of traditionally ruling authorities, such as medical experts, and a stronger alignment with healthy lifestyles (Hoving et al. 2010). The shift towards the patients' abilities to help themselves and make informed choices has also been promoted by the reorganisation of healthcare systems and pressures of healthcare costs. In addition, it has been paralleled by an increase in the importance of evidence-based medicine that reflects the pronounced call for quality assurance of health-related information (Eysenbach et al. 2002). The call for more evidence-based approaches responds to the issue of the varying quality of health information in an online environment as a result of the absence of restrictions on the publishing of content and the lack of consensus for guidelines to evaluate the quality of health information.

Since the volume of health information available is vast and continues to grow, there is an even greater desideratum to explore perspectives addressing the risks or "pathologies" of information. Such perspectives make references to issues such as information overload, paradox of choice, information anxiety, or to coping strategies such as information avoidance, information withdrawal, or satisficing (Bawden and Robinson 2009). Other issues related to the information environment Web 2.0 are the anonymity of contributors, the loss of identity and authority, the replacement of objectivity by subjectivity, impermanence of information, or the expectation of constant novelty (Hardey 2008).

9   Transitions in Population Health and the Transformation of Health to an All-Pervasive Value

Another wider context in which the topic of health literacy has evolved can be framed by a mix of interrelated processes which have been referred to as demographic, epidemiological or risk transition. These movements share the focus on disease patterns and the health status of populations and have significantly contributed to understanding the determinants of health (Young 2004). The insights gained about the web of causation of diseases and health have, in turn, promoted processes of the transformation in healthcare provision and have resulted in redefining ideas about the nature of health (Warwick-Booth et al. 2012). The demographic, epidemiologic and risk transition have been traced back to advances in health technologies in the early to mid-20th century, which in combination with socioeconomic innovations have led to a dramatic reduction in the mortality from infectious diseases and the raise of life expectancies. As regards the understanding of health, there has also been a shift of definitions away from the traditional focus on pathogenic perspectives. A major impetus has regularly been ascribed to key statements of health care organisations (in particular the World Health Organization WHO) which defined health as not just the absence of disease, which can be mainly controlled by medical technology, but the complete physical, social and psychological well-being which is amenable to a range of non-medical perspectives and professions. The improved expectations of longevity and health status were questioned by the rise of chronic disease conditions which significantly impacted on the quality rather than the quantity of life and brought health care systems and technologies to their limits (Omran 2005). One response to this was a reorientation towards prevention and health promotion. These changes coincided with socioeconomic advances in Western societies which paved the way for the rise of the consumerist movement that was predominantly connected with anti-authoritarianism and civil rights perspectives in the 1960s and 70s, and with neoliberal and free-market ideas in the 1980s and 90s. Another cultural trend in Western societies was the move towards reflexivity, self-awareness, and self-help, leading to expectations of self-fulfilment and heightened consciousness of health, well-being and quality of life. This was accompanied by a series of other trends: A growing commercialisation of health, a progressive medicalisation of core aspects of daily life such as food choices, leisure activities, mood changes and coping with life events, increased media interest in health topics leading to higher levels of awareness and uncertainties about the conditions for diseases, health, and well-being (Greenhalgh and Wessely 2004). As a result, many health problems have increasingly been linked with individual acts and malpractices, and responsibilities for achieving well-being have been shifted to the individuals' side. Overall, these trends have also reinforced the notion of health as a central social value and a metaphor for well-being and quality of life. Consequently, any decision has now become at the same time a decision about health. In this way, health exerts a significant influence over social developments and decisions, which is reflected by a culture in which the needs and worries associated with caring for health increasingly shape the living arrangements, well-being and mental states of individuals.

Direct connections between fundamental social changes, the health status of populations and the topic of health literacy have been established by Kickbusch (2006) and Nefiodow (2011). The reasoning in both contributions is based on historical retrospect, with Kickbusch focusing on the development of the health of populations and Nefiodow focusing on macroeconomic and cyclical perspectives. Kickbusch's perspective presumes that the current situation in society has been shaped by three health revolutions. The first health revolution (in the 19th and early 20th centuries), which contributed to safeguarding public health, was followed by a second health revolution (in the course of the 20th century), which led to the expansion of the health care system and to population-wide safeguarding against illness, disability and ageing. For the 21st century, Kickbusch then proposes a third health revolution in which the focus is on promoting health in the multifarious living environments of everyday life, thus focusing on population groups and settings instead of diseased individuals. Here, references are also made to the increasingly pivotal role and promising prospects of the health sector as an economic growth sector. Health promotion is to be achieved through an emancipatory overall policy that focuses on information, education and empowerment. At the same time, however, the people are also exposed to a growing flow of information, which is considered a risk to health and, therefore, makes it vital to promote the citizens' ability to act. Health literacy is here defined as the means by which empowerment is achieved (Kickbusch 2006). Accordingly, health literacy strengthens the autonomy to define and make decisions about health and enables people to take responsibility for their own health. The self-determined, health literate and self-responsible citizen, who cares for their own health for their own sake as a rationally acting entrepreneur, can be regarded as the model individual in such a society.

Nefiodow refers to Kondratiev cycles in his demonstration of the relevance of health literacy, making his reasoning explicitly an economic one. Kondratiev cycles are at the core of a theoretical approach to cyclical economic development, which is also known as the theory of long waves. The origins of long waves are innovation-driven shifts in paradigm and the related investments in new technologies that trigger social change and development. The broad implementation of an innovation is then accompanied by a decrease in investment and stimulates an economic downswing and the emergence of a new paradigm. According to this theory, five long waves can be identified in retrospect, with the ongoing fifth Kondratiev cycle being stimulated and perpetuated by information and communication technology as the basic innovation (Nefiodow 2011). Nefiodow connects his work with the fifth cycle and provides considerations on the technology that will dominate a possible sixth Kondratiev cycle. He argues that the driving forces for economic growth and structural development will no longer be labour and capital, but rather productivity gains, which in turn will be determined by competencies. Based on the premise that physical, mental and social disorders and diseases are currently the greatest barriers to growth, he concludes that future advances in productivity will result primarily from the strengthening of health literacy (Nefiodow 2011).

The juxtaposition of health literacy with the broader movements that have constantly redefined the subject of health shows that the health literacy discourse should become aware of how health can be related to literacy in different ways. References to health can specifically address the management or prevention of diseases. In such biomedical or pathogenic approaches, health is about treatment and risk management of diseases in order to restore health or to avoid disease, and health literacy processes instruct how to avoid life-threatening situations. Health can also be addressed in a way that is decoupled from any specific disease, through social models of health that address the social determinants of health and the impact of the social environment on individual health and well-being. Social models of health overlap with pathogenic health models but also connect to salutogenic approaches that are concerned with the origins of health and well-being. They address factors and processes that support individuals in responding to stimuli from internal and external environments in ways which promote their own quality of life (see Saboga-Nunes et al. 2019).

Another aspect that becomes apparent from the previous two sections is that the topic of health literacy has been considered to be relevant to a selection of ongoing processes of social change and the challenges or uncertainties associated with these processes. On the one hand, references are made to processes of social reorganization that are initiated and catalysed by digitalization. Here, fields of tension are described for a number of issues related to the topic of knowledge. Health literacy is incorporated into such considerations as a potential way to cope with challenges associated with health-related knowledge. On the other hand, the topic of health literacy has also been integrated with a high profile into the political discourses on the promotion of health and the redefinition of the health care systems and agents in charge of it. In this context, health literacy has been embodied as a personal or organisational quality that contributes to more empowerment and health-friendly decision-making. The brief glimpse into deliberations on the development of a population's health from the socio-political angle suggests that health literacy holds a high potential for social innovation, which sustains the promotion of population health and is seen in addition as a driver of economic growth. It is worth highlighting that the outlined discussions on the social significance of health literacy have taken place particularly in policy fields relating to health, the economy or social issues and have succeeded in placing health literacy on the political agenda. However, a scientific debate that systematically addresses the topic from a socio-economic perspective is still pending. The way in which the question of the relevance of health literacy to society has been addressed in the scientific field appears to be such that any assessment that has primarily been made within public policy discourses for setting the political agenda has been considered appropriate, and that the premises and conclusions of the predominantly political arguments have hardly been questioned or contested. However, if the topic—as has been increasingly proposed—is credited with major relevance to society as a whole and if any such assessment is not to be mere rhetoric, then it appears imperative to call for discussing health literacy more systematically and comprehensively against the background of approaches to social and agency theory.

10   Conclusions and Outlook

As can be concluded from the review of current research, focusing on the theoretical-conceptual perspectives on health literacy continues to be a highly relevant and promising approach that provides innovative stimuli for future research as well as for the translation of research results into the various fields of application. An overall and integrated approach would benefit most from the establishment of research structures that facilitate more interdisciplinary work and create the conditions for a concerted multidisciplinary approach to make a significant contribution to the further development of health literacy. One major goal of such a concerted multidisciplinary approach should not be to arrive at a universally valid uniform concept, but rather to break down and illuminate current conceptualisations in order to make them accessible for the range of different disciplinary perspectives that have been involved with the topic. Such an approach does not intend to contribute to a prioritisation and harmonisation of different disciplinary perspectives, but rather to establish a framework in which disciplinary perspectives communicate and interact with each other. In this way, it is initially associated with an openness to results. This means that it will be open to movements both in the direction of a synthesis of perspectives, but also in the direction of positions that cannot easily be matched. The priority is thus to establish a culture that recognizes a maximum of disciplinary autonomy and creates spaces for mutual forms of communication, critical interaction and reciprocal share of innovative perspectives.

Concerted and comprehensive multidisciplinary research on health literacy could be guided and organised at the onset by three major fields of action: (a) work on the definitions and concepts of health literacy, i.e. on theoretical and conceptual frameworks whose subject matter is to explore the topic and aim to define and shape health literacy, (b) work on the theories and concepts to which references are made in the definitions of health literacy, i.e. theoretical and conceptual frameworks in which the subject matter is embedded, and (c) work on the research on practice and policy transfer, i.e. the identification and discussion of approaches by which theoretical research knowledge could be transferred into health literacy practice and policy.

Research focusing on the definitions and concepts of health literacy is concerned with the topic to be explored and aims to clarify two issues: What represents health literacy? What determines health literacy? Open issues can, for instance, be linked to the current discourse in health literacy and based on the premise that health literacy is a skill-based concept. An emergent desideratum that can be taken up from the ongoing research as a goal are open questions about the definition and categorisation of the broad range of skill dimensions or defined skills as well as the domains of knowledge that have been suggested for the health literacy construct or can be considered as candidates for such a framework. Therefore, the primary concern would be to clarify and specify existing and predominant definitions and concepts. Another open issue connects to views that see health literacy as a relational concept. According to these views, health literacy is a function of personal abilities, but also depends on the demands of organisations or systems on personal abilities. There is, however, a need to address the perspective of organisational health literacy and to identify what characteristics and competencies are attributable to organisations or systems on the level of structures, processes and outputs in order to qualify an organisation or system to be health literate. Other alternative approaches can be stimulated by the definition that "health literacy is linked to literacy" and be guided by the goal to explore to what extent and in what form health literacy is linked to literacy. This project could be started off by contrasting the two research discourses (health literacy and literacy) and by focusing on the perspectives of literacy which see in literacy a socio-cultural practice with the aim to study to what extend they are transferable to health literacy. Therefore, this kind of research could first explore whether and how socio-cultural perspectives of literacy that have been poorly addressed by literacy research can also be considered in the conceptual frameworks of health literacy. This also includes questions about the implications of such redefinitions. Addressing the determinants of health literacy is another issue of paramount relevance because of its contribution to understanding causal pathways. Research on this should involve the analysis of both personal and social determinants, their interplay and the directions of their effects. Other gaps in the current discourse are related to the emergence of health literacy and the call for a target-group-specific perspective that involves the growing-up populations. Here, research should pursue the question of how health literacy develops during childhood and adolescence.

Another analytical dimension aims at the theoretical and conceptual frameworks to which references are made by the definitions and concepts of health literacy. Research on this primarily addresses the multifaceted and mixed premises underlying the construct of health literacy. Future research on this should focus on both, explicitly articulated assumptions on which health literacy constructions are based as well as underlying tacit assumptions that can be inductively derived from an analysis of the current constructions of health literacy. Such an approach can be informed by research work that, for instance, connects health literacy with choice and rational decision-making or with health lifestyle approaches. It also includes the call for considering the agency-structure debate as another theoretical and conceptual framework. Last but not least, there is the need to subject the ascription of significance that health literacy has recently experienced in scientific and public discourses to a critical analysis. Here, research should be guided by the question why the concept of health literacy has gained significant importance and acceptance in a relatively short period of time. An analytical approach could be framed by social-theoretical considerations of social change with regard to topics such as digitalisation, knowledge, health promotion and social inequalities. One overall goal of such research could be the integration of health literacy into patterns of social dynamics in health and education. Another desideratum that can be approached by means of relevant social theories addresses socially determined inequalities in health and education and subjects descriptions of health literacy as a social determinant to an equity-focused analysis. This includes a review of both, the evidence base of the claim that health literacy is a social determinant, and the alleged impact of health literacy on inequalities in health and education. Another neglect within the current discussions on health literacy arises from the finding that the concept is a result of Western thinking and inevitably evokes questions as to the legitimacy of the assertion that health literacy concepts have global and universal validity. This implies taking socio-spatial conditions into consideration more pronouncedly, as well as addressing and discussing ethical questions regarding the implementation of health literacy in different settings within and across societies.

A considerable increase in insights on a theoretical-conceptual and methodological level can be expected from such a comprehensive and multidisciplinary approach. The ongoing development of the topic will be enriched by the review, revision and widening of current perspectives on health literacy, a systematic integration of perspectives from literacy research and research on choice, decision-making, or healthy life styles as well as from an inequality-sensitive contextualisation with social theories. In this way, a significant contribution can be made to the clarification of the theoretical and conceptual frameworks that underly the construction of health literacy. The comprehensive exploration and redefinition of the theoretical and conceptual frameworks also goes hand in hand with an improved understanding of the modes of operationalisation. Revisions and extensions of the methodological repertoires, in which the health literacy construct is made visible both qualitatively and quantitatively, are to be expected here. This has further implications for the transfer of research findings into policy and practice, such that strategies and programmes become more sensitive to social inequalities, go beyond the focus on personal skills and are backed up by a range of valid evaluation tools.

References

Bankson, H. L. (2009). Health literacy: An exploratory bibliometric analysis, 1997–2007. *Journal of the Medical Library Association, 97*(2), 148–150.

Barton, D., & Hamilton, M. (1998). *Local literacies: Reading and writing in one community*. New York: Routledge.

Barton, D., & Hamilton, M. (2000). Literacy practices. In D. Barton, M. Hamilton, & R. Ivanič (Eds.), *Situated literacies: Reading and writing in context* (pp. 7–15). London: Routledge.

Bauer, U. (2019). The social embeddedness of health literacy. In O. Okan, U. Bauer, D. Levin-Zamir, P. Pinheiro, & K. Sørensen (Eds.), *International handbook of health literacy* (pp. 573–587). Bristol: Policy Press.

Bauer, U., Okan, O., & Hurrelmann, K. (2018). Stärkung der Gesundheitskompetenz im Bildungssektor. *Monitor Versorgungsforschung, 05,* 47–49.

Bawden, D., & Robinson, L. (2009). The dark side of information: Overload, anxiety and other paradoxes and pathologies. *Journal of Information Science, 35*(2), 180–191.

Berkman, N. D., Sheridan, S. L., Donahue, K. E., Halpern, D. J., & Crotty, K. (2011). Low health literacy and health outcomes: An updated systematic review. *Annals of Internal Medicine, 155*(2), 97–107.

Bittlingmayer, U. H. (2016). Strukturorientierte Perspektiven auf Gesundheit und Krankheit. In K. Hurrelmann & M. Richter (Eds.), *Soziologie der Gesundheit und Krankheit. Ein Lehrbuch* (pp. 23–40). Wiesbaden: Springer VS.

Borzekowski, D. (2009). Considering children and health literacy: A theoretical approach. *Pediatrics, 124,* 282–288.

Brach, C. (2017). The journey to become a health literate organization: A snapshot of health system improvement. *Studies in Health Technology and Informatics, 240,* 203–237.

Brijnath, B., & Antoniades, J. (2016). "I'm running my depression:" Self-management of depression in neoliberal Australia. *Social Science and Medicine, 152,* 1–8.

Bröder, J., Okan, O., Bauer, U., Schlupp, S., Bollweg, T., Saboga-Nunes, L., et al. (2017). Health literacy in childhood and youth: A systematic review of definitions and models. *BMC Public Health, 17*(1), 1–25.

Chall, J. S. (1983). *Stages of reading development.* New York: Harcourt Brace.

Clarke, A., Shim, J., Mamo, L., Fosket, J., & Fishman, J. (2003). Biomedicalization: Technoscientific transformations of health, illness, and U.S. biomedicine. *American Sociological Review, 68*(2), 161–194.

Cline, R. J., & Haynes, K. M. (2001). Consumer health information seeking on the Internet: The state of the art. *Health Education Research, 16*(6), 671–692.

Cockerham, W. C. (2005). Health lifestyle theory and the convergence of agency and structure. *Journal of Health and Social Behavior, 46*(1), 51–67.

Collyer, F. M., Willis, K. F., Franklin, M., Harley, K., & Short, S. D. (2015). Healthcare choice: Bourdieu's capital, habitus and field. *Current Sociology, 63*(5), 685–699.

Davidson, K. (2010). The integration of cognitive and sociocultural theories of literacy development: Why? How? *The Alberta Journal of Educational Research, 56*(3), 246–256.

Eysenbach, G., Powell, J., Kuss, O., & Sa, E. R. (2002). Empirical studies assessing the quality of health information for consumers on the world wide web: A systematic review. *Journal of the American Medical Association, 287*(20), 2691–2700.

Fairbrother, H., Curtis, P., & Goyder, E. (2016). Making health information meaningful: Children's health literacy practices. *SSM Population Health, 2,* 476–484.

Gaffney, J. S., & Anderson, R. C. (2000). Trends in reading research in the United States: Changing intellectual currents over three decades. In M. L. Kamil, P. B. Mosenthal, P. D. Pearson, & R. Barr (Eds.), *Handbook of reading research* (Vol. III, pp. 53–74). New York: Erlbaum.

Greenhalgh, T. (2009). Patient and public involvement in chronic illness: beyond the expert patient. *British Medical Journal, 338,* b49.

Greenhalgh, T., & Wessely, S. (2004). "Health for me": A sociocultural analysis of healthism in the middle classes. *British Medical Bulletin, 69*(1), 197–213.

Hamilton, M. (2010). The social context of literacy. In N. Hughes & I. Schwab (Eds.), *Teaching adult literacy: Principles and practice* (pp. 7–27). Maidenhead UK: McGraw-Hill Education.

Hardey, M. (2008). Public health and Web 2.0. *The Journal of the Royal Society for the Promotion of Health, 128*(4), 181–189.

Heijmans, M., Uiters, E., Rose, T., Hofstede, J., Devillé, W., van der Heide, I., et al. (2015). *Study on sound evidence for a better understanding of health literacy in the European Union.* Brussels: European Commission.

Hoving, C., Visser, A., Mullen, P. D., & van den Borne, B. (2010). A history of patient education by health professionals in Europe and North America: From authority to shared decision making education. *Patient Education and Counseling, 78*(3), 275–281.

Hurrelmann, K., & Bauer, U. (2018). *Socialisation during the life course.* London: Routledge.

Kennedy, E., Dunphy, E., Dwyer, B., Hayes, G., McPhillips, T., Marsh, J., O'Connor, M., & Shiel, G. (2012). *Literacy in early childhood and primary education (3–8 years). NCCA Research Report No. 15.* Dublin: National Council for Curriculum and Assessment.

Kickbusch, I. (2006). *Die Gesundheitsgesellschaft. Megatrends der Gesundheit und deren Konsequenzen für Politik und Gesellschaft.* Gamburg: Verlag für Gesundheitsförderung.

Nefiodow, L. A. (2011). Die Gesundheitswirtschaft. In P. Granig & L. A. Nefiodow (Eds.), *Gesundheitswirtschaft – Wachstumsmotor im 21. Jahrhundert* (pp. 25–41). Wiesbaden: Gabler.

Lee, K., Hoti, K., Hughes, J. D., & Emmerton, L. M. (2015). Consumer use of "Dr Google": A survey on health information-seeking behaviors and navigational needs. *Journal of Medical Internet Research, 17*(12), e288.

Lyytinen, K. J. (1985). Implications of theories of language for information systems. *MIS Quarterly, 9*(1), 61–74.

Malloy-Weir, L. J., Charles, C., Gafni, A., & Entwistle, V. (2016). A review of health literacy: Definitions, interpretations, and implications for policy initiatives. *Journal of Public Health Policy, 37*(3), 334–352.

McDaid, D. (2016). *Investing in health literacy. What do we know about the co-benefits to the education sector of actions targeted at children and young people?.* Copenhagen: World Health Organization.

Moreira, L. (2018). *Health literacy for people-centred care: Where do OECD countries stand? OECD Health Working Papers, No. 107.* Paris: OECD Publishing.

Nordgren, L. (2010). Mostly empty words – What the discourse of 'choice' in health care does. *Journal of Health Organization and Management, 24*(2), 109–126.

Okan, O. (2019). From Saranac Lake to Shanghai: A brief history of health literacy. In O. Okan, U. Bauer, D. Levin-Zamir, P. Pinheiro, & K. Sørensen (Eds.), *International handbook of health literacy* (pp. 21–39). Bristol: Policy Press.

Okan, O., Lopes, E., Bollweg, T. M., Bröder, J., Messer, M., Bruland, D., et al. (2018). Generic health literacy measurement instruments for children and adolescents: A systematic review of the literature. *BMC Public Health, 18*(1), 1–19.

Omran, A. R. (2005). The epidemiologic transition: A theory of the epidemiology of population change. *The Milbank Quarterly, 83*(4), 731–757.

Parikh, N. S., Parker, R. M., Nurss, J. R., Baker, D. W., & Williams, M. V. (1996). Shame and health literacy: The unspoken connection. *Patient Education and Counseling, 27*(1), 33–39.

Parker, R., & Ratzan, S. C. (2010). Health literacy: A second decade of distinction for Americans. *Journal of Health Communication, 15*(Suppl. 2), 20–33.

Peacock, M., Bisselly, P., & Owen, J. (2014). Dependency denied: Health inequalities in the neo-liberal era. *Social Science and Medicine, 118*, 173–180.

Perry, K. H. (2012). What is literacy? A critical overview of sociocultural perspectives. *Journal of Language and Literacy Education, 8*(1), 50–71.

Pescosolido, B. A. (1992). Beyond rational choice: The social dynamics of how people seek help. *American Journal of Sociology, 97*(4), 1096–1138.

Reeve, C. L., & Basalik, D. (2014). Is health literacy an example of construct proliferation? A conceptual and empirical evaluation of its redundancy with general cognitive ability. *Intelligence, 44*, 93–102.

Rothman, R. L., Yin, H. S., Mulvaney, S., Homer, C., & Lannon, C. (2009). Health literacy and quality: Focus on chronic illness care and patient safety. *Pediatrics, 124*(Suppl 3), 315–326.

Rowlands, G., Russell, S., O'Donnell, A., Kaner, E., Trezona, A., Rademakers, J., et al. (2018). *What is the evidence on existing policies and linked activities and their effectiveness for improving health literacy at national, regional and organizational levels in the WHO European Region?*. Copenhagen: World Health Organization.

Saboga-Nunes, L., Bittlingmayer, U. H., & Okan, O. (2019). Salutogenesis and health literacy: The health promotion simplex! In O. Okan, U. Bauer, D. Levin-Zamir, P. Pinheiro, & K. Sørensen (Eds.), *International handbook of health literacy* (pp. 21–39). Bristol: Policy Press.

Schaeffer, D., Hurrelmann, K., Bauer, U., & Kolpatzik, K. (Eds.). (2018). *National action plan health literacy. Promoting health literacy in Germany*. Berlin: KomPart.

Sentell, T., Pitt, R., & Buchthal, O. V. (2017). Health literacy in a social context: Review of quantitative evidence. *Health Literacy Research and Practice, 1*(2), e41–e70.

Sørensen, K., Pelikan, J. M., Röthlin, F., Ganahl, K., Slonska, Z., Doyle, G., et al. (2015). Health literacy in Europe: comparative results of the European health literacy survey (HLS-EU). *European Journal of Public Health, 25*(6), 1053–1058.

Sørensen, K., van den Broucke, S., Fullam, J., Doyle, G., Pelikan, J., Slonska, Z., et al. (2012). Health literacy and public health: A systematic review and integration of definitions and models. *BMC Public Health, 12*(80), 1–13.

Sperlich, S. (2016). Handlungsorientierte Perspektiven auf Gesundheit und Krankheit. In K. Hurrelmann & M. Richter (Eds.), *Soziologie der Gesundheit und Krankheit. Ein Lehrbuch* (pp. 41–54). Wiesbaden: Springer VS.

Street, B. (1984). *Literacy in theory and practice*. Cambridge: Cambridge University Press.

Street, B. (2005). At last: Recent applications of new literacy studies in educational contexts. *Research in the Teaching of English, 39*(4), 417–423.

Teghtsoonian, K. (2009). Depression and mental health in neoliberal times: A critical analysis of policy and discourse. *Social Science and Medicine, 69*, 28–35.

Tracey, D. H., & Morrow, L. M. (2006). *Lenses on reading*. New York: Guilford Press.

Trezona, A., Rowlands, G., & Nutbeam, D. (2018). Progress in implementing national policies and strategies for health literacy – What have we learned so far? *International Journal of Environmental Research and Public Health, 15*(7), 1554.

United Nations Economic and Social Council ECOSOC. (2010). Health literacy and the Millennium Development Goals: United Nations Economic and Social Council (ECOSOC) regional meeting background paper (abstracted). *Journal of Health Communication., 15*(Suppl. 2), 211–223.

Warwick-Booth, L., Cross, R., & Lowcock, D. (2012). What is health? In L. Warwick-Booth, R. Cross, & D. Lowcock (Eds.), *Contemporary health studies: An introduction* (pp. 7–29). Cambridge: Polity Press.

Weishaar, H., Hurrelmann, K., Okan, O., Horn, A., & Schaeffer, D. (2018). Framing health literacy: A comparative analysis of national action plans. *Health Policy, 123*(1), 11–20.

WHO. (2013). *Health literacy. The solid facts.* Copenhagen: World Health Organization.

WHO & UNICEF. (2018). Declaration of Astana. Global Conference on Primary Health Care in Astana, Kazakhstan. https://www.who.int/docs/default-source/primary-health/declaration/gcphc-declaration.pdf. Accessed 07 Oct 2019.

Young, T. K. (2004). *Population health: Concepts and methods.* New York: Oxford University Press.

CPSIA information can be obtained
at www.ICGtesting.com
Printed in the USA
LVHW081338131220
674072LV00003B/76